AF478922

Schistosomiasis
Epidemiology, Treatment and Control

Schistosomiasis

Epidemiology, Treatment and Control

PETER JORDAN, C.M.G., M.D., F.R.C.P., M.F.C.M., D.T.M.&H.

External Staff Medical Research Council; Member of Expert Advisory Panel on Parasitic Diseases, World Health Organization; formerly Director Research & Control Department, St. Lucia and Director, East African Institute for Medical Research, Tanzania

GERALD WEBBE, D.Sc., M.Sc., F.I.BIOL.

Professor of Applied Parasitology and Head of the Department of Medical Helminthology, London School of Hygiene and Tropical Medicine, University of London; Member of Expert Advisory Panel on Parasitic Diseases, World Health Organization

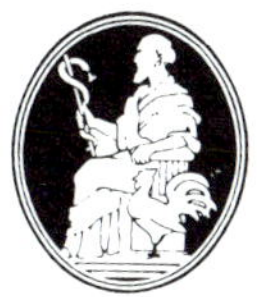

WILLIAM HEINEMANN MEDICAL BOOKS LTD
LONDON

First published 1982

ISBN 0-433-17581-8

Text set in 11/12 pt Linotron 202 Baskerville, printed and bound in
Great Britain at The Pitman Press, Bath

Contents

Contributors

Andrew Davis MD, FRCP(E), FFCM, DTM&H
Director, Parasitic Diseases Programme, WHO, Geneva

Herbert M. Gilles KOSJ, MD, FRCP, FFCM, DTM&H
Professor of Tropical Medicine, Liverpool School of Tropical
Medicine

Michael Goddard PhD
Faculty of Mathematics, Department of Statistics, University of
Waterloo, Ontario, Canada

Peter Jordan CMG, MD, FRCP, MCFM, DTM&H
External Staff, Medical Research Council

Kenneth E. Mott MD, MPH
Medical Officer, Special Programme for Research and Training
in Tropical Diseases, Division of Schistosomiasis and other
Helminthic Infections, WHO, Geneva

Aluizio Prata MD
Professor of Tropical Medicine, Head of the Nucleo de Medicina
Tropical a Nutrição, Universidade de Brasilia, Brasil

Kenneth S. Warren MD
Director, Health Sciences Division, Rockefeller Foundation,
New York

Gerald Webbe DSc, MSc, FIBiol
Professor of Applied Parasitology, London School of Hygiene
and Tropical Medicine

Preface

This book is the successor to our *Human Schistosomiasis*, published in 1969, since which time major changes have occurred in this field of study. The schistosomiasis problem associated with man-made lakes was then only becoming evident, but 10 years later research by the World Health Organization led to the introduction of successful measures to control transmission in Lake Volta.

In 1969 hycanthone—the first effective single-dose schistosomicidal drug—was comparatively new, likewise the low cost metrifonate. Now two other highly effective single-dose drugs with minimal side effects are available. These drugs have changed the whole outlook for the infected individual and the prospects of control. However, though the drugs now available may approach the ideal, problems of their delivery may limit the extent to which they can be used for control in some endemic areas. But chemotherapy is now a potential method of controlling transmission and disease.

Transmission has also been shown to be reduced if entry into infected water is limited by provision of alternative safe water, thus providing an additional benefit and further reason for development of water supplies in rural areas. This emphasises the need for greater involvement of engineers in health programmes and indeed a society for engineers, biologists and physicians has been formed to exchange ideas on engineering aspects of control.

An appreciation of the potential role of water supplies in control has led to an increased interest in details of water contact and these are now being studied by sociologists in many areas.

With improved control strategies has come a better understanding of their limitations and methods for assessing their effects.

Developments in immunology have necessitated a separate

chapter on this subject. It has been said that schistosomiasis has given more to the immunologist than the immunologist has given to schistosomiasis but, while knowledge of the complex immunological reactions is slowly being unravelled, a vaccine is still a long way off.

While emphasis is on epidemiology and control and these chapters have been written essentially for the man in the field, the chapters on the parasite, the snail as intermediate host and the relationship between them provide detailed information for students of parasitology; chapters on the clinical picture and treatment, all written by experts in their own fields, should provide sufficient data for medical students and physicians.

Each chapter has an extensive bibliography to assist in further reading.

Peter Jordan
Gerald Webbe
1982

Acknowledgements

We wish to thank the contributors to this volume and the many others who have helped in various ways with photographs, figures or information—Dr J. A. Cook, Mr C. England, Dr A. Fenwick, Dr D. M. Forsyth, Professor A. E. M. Lees, Miss Jane Lillywhite, Dr F. von Lichtenberg, the late Dr David Scott, Dr Andrew Wilkins and Dr D. H. Connor.

We wish to thank staff of our respective departments who have helped in many ways—Mr M. A. Prentice, Mr G. Barnish, Mr R. K. Bartholomew and Miss Verne Henry (secretarial assistance) of the Research and Control Department and Dr C. James, Dr M. G. Taylor and Mrs D. Mulholland of the London School of Hygiene and Tropical Medicine.

Thanks are due to the Editors of the *Bulletin of the World Health Organization*, of the *International Journal for Parasitology* and the Royal Society of Tropical Medicine and Hygiene for permission to reproduce published material.

We wish also to thank Mr R. S. Emery of Heinemann Medical Books for his patience, encouragement and help.

1 The Parasites

Gerald Webbe

DISCOVERY

In 1851 Theodor Bilharz first recovered *S. haematobium* worms
from the mesenteric veins during the post-mortem examination of
a patient in Cairo, and shortly afterwards he demonstrated their
relationship to the haematuria seen in Egyptians passing terminal-spined eggs of the parasite in their urine. Unfortunately,
Bilharz reported the presence of both lateral and terminal-spined
eggs in the uterus of the same worm and many years passed before
it was realised that there were two different parasites infecting
man in Egypt, one involving the bladder—*S. haematobium*—the
other the bowel and liver—*S. mansoni*. Urinary schistosomiasis
was reported from South Africa by Harley (1864) and he believed
that he was dealing with a distinct species which he named
Bilharzia capensis. Like Bilharz, Harley suggested that a mollusc
was a necessary intermediate host. However, Looss (1894)
considered there was no such phase in the life-cycle. With the
discovery of infections with lateral-spined eggs in the faeces in the
West Indies and Uganda by Manson (1902) and Castellani
(1903), it became obvious that there were at least two species of
blood flukes infecting man. However, Looss, who was an
outstanding authority, disagreed with this and considered that
the lateral-spined eggs were those of *S. haematobium* produced
parthenogenetically. Sambon, who was always keen to enter into
a controversy, disagreed with Looss. He collected all the available
data and in 1907 designated the species with lateral-spined eggs
S. mansoni. The work of Leiper (1915) in Egypt provided final
proof of the existence of two distinct species. He showed that the
adult and eggs were different: they had a different distribution in
the definitive host, and they developed in snail intermediate hosts
belonging to different genera. He also showed that infection was
acquired by a cutaneous route.

In retrospect, it seems likely that the first account of disease caused by *S. japonicum* was given by Fujii in 1847, Baelz apparently carried out the first epidemiological survey in Japan but attributed the disease to *Clonorchis sinensis* Cobbold. Yamagiwa (1890), Kurimoto (1893) and Fujinami (1904) found eggs in various organs of patients and ascribed to these eggs the aetiological role in the infection. Kasai (1908) first found the eggs in faeces but Katsurada (1904), having recovered worms from the portal system of a cat, first established the relationship of the true parasite to the disease. He described the worms and the acute infection in dogs and cats and named the parasite *S. japonicum*. Logan (1905) first diagnosed the infection in China. The route of infection from the skin was established in animal experiments by Fujinami and Nakamura (1909), while the life-cycle of the parasite was established by the experimental work of Fujinami (1910), Miyagawa (1912, 1913), Miyairi and Suzuki (1913, 1914) and by Leiper and Atkinson (1915).

GEOGRAPHICAL DISTRIBUTION

S. haematobium is found in North Africa, including Morocco, Algeria, Libya, Tunisia and Egypt; it is widely distributed throughout most of the African continent, including the east coast from Somalia to the Cape; the islands off the east coast, Zanzibar, Republic of Malagasy, Mauritius, Reunion; large areas of Central Africa, and in West Africa from Nigeria as far south as Angola. It has been reported in Aden, Saudi Arabia, Yemen, Israel, Lebanon, Syria, Turkey, Iran and Iraq, and limited foci have been recorded in Portugal and India.

S. mansoni is reported in Libya, and is endemic in the Nile Delta. There is now evidence of the spread of *S. mansoni* to Middle and Upper Egypt, and it is widespread south of Khartoum in southern Sudan. It occurs in Somalia, Eritrea, Kenya, Uganda, Tanzania (mainland) and Mozambique, in the Transvaal, Zimbabwe, Zambia and the Congo. In West Africa its distribution extends from Senegal and Gambia to the Cameroons and inland to Lake Chad, throughout the Congo Basin, Sierra Leone and Liberia. In the Middle East, *S. mansoni* also occurs in Israel, Yemen, Aden and Saudi Arabia. In the western hemisphere, *S. mansoni* is endemic in Brazil, Venezuela, Surinam, Dominican Republic, Puerto Rico, Montserrat, Guadeloupe, Martinique and St Lucia, and has been reported in Antigua, St Kitts and French St Martin, but has probably disappeared from these islands with the canalisation of streams and deforestation leading to less rainfall.

S. japonicum is endemic in many provinces of mainland China (Faust and Russell, 1964; Anon, 1965), but in Japan the infection has almost disappeared (Yokogawa, 1976). There is a long-standing focus in the Celebes (Central Sulawesi), and in the Philippines this species occurs in the islands of Luzon, Leyte, Samar, Mindoro, Mindanao and Bohol. *S. japonicum* was found in lower animals in Taiwan (Formosa), but no human cases have been recorded; this focus, however, no longer exists (Cross, 1976). In Malaysia a small focus of *S. japonicum* exists among aborigines (Sornmani, 1976). It is now considered that *S. mekongi* (Voge *et al.*, 1978) is responsible for the Mekong focus of schistosomiasis in Laos, Cambodia and Thailand.

HUMAN SCHISTOSOMES

The human schistosomes or blood flukes are digenetic trematodes belonging to the super family *Schistosomatoidea*; they have no muscular pharynx and they produce non-operculated eggs. The three species of schistosomes commonly affecting man have similar life-cycles and develop over a succession of stages—egg, miracidium, first-stage sporocyst, second-stage sporocyst, cercaria, schistosomulum and adult. The basic life-cycle has an alternation of generations, with the sexual generation of adult schistosomes in the definitive vertebrate host and an asexual stage in a molluscan host. A relatively short-lived, free-swimming stage, the miracidium, hatches from the egg and is infective to the snail intermediate host. In the appropriate snail host the miracidium becomes a first-stage sporocyst; this gives rise to second-stage sporocysts which produce numerous free-swimming cercariae which are infective to the vertebrate host. The usual portal of entry is the skin and the cercariae, after penetration, are known as schistosomula. These migrate and develop into mature adult schistosome worms (Fig. 1.1).

While the species of human schistosomes are similar in their basic life-cycles, they differ in the morphology of the adults, the shape and size of their eggs and the larvae hatched from the eggs. They also show marked differences in their infectivity to

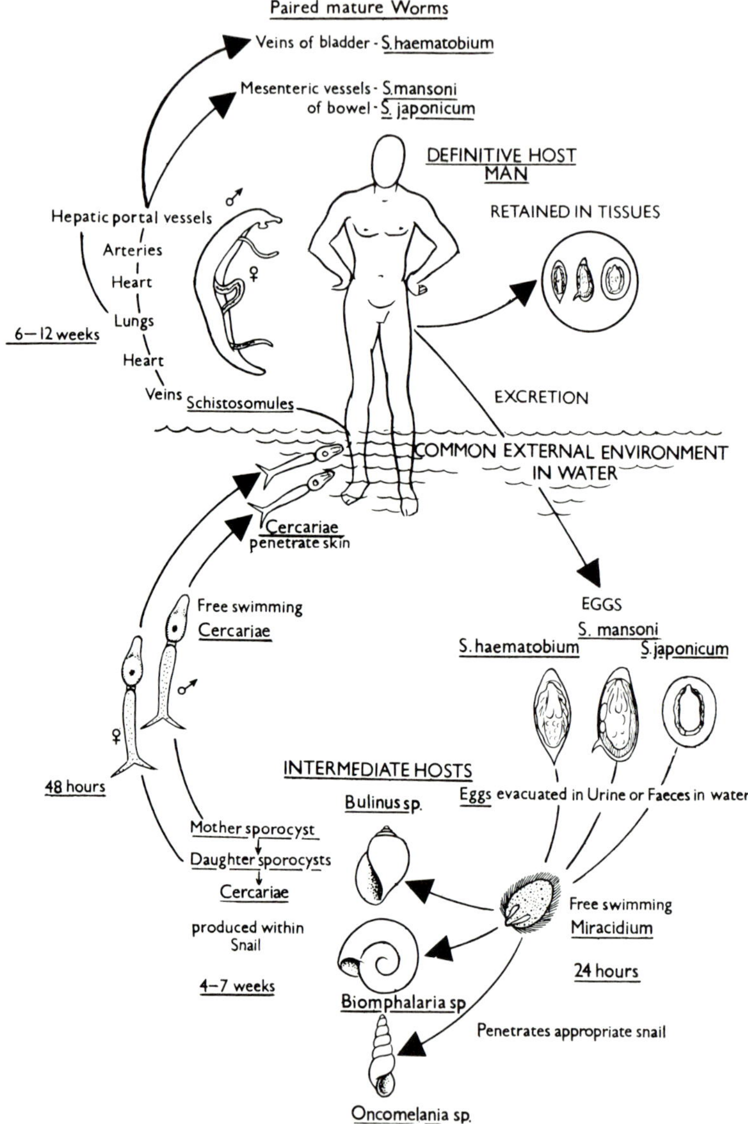

Fig. 1.1 The life-cycle.

the particular groups of snails which they utilise as intermediate hosts and in their infectivity to other mammalian hosts. The adult schistosomes are an unusual group of trematodes in that they are elongated and superficially resemble roundworms. This is an adaptation to their habitat, which is inside blood vessels.

The female worm is held in the 'schist' or gynaecophoric canal of the male during copulation and oviposition, and both sexes have oral and ventral suckers (Dawes, 1946; Faust and Russell, 1964).

S. haematobium

The adult worms inhabit the veins of the vesical plexus of the mammalian host, although some parasites may live in the portal vein and its mesenteric branches.

The male worm is short and cylindrical (due to ventral infolding of its sides to form the gynaecophoric canal) and measures 10–15 mm in length and 0·75–1 mm in breadth. The cuticle is covered with fine tubercles. The single posterior caecum extends about half way along the body. Four or five testes are present. The female is long and slender and measures 20–26 mm by 0·25 mm and is usually darker than the male with relatively more blood pigment in the gut. The small cuticular tubercles are usually confined to the extremity of the worm. The ovary is in the posterior third of the body and the uterus is long; 10–100 eggs develop *in utero* at one time. Oviposition normally occurs in the small terminal venules of the vesical plexus, but occasionally in the rectal venules, the mesenteric portal system and ectopic sites (Faust, 1948). Eggs are partly mature when laid, and migrate through the bladder wall to be discharged in the urine. They have a yellowish-brown transparent shell with a prominent terminal spine and measure 83–187μ in length (Pitchford, 1965). One female probably produces between 20 and 290 eggs per day.

S. mansoni

The adult worms of *S. mansoni* resemble those of *S. haematobium* but they are smaller, the male measuring 6–13 mm in length and the female 7–17 mm. The posterior caecum occupies two-thirds of the body length. In addition to the cuticular tubercles on the male being more conspicuous than those of *S. haematobium*, the cuticle has small sensory papillae with microscopic tufts of hair on its surface. The lateral margins of the male interlock and are held in position by acuminate spines longer than those found on the cuticle (Gonnert, 1948). The male has 4 to 13 testes. In the female the ovary is situated anteriorly and the short uterus occupies the anterior third of the body and usually contains only one or two eggs at a time.

The mature worms are normally found in the inferior mesenteric vein and its tributaries and the eggs pass into the lumen of the bowel and are discharged in the faeces. The eggs have a yellowish-brown transparent shell with a characteristic lateral spine. They measure 112–175μ in length by 45–70μ in diameter, and are usually mature when passed in the faeces. A single female produces from 100 to 300 eggs per day.

S. japonicum

The male worms have 6 to 7 testes and measure 12–20 mm in length by 0·5–0·55 mm in the greatest diameter. The cuticle is covered with small acuminate spines which are prominent in the regions of the suckers and the gynaecophoric canal, but there are no cuticular tubercles. The female worm measures 12–28 mm in length and is about 0·3 mm at its greatest diameter. The cuticle is covered with minute spines. The posterior caecum occupies one-third of the body length. The ovary is situated in the middle of the worm; the uterus is long and straight, it occupies the anterior half of the body and it contains 50 or more eggs at one time.

The mature worms live mainly in the capillaries of the superior mesenteric vein or its tributaries in the wall of the small intestine, but they may be present in the portal vein and the inferior mesenteric veins and eggs are passed into the lumen of the bowel. The eggs are pale yellow, oval in shape and have a rudimentary spine in a small depression of the shell. The eggs *in utero* measure 60–80μ in length by 40–60μ in breadth, but 70–100μ by 50–60μ when present in the faeces (Faust and Russell, 1964). A single female produces 1500–3500 eggs per day.

S. mekongi **sp. n. (Voge** *et al.***, 1978)**

The male worm measures some 15 mm in length by 0·41 mm at the widest point, with the gynaecophoric canal extending from the anterior to the posterior end. The integument is covered with spines from the anterior level of the gynaecophoric canal to the posterior end of the body, then ventrally between the suckers only. The male worm has 6 to 7 testes. The female worm measures some 12 mm in length by 0·23 mm at the widest point and the integument is completely spined. The ovary is situated in the anterior five-eighths of the body, being unlobed and oblong in shape (0·76 mm long by 0·15 mm wide). The embryonated eggs measure $50-65\,\mu$ by $30-35\,\mu$ (taken from mouse liver 35-day old infection). When first discovered, *S. mekongi* was considered to be a strain of *S. japonicum*, but the size as well as the shape of the eggs differ from those of *S. japonicum*, whatever the host species in which they develop. While the size range of other structures in the two species differs, it is considered that body size, the size of the gonads and of the suckers are not useful characters in the differentiation of Asian schistosomes, the only useful measurement being that of the embryonated egg.

An important difference between *S. mekongi* and *S. japonicum* is the length of the prepatent period in the mammalian host. It was found that on average the prepatent period of *S. mekongi* is 7 to 8 days longer than that of *S. japonicum* in the mouse. The two parasites develop in different snail intermediate hosts—*S. mekongi* in *Tricula aperta*, and *S. japonicum* in *Oncomelania* spp. (Voge *et al.*, 1978).*

OTHER SPECIES WHICH MAY PARASITISE MAN

S. bovis Sonsino (1876), Blanchard (1895)

This is a member of the *S. haematobium* complex, and was first described from cattle in Egypt. It is a common parasite of the mesenteric portal system of cattle and sheep of Southern Europe, Africa and Iraq. The adult worms are larger than those of *S. haematobium* and the eggs are longer and narrower with a prominent central bulge and terminal spine, and measure 130–260 μ in length (Pitchford, 1965). There appear to be few authentic records of *S. bovis* in man, but cases have been described from Uganda (Raper, 1951), Zimbabwe (Blair, 1966) and South Africa (Kisner *et al.*, 1953). An attempt to infect a human volunteer failed (MacHattie *et al.*, 1933). In Kenya, *S. bovis* cercariae are commonly found in waters used by the local inhabitants; no human infections have been seen (Teesdale and Nelson, 1958). Of some importance, however, is the finding that in Sardinia positive reactions were obtained with the fluorescent antibody test in persons exposed to the infection (Sadun and Biocca, 1962).

** See also* The Mekong Schistosome (1980), Malacological Review Suppl. 2. Eds. J. I. Bruce, H. L. Asch, K. A. Crawford.

There have been recent studies on the parasitology of *S. bovis* and of the pathology of the disease in sheep and cattle (Hussein, 1973; Massoud, 1973; Hussein *et al.*, 1976; Southgate and Knowles, 1976) and on immunisation in sheep and cattle (Massoud and Nelson, 1972).

Heterologous immune interactions involving *S. bovis* in primates and rodents have also been studied (Massoud and Nelson, 1972; Taylor *et al.*, 1973).

S. mattheei Veglia and Le Roux (1929)

In southern Africa, this parasite apparently replaces *S. bovis* in domestic and wild animals (Dinnik and Dinnik, 1965). The hosts include the horse, sheep, cow, zebra, baboon and a wide variety of antelopes (Le Roux, 1957; Pitchford, 1961). Man is more susceptible to *S. mattheei* than to *S. bovis* and a prevalence rate of 40% in the human population has been reported (Pitchford, 1959). *S. mattheei* has nearly always been found in patients infected with either *S. mansoni* or *S. haematobium*, suggesting that it may not be well adapted to humans and the female may require the males of the other schistosomes to transport it to a site for egg laying (Nelson *et al.*, 1962). Eggs which are seen in the faeces or urine measure 120–280 μ in length (Pitchford, 1965) and have a terminal spine.

The ecology and parasitology of *S. mattheei* and the pathology of the disease in sheep and cattle have been extensively studied in recent years (Haenens and Santele, 1955; Pitchford and Visser, 1975; Van Wyk *et al.*, 1976; Dargie *et al.*, 1977; Lawrence, 1977) and studies on immunity and the possibilities of vaccination in sheep and cattle have also been made (Lawrence, 1973; Preston and Webbe, 1974; Taylor *et al.*, 1976; Dargie *et al.*, 1977; Taylor *et al.*, 1979).

S. intercalatum Fisher (1934)

This species was described following the recovery of terminal-spined eggs exclusively from the faeces of man in the Stanleyville district of the Congo (Fisher, 1934). The eggs measure 140–240 μ by 50–85 μ. The evidence suggests that this is a distinct schistosome. It is morphologically similar to *S. mattheei* but differs markedly in its infectivity to man. In view of its high infectivity to man and its low pathogenicity, it may be of value in

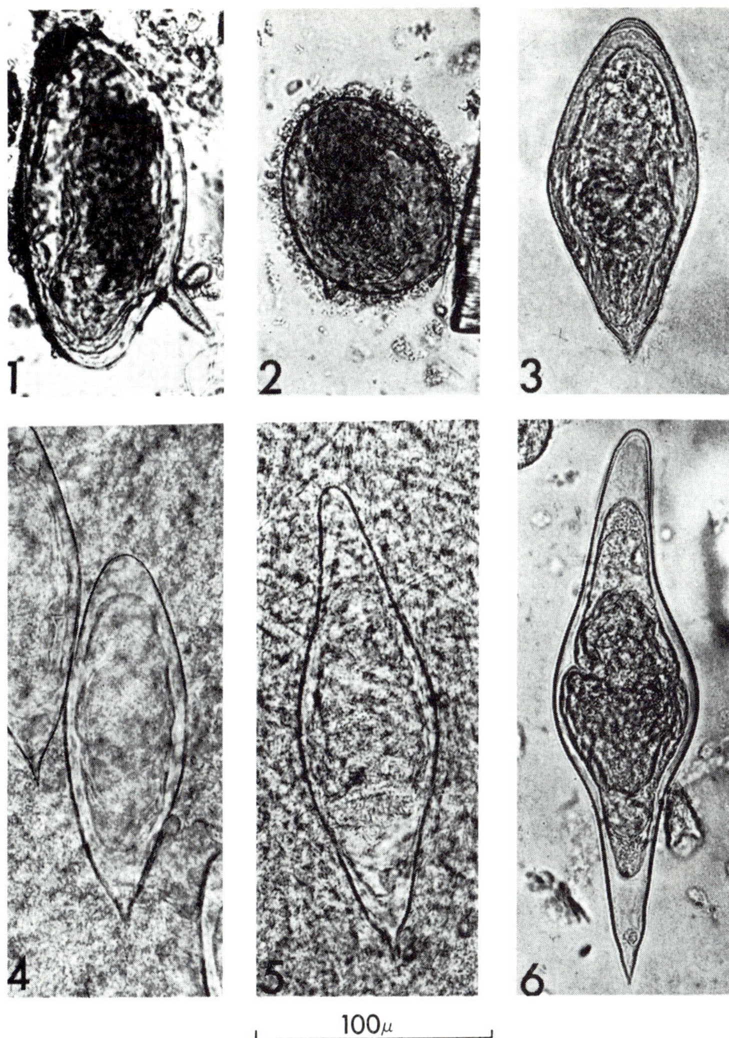

Fig. 1.2 Eggs of (1) *S. mansoni*, (2) *S. japonicum*, (3) *S. haematobium*, (4) *S. intercalatum*, (5) *S. mattheei*, (6) *S. bovis*. (Material from the Department of Helminthology, London School of Hygiene and Tropical Medicine.)

immunological studies (Nelson *et al.*, 1962). Apart from the human infection, this parasite has been found only in a *Hybomys* rat (Schwetz, 1956) but it has been suggested that sheep and goats may be important reservoirs in the Congo since sheep have been successfully infected experimentally (Chesterman, 1960).

It has been demonstrated that *S. intercalatum* is not a homogeneous entity (Wright *et al.*, 1972) and that there are two distinct forms of the parasite which are transmitted by snail intermediate hosts of two species groups: *S. intercalatum* Cameroon (Lower Guinea), being compatible with snails of the *forskali* group, and only very slightly compatible with snails of the *africanus* complex; and *S. intercalatum* (Zaire) being compatible with snails of the *africanus* complex. Parasites are generally restricted by the distribution of their hosts, but in the case of *S. intercalatum* the known snail intermediate hosts and definitive hosts have a far greater range than that of the parasite and the question, therefore, arises—why is *S. intercalatum* not more widespread in distribution (Southgate, 1978)? *S. intercalatum* also affects man in Gabon and Central Africa Republic, and there have been other isolated and unconfirmed case reports of the infection in Senegal, Mali, Upper Volta, Nigeria and Angola (Van Wyk, 1975).

S. margrebowiei Le Roux (1933)

This is a parasite common in antelopes in Central Africa. The egg is smaller than that of *S. mansoni* (65μ by 43μ), and lacks a lateral spine (Le Roux, 1933). It is practically indistinguishable from *S. japonicum* and may account for the occasional report of this infection in Africa (Fig. 1.2). Similar eggs were recovered from human faeces in the Congo (Walkiers, 1928) and named as those of a new species—*S. faradjei*.

S. rodhaini Brumpt (1931)

This is a distinct species which is closely related to *S. mansoni*. It has been found in wild rodents and carnivores in the Congo, Uganda and Kenya. There appears to be only one record of *S. rodhaini* from man (Haenens and Santele, 1955). The eggs have a sub-terminal spine and at the opposite pole the shell has a slight curvature in the opposite direction. *S. rodhaini* and *S. mansoni* have been hybridised (Taylor, 1970) and the offspring produced eggs which resembled eggs seen in wild rodents and described under the name *S. mansoni var rodentorum* by Schwetz (1953). This is a dubious form and is considered to be nothing more than *S. mansoni* in rodents (Nelson *et al.*, 1962). The shape of *S. mansoni* ova depends to some extent upon the host species and its diet (Pitchford and Visser, 1960).

The veterinary aspects of several species of schistosomes found in domestic animals in Asia have recently been studied, including *S. spindale*, *S. indicum*, *S. incognitum* and *S. nassale* (Rao and Devi, 1971; Ahluwalia and Dutt, 1972; Chaudan *et al.*, 1973; Rajanohanan and Peter, 1975; Sharma and Dwivedi, 1976).

HYBRIDISATION

All the species of schistosomes which have been studied have the same chromosome number (2n = 16) and very similar chromosome morphologies. Interspecific hybridisation experiments have been carried out on African (but not Asian) schistosomes in rodents using sibling species combinations, and in many cases viable hybrids were produced which in some cases were selfed for many generations (Taylor, 1970; Taylor and Andrews, 1973; Taylor *et al.*, 1973; Wright and Southgate, 1976). No evidence of reproductive isolation has been shown by hybridisation experiments between geographical 'strains' of *S. japonicum*, but some reproductive barriers apparently occur in the case of *S. intercalatum* (Frandsen, 1978). *S. bovis* and *S. mattheei* do not hybridise in cattle, although mixed infections are common in some parts of Central Africa (Dinnik and Dinnik, 1965). In South Africa, however, there is evidence of hybridisation between *S. mattheei* and *S. haematobium* (Pitchford, 1961), and it has been suggested that such a hybrid might eventually replace the 'parental' species with a schistosome equally infecting both man and cattle.

It has been shown conclusively that *S. intercalatum* and *S. haematobium* hybridise in the laboratory and in nature (Wright *et al.*, 1974; Southgate *et al.*, 1976; Southgate and Wright, 1976). It is considered that this hybrid, together with *S. haematobium*, is displacing *S. intercalatum* at Loum, Cameroun, and that its 'hybrid vigour' is enhanced by greater snail host specificity (*B. rohlfsi* and *B. forskali*); and, like *S. haematobium*, the hybrid eggs are voided in the urine. As the result of introgressive hybridisation, therefore, it seems likely that a new strain of *S. haematobium* may evolve which could halt the spread of *S. intercalatum* (Southgate, 1978).

Although the animal schistosomes are of relatively little importance as direct pathogens in man, they may be of some significance as immunising agents conferring some degree of heterologous immunity against *S. mansoni* and *S. haematobium* (Amin *et al.*, 1968).

The question of whether the exposure of man to the cercariae of animal schistosomes in nature can prevent or limit the spread of human schistosomiasis—'zooprophylaxis' (Nelson *et al.*, 1962)—has again been considered as the result of recent studies on *S. margrebowiei* (Pitchford, 1976). It was found that there was little overlap in the distribution of *S. margrebowiei* and *S. leiperi* (Le Roux), and that of *S. haematobium* and *S. mansoni*, and no overlap with *S. mattheei* in the area studied. The theory was therefore advanced that the presence of either or both the antelope species of schistosomes restricts the spread of the human parasites and of *S. mattheei* (Pitchford, 1976).

Recent investigations have shown that baboons infected with *S. haematobium* can develop a marked degree of acquired immunity to *S. mansoni*, and that while the challenge infection may become established, the worm load is considerably reduced and the pathogenicity of the infection ameliorated (Webbe *et al.*, 1979). It was considered that these findings may have profound immunological and epidemiological implications in endemic areas where man is exposed to the transmission of both parasites.

Cercarial dermatitis and 'swimmer's itch' are terms used to describe a condition of the skin in man caused by the penetration of the cercariae of certain non-human schistosomes. *Trichobilharzia ocellata* (La Valette) was shown to be responsible for this condition in persons bathing in infested waters in Lake Douglas, Michigan (Cort, 1928). The dermatitis is regarded as a sensitisation phenomenon which may build up to a severe reaction following repeated exposure (Macfarlane, 1949; Olivier, 1949). Cercariae-infested freshwater may be responsible for dermatitis acquired after contact with water in almost any part of the world (Faust and Russell, 1964), including Wales (Manson-Bahr, 1966). Cercariae of the avian blood flukes—*Trichobilharzia* (McMullen and Beaver, 1945), *Gigantobilharzia* (Cort, 1950; Hunter *et al.*, 1951), and *Ornithobilharzia* (Szidat, 1951)—have been incriminated as causes of dermatitis. The molluscan hosts include species of *Lymnaea*, *Physa*, *Planorbis*, *Polyplis* and *Chilina*.

A dermatitis in people working in rice fields in Malaya was caused by cercariae of *S. spindale* (Montgomery, 1906), a mammalian species of blood fluke for which man is not a compatible definitive host (Buckley, 1938).

Cercarial dermatitis has also been reported from certain salt-water beaches where marine molluscs are the intermediate hosts of trematodes of salt-water and migratory birds. The adult worms of a species of *Microbilharzia* were identified from studies of the cercariae (Stunkard and Hinchliffe, 1952).

REFERENCES

Ahluwalia, S. S. and Dutt, S. C. (1972). *Indian Vet. J.* **49,** 863.

Amin, M. A., Nelson, G. S. and Saoud, M. F. A. (1968). *Bull. Wld Hlth Org.* **38,** 19.

Anon. (1965). *WHO Monograph Series* No. 50, p. 12, World Health Organization, Geneva.

Blair, D. M. (1966). *Cent. Afr. J. Med.* **12,** 103.

Buckley, J. J. C. (1938). *J. Helminth.* **16,** 117.

Castellani, A. (1903). *Ann. Med. Nav.* **2,** 354.

Chauhan, A. S., Srivastava, C. B. and Chauhan, B. S. (1973). *J. Zool. Soc. Ind.* **25,** 83.

Chesterman, C. C. (1960). *Trans. R. Soc. Trop. Med. Hyg.* **54,** 319.

Cort, W. W. (1928). *J. Am. Med. Ass.* **90,** 1027.

Cort, W. W. (1950). *Am. J. Hyg.* **52,** 251.

Cross, J. H. (1976). *S.E. Asian J. Trop. Med. Publ. Hlth.* **7,** 167.

Dargie, J. D., Berry, C. I., Holmes, P. H., Reid, J. F. S., Breeze, R., Taylor, M. G., James, E. R. and Nelson, G. S. (1977). *J. Helminth.* **57,** 347.

Dawes, B. (1946). *The Trematoda.* Cambridge University Press, Cambridge.

Dinnick, J. A. and Dinnik, N. N. (1965). *Bull. Epizoot. Dis. Afr.* **13,** 341.

Faust, E. C. (1948). *Am. J. Trop. Med.* **28,** 175.

Faust, E. C. and Russell, P. F. (1964). In *Craig and Faust's Clinical Parasitology,* pp. 530, 533, 555, 566, Henry Kimpton, London.

Fisher, A. C. (1934). *Trans. R. Soc. Trop. Med. Hyg.* **28,** 277.

Frandsen, F. (1978). *J. Helminth.* **52,** 11.

Fujii, Y. (1847). *Chugai Iji Shimpo* **691,** 55.

Fujinami, K. (1904). *Hiroshima Eisei Iji Geppo* **69,** 1.

Fujinami, K. (1910). *Tokyo Iji Shinshi. Tokyo Med. J.* **2,** 3.

Fujinami, K. and Nakamura, D. (1909). *Hiroshima Eisei Iji Geppo* **132,** 324.

Gönnert, R. (1948). *Ttschr. Tropenmed. Parasit.* **1,** 105.

Haenens, G. D. and Santele, A. (1955). *Ann. Soc. Belg. Méd. Trop.* **35,** 497.

Harley, J. (1864). *Med. Chir. Trans.* **47,** 55.

Hunter, G. W. III, Ritchie, L. S. and Tanabe, H. (1951). *Trans. R. Soc. Trop. Med. Hyg.* **45,** 103.

Hussein, M. F. (1973). *Vet. Bull.* **43,** 341.

Hussein, M. F., Bishara, J. O. and Ali, K. E. (1976). *J. Helminth.* **50,** 235.

Kasai, K. (1908). *Chugai Iji Shimpo* **673,** 488.

Katsurada, F. (1904). *Annot. Zool. Japan* **5,** 146.

Kisner, C. D., Stoffberg, N. and de Meillon, B. (1953). *S. Afr. Med. J.* **27,** 357.

Kurimoto, T. (1893). *J. Tokyo Med. Ass.* **7,** 22.

Lawrence, J. A. (1973). *Res. Vet. Sci.* **14,** 400.

Lawrence, J. A. (1977). *J.S. Afr. Vet. Assoc.* **48,** 77.

Leiper, R. T. (1915). *J.R. Army Med. Corps.* **25,** 1.

Leiper, R. T. and Atkinson, E. L. (1915). *China Med. J.* **29,** 143.

Le Roux, P. L. (1933). *J. Helminth.* **11,** 57.

Le Roux, P. L. (1957). *Rep. F.A.O., U.K.* **696,** 1.

Logan, O. T. (1905). *China Med. Miss. J.* **19,** 268.

Looss, A. (1894). *Zbl. Bakt.* **16,** 286.

Macfarlane, W. V. (1949). *Am. J. Hyg.* **50,** 143.

MacHattie, C., Mills, E. A. and Chadwick, C. R. (1933). *Trans. R. Soc. Trop. Med. Hyg.* **27,** 173.

McMullen, D. E. and Beaver, P. C. (1945). *Am. J. Hyg.* **42,** 128.

Manson, P. (1902). *J. Trop. Med.* **5,** 384.

Manson-Bahr, P. H. (1966). *Manson's Tropical Diseases*, p. 605. Baillière Tindall and Cassell, London.

Massoud, J. (1973). *J. Helminth.* **47,** 155.

Massoud, J. and Nelson, G. S. (1972). *Bull. Wld Hlth Org.* **47,** 591.

Miyagawa, Y. (1912). *J. Tokyo Med. Ass.* **26,** 385.

Miyagawa, Y. (1913). *Zbl. Bakt.* **69,** 132.

Miyairi, K. and Suzuki, M. (1913). *Tokyo Iji Shinshi, Tokyo Med. J.* **1836,** 1.

Miyairi, K. and Suzuki, M. (1914). *Mitteil, Med. Fak. Kaiserl. Univ. Kyushu* **1,** 187.

Nelson, G. S., Teesdale, C. and Highton, R. B. (1962). *Ciba Foundation Symposium on Bilharziasis*, p. 127, Eds C. E. W. Wolstenholme and M. O'Connor, J. and A. Churchill, London.

Olivier, L. (1949). *Am. J. Hyg.* **49,** 290.

Pitchford, R. J. (1959). *Trans. R. Soc. Trop. Med. Hyg.* **53,** 213.

Pitchford, R. J. (1961). *Trans. R. Soc. Trop. Med. Hyg.* **55,** 44.

Pitchford, R. J. (1965). *Bull. Wld Hlth Org.* **32,** 105.

Pitchford, R. J. (1976). *J. Helminth.* **50,** 111.

Pitchford, R. J. and Visser, P. S. (1960). *Ann. Trop. Med. Parasit.* **54,** 247.

Pitchford, R. J. and Visser, P. S. (1975). *J. Helminth.* **49,** 137.

Preston, J. M. and Webbe, G. (1974). *Bull. Wld Hlth Org.* **50,** 566.

Rajanohanan, K. and Peter, C. T. (1975). *Kerala J. Vet. Sci.* **6,** 94.

Rao, P. V. R. and Devi, T. I. (1971). *Kerala J. Vet. Sci.* **2,** 94.

Raper, A. B. (1951). *E. Afr. Med. J.* **28,** 50.

Sadun, E. H. and Biocca, E. (1962). *Bull. Wld Hlth Org.* **27,** 810.

Schwetz, J. (1953). *Ann. Trop. Med. Parasit.* **47,** 183.

Schwetz, J. (1956). *Trans. R. Soc. Trop. Med. Hyg.* **50,** 275.

Sharma, D. N. and Dwivedi, J. N. (1976). *J. Comp. Pathol.* **86,** 449.

Sornmani, S. (1976). *S.E. Asian J. Trop. Med. Publ. Hlth* **7,** 149.

Southgate, V. R. (1978). *Ztschr. Parasitkde* **56,** 183.

Southgate, V. R. and Knowles, R. J. (1976). *J. Nat. Hist.* **9,** 273.

Southgate, V. R., Van Wyk, J. B. and Wright, C. A. (1976). *Ztschr. Parasitkde* **49,** 145.

Stunkard, H. W. and Hinchliffe, M. C. (1952). *J. Parasit.* **38,** 248.

Szidat, L. (1951). *Communic. Inst. Mac. Investig. Giencias Nat.* **2,** 129.

Taylor, M. G. (1970). *J. Helminth.* **44,** 253.

Taylor, M. G. and Andrews, B. J. (1973). *J. Helminth.* **47,** 439.

Taylor, M. G., James, E. R., Bickle, Q. D., Hussein, M. F., Andrews, B. J., Dobinson, A. R. and Nelson, G. S. (1979). *J. Helminth.* **53,** 1.

Taylor, M. G., James, E. R., Nelson, G. S., Bickle, Q. D., Dunne, D. W. and Webbe, G. (1976). *J. Helminth.* **50,** 1.

Taylor, M. G., Nelson, G. S., Smith, M. and Andrews, B. J. (1973). *Bull. Wld Hlth Org.* **49,** 59.

Teesdale, C. and Nelson, G. S. (1958). *E. Afr. Med. J.* **35,** 427.

Van Wyk, J. A. (1975). Thesis, University of Amsterdam.

Van Wyk, J. A., Rensburg, L. J. van and Heitman, L. P. (1976). *Onderstepoort J. Vet. Res.* **43,** 43.

Voge, M., Bruckner, D. and Bruce, J. I. (1978). *J. Parasit.* **64,** 577.

Walkiers, J. (1928). *Ann. Soc. Belg. Méd. Trop.* **8,** 21.

Webbe, G., James, C., Nelson, G. S., Ismail, M. M. and Shaw, J. R. (1979). *Trans. R. Soc. Trop. Med. Hyg.* **73,** 43.

Wright, C. A. and Southgate, V. R. (1976). In Genetic aspects of host–parasite relationships. *Symposia of the British Society for Parasitology* **14,** 55. Blackwell Scientific, London, Melbourne.

Wright, C. A., Southgate, V. R. and Knowles, R. J. (1972). *Trans. R. Soc. Trop. Med. Hyg.* **66,** 28.

Wright, C. A., Southgate, V. R., Van Wyk, J. A. and Moore, P. J. (1974). *Trans. R. Soc. Trop. Med. Hyg.* **68,** 413.

Yamagiwa, K. (1890). *Virchows Arch. Path. Anat.* **119,** 447.

Yokogawa, M. (1976). *S.E. Asian J. Trop. Med. Publ. Hlth* **7,** 322.

2 The Intermediate Hosts and Host–Parasite Relationships

Gerald Webbe

GENERAL CLASSIFICATION

The sub-classes *Pulmonata* and *Prosobranchiata*, contained within the class *Gastropoda*, embrace all the intermediate hosts of *Schistosoma*. Two families of the sub-class *Pulmonata—Planorbidae* and *Lymnaeidae*—contain natural snail hosts of schistosomes, while a third family—*Ancylidae*—contains one species, *Ferrissia tenuis* (Bourguignat), which has been experimentally infected with *S. haematobium* (Gadgil and Shah, 1956). The natural transmission of the parasite by this snail in the Bombay area of India, however, has not been fully established. In the family *Planorbidae*, certain groups of the sub-family *Bulininae* have been classified within a single genus—*Bulinus*—with sub-genera *Bulinus* and *Physopsis* (Mandahl-Barth, 1958) containing most of the intermediate hosts of *S. haematobium*.

The sub-family *Helisomatinae* contains the species *Planorbarius metidjensis* (Forbes), the intermediate host of *S. haematobium* in the Algarve Province of Portugal, though it has been reported that this focus of transmission has been eliminated. The species is also found in Spanish Morocco, but apparently is not susceptible to African strains of *S. haematobium*.

The intermediate hosts of *S. mansoni* in Africa have all been classified within one genus, *Biomphalaria*, of the sub-family *Planorbinae*, and snails of the genera *Australorbis*, *Tropicorbis* and *Taphius*, which transmit *S. mansoni* in the Americas, are anatomically indistinguishable from *Biomphalaria* (Hubendick, 1955). The name is now given precedence over all other synonyms, so that all snail hosts of *S. mansoni* now belong to this genus. (Ruling by the International Commission on Zoological Nomenclature 1966, Opinion 735; see Wright, 1962a.)

The snail intermediate hosts of *S. japonicum* belong to the family *Pomatiopsidae*, sub-family *Pomatiopsinae*, of the sub-class *Prosobranchiata*, and are contained within the genus *Oncomelania* (Gredler, 1881). The intermediate host of *S. mekongi* belongs to the genus *Tricula* (Benson, 1893) of the sub-family *Triculinae* (Davis, 1979).

EXPERIMENTAL TAXONOMY OF MOLLUSCS

The taxonomic status and classification of the snail intermediate hosts of schistosomes, based upon morphological criteria (conchological and anatomical), continue to present equivocal data, and other methodologies including chromosome, biochemical and immunological studies have been developed in order to resolve problems of doubtful affinities and the identification of variations both between and within different populations. At the species group level, karyotypic studies have provided interesting results and there is evidence that the susceptibility of certain bulinids to schistosomes is associated with polyploidy. The species of *Biomphalaria* which have been examined all have the haploid chromosome number of 18, typical of the *Planorbidae*. This number, with a few exceptions ranging up to 21, is also found in all species of *Bulinus* except those belonging to the *truncatus* group, in which the basic number is 36, although populations with 54 and 72 pairs of chromosomes have been recorded (Brown and Burch, 1967; Brown *et al.*, 1967; Burch and Lindsay, 1970; Burch, 1972).

Wright reviewed the application of experimental biochemical and immunological techniques to the taxonomy of the *Mollusca* and stated that emphasis has been placed upon species discrimination and the characterisation of infraspecific categories rather than on the relationships of the phylum and of classes and orders within the phylum (Wright, 1974). It is clear that no single method is available which serves to answer every taxonomic question and such experimental data must be evaluated in conjunction with basic morphological information.

Some techniques, however, have now been developed as routine taxonomic procedures. These include the electrophoresis of egg-proteins on cellulose acetate, paper chromatography of body surface mucus, Ouchterlony immunodiffusion in agar using egg-proteins and anti-sera raised against them, and iso-electric focusing of digestive-gland enzymes. These techniques are of value in relation to the planorbid snail hosts of schistosomes but require modification in some cases for application to the prosobranchs (Davis and Lindsay, 1967; Coles, 1970; Saladin *et al.*, 1976; Jelnes, 1977).

During the past five years, certain techniques have proved of great value in determining relationships and distribution patterns within the genus *Bulinus*. Wright (1977) pointed out, however, that no enzyme system has been discovered which can be associated directly with the susceptibility of snails to parasite infection, and that the complexity of the host–parasite relationship between snails and schistosomes is so great that correlations of this kind are unlikely to occur. This author considers, however, that where heterogeneity is detectable within a snail population by enzyme analysis, it may be possible to relate that heterogeneity to infection susceptibility within the context of local transmission, and that this is possibly the most significant potential contribution of the experimental taxonomy approach to schistosomiasis epidemiology and control programmes.

Identical methods of enzyme analysis have been applied to the schistosomes, and recently it has been shown that larval trematode infections in snails can be identified by distinctive enzyme patterns, which are usually different from those of the snail hosts (Wright and Rollinson, 1979). Such data could, of course, provide important information on the effects of control measures on transmission through the changes which may occur in both the parasites and snail intermediate hosts in the course of a control programme.

INTERMEDIATE HOSTS OF *S. HAEMATOBIUM*

Mandahl-Barth (1958) revised the African species of the genera *Biomphalaria* and *Bulinus*, which he classified within a species-group system, the recognised species and sub-species being largely divided according to the shape and sculpture of the shell, and to certain anatomical structures. In the past 20 years it has become apparent that morphological characteristics are not always adequate for a complete species determination and that knowledge of the compatibility of different geographic strains of *S. haematobium* with different intermediate hosts is incomplete. During the last decade, however, there has been a considerable advance in the knowledge of the basic relationships between

Bulinus, S. haematobium and other terminal-spined schistosomes to which different species are adapted. The genus *Bulinus*, which contains most of the snail intermediate hosts of *S. haematobium*, has been divided into four species-groups, three of which are contained in the sub-genus *Bulinus*, and one which contains the remaining members in the sub-genus *Physopsis* (Krauss) (see Table 2.1).

The bulinid shell is sinistral and higher than it is wide, being ovate or almost cylindrical in some forms and turreted according to the height of the spire. The height varies between 4 mm and 23 mm and there are usually four or five whorls, but there may be as many as seven. In shells having a low spire, the aperture is high and wide, being relatively narrower in shells with a high spire. The colour of the shell varies from almost pure white to 'dark chestnut brown' but usually it is a lighter or darker brown and is frequently concealed by a grey or black coating. The shell has a sculpture consisting of growth lines which are transversely arranged and in some forms 'pronounced transverse ribs' are apparent (Mandahl-Barth, 1958). It has been pointed out that conditions of life in African inland waters favour the evolution of microgeographic races but the formation of new species is generally hindered since the 'isolation' and 'variation' of different habitats, which tend to result in the formation of new species, is countered by another aspect of freshwaters—their 'unstable' nature and usually short duration. The differences between many of the intermediate hosts of schistosomes are therefore indistinct, and recent examination of new material has apparently shown that several of the specific and sub-specific characters are less constant and therefore less reliable than hitherto assumed (Mandahl-Barth, 1965). Most species are therefore linked by intermediate forms which normally occur only in limited areas, and which may be expected in the centres of evolution of the species concerned (Wright, 1961).

The sub-genus *Physopsis* differs from *Bulinus sensu stricto* in having a shell with a 'truncate columella' which is often provided with a 'lamella', by the interrupted 'spiral sculpture' which consists of small nodules or a 'punctation' on the upper whorls—which should not be confused with the very delicate punctation which is present on the embryonic whorls of all *Bulinus*, and by the ridge on the kidney. While those characters may not be present in all the individuals, the microsculpture is the only one found lacking in all specimens of a population

Table 2.1 The recognised species of *Bulinus* arranged within groups in alphabetical order. (After Brown, D. S., 1980.)

1. Sub-genus *Physopsis* Krauss, 1848
   1.1 *Bulinus africanus* group
     ***B. abyssinicus* (Martens, 1866)
     ***B. africanus* (Krauss, 1848)
     ***B. globosus* (Morelet, 1866)
      **B. hightoni* Brown & Wright, 1978
     ***B. jousseaumei* (Dautzenberg, 1890)
     ***B. nasutus* (Martens, 1879)
     ***B. obtusispira* (Smith, 1886)
       B. obtusus Mandahl-Barth, 1973
       B. ugandae Mandahl-Barth, 1954
       B. umbilicatus Mandahl-Barth, 1973

2. Sub-genus *Bulinus*
   2.1 *B. forskali* group
      **B. bavayi* (Dautzenberg, 1894)
     ***B. beccarii* (Paladilhe, 1872)
     ***B. camerunensis* Mandahl-Barth, 1957
       B. canescens (Morelet, 1868)
     ***B. cernicus* (Morelet, 1867)
      **B. crystallinus* (Morelet, 1868)
      **B. forskali* (Ehrenberg, 1831)
       B. scalaris (Dunker, 1845)
     ***B. senegalensis* Müller, 1781

   2.2 *B. reticulatus* group
      **B. reticulatus* Mandahl-Barth, 1954
     ***B. wrighti* Mandahl-Barth, 1965

   2.3 *B. truncatus/tropicus* complex
       B. angolensis (Morelet, 1866)
      **B. coulboisi* (Bourguignat, 1888)
      **B. depressus* Haas, 1936
     ***B. guernei* (Dautzenberg, 1890)
       B. hexaploideus Burch, 1972
       B. liratus (Tristram, 1863)
      **B. natalensis* (Küster, 1841)
       B. nyassanus (Smith, 1877)
      **B. octoploideus* Burch, 1972
       B. permembranaceus (Preston, 1912)
     ***B. rohlfsi* (Clessin, 1886)
       B. succinoides (Smith, 1877)
       B. transversalis (Martens, 1897)
       B. trigonus (Martens, 1892)
       B. tropicus (Krauss, 1848)
     ***B. truncatus* (Audouin, 1827)

---

 * Compatible with this parasite to some extent in the laboratory.
** Known to serve as natural intermediate host of *S. haematobium*.

(Mandahl-Barth, 1965). A good distinguishing character in live specimens is the pointed 'tail' of *Physopsis* and the blunter one of *Bulinus s.s.*

The *africanus* group (= sub-genus *Physopsis*)

This is a very important group medically as most of the species contained in it serve as intermediate hosts of *S. haematobium* in Africa south of the Sahara and of some cattle schistosomes as well. It includes: *Bulinus (Physopsis) abyssinicus* in south-east Ethiopia and Somalia; *B. (P.) africanus africanus (Krauss)* and *B. (P.) africanus ovoideus* (Bourguignat) in southern and eastern Africa; *B. (P.) globosus* widely distributed in all of Africa south of the Sahara; the recently discovered *B. (P.) hightoni* from north-east Kenya—referred to as the *africanus-species group* on the basis of immunological cross-sections of the egg-proteins (Brown and Wright, 1978); *B. (P.) jousseaumei* from Chad and Senegal; *B. (P.) obtusispira* (Smith) intermediate host in Madagascar, assigned to the *africanus* group on the basis of immunological reactions, although it sometimes resembles *B. liratus* of the *truncatus/tropicus* complex. *B. (P.) obtusus* in Chad and *B. (P.) ugandae* found in Uganda, Kenya, mainland Tanzania and the Sudan are not susceptible to infection, while *B. (P.) umbilicatus* found in Sudan, Mali and Mauritania is thought to be an intermediate host, but the 'renal ridge' is lacking in young snails which suggests a relation with the *truncatus/tropicus* complex (Mandahl-Barth, 1973).

Certain other taxonomic difficulties are presented by the *africanus-species group*, including the occurrence of morphological intermediates among *africanus, globosus* and *nasutus* in the East African coastal belt and between *globosus* and *ugandae* in the Kisumu area of Kenya. Difficulties have also been experienced in identifying *globosus* and *jousseaumei* in West Africa, while intermediates between *africanus* and *globosus* have been found in Zambia–Angola. Some of these taxonomic difficulties have been clarified by electrophoretic analysis of egg-protein and immuno-logical studies.

The sub-genus *Bulinus*

This sub-genus contains three species-groups, the compositions of which have been changed during the past seven years as the result of morphological, biochemical and cytological studies (Brown, 1980).

The reticulatus *group*

Bulinus (*Bulinus*) *reticulatus* has distinct morphological characteristics and occurs between Ethiopia and South Africa. It does not appear to be of importance in the transmission of *S. haematobium* although it is susceptible to the parasite in the laboratory and can be infected with a large number of different schistosomes. In Aden and Arabia *B. (P.) wrighti* Mandahl-Barth is a natural intermediate host of *S. haematobium*.

The forskali *group*

B. (B.) forskali (Ehrenberg) is a common and ubiquitous species in Africa, but earlier evidence of its natural role as an intermediate host of *S. haematobium* in the Gambia (Smithers, 1956) has not been confirmed, although it is an intermediate host of *S. intercalatum* in Cameroon and Gabon (Wright *et al.*, 1972), and of *S. bovis* in western Kenya (Southgate and Knowles, 1975). It has been shown that *S. intercalatum* breeds successfully with *S. haematobium* in the laboratory and in nature (Wright, 1974; Southgate *et al.*, 1976), and that hybrid miracidia under laboratory conditions are capable of developing in snails of both the *forskali* and *truncatus* species-groups. There is a possibility that such a parasite strain could be established in nature, thus emphasising the necessity for continuing surveillance of *B. forskali* throughout its range (Brown, 1980). *B. (B.) bavayi* is a potential host of *S. haematobium* in the Malagasy Republic where *B. (B.) mariei* (Crosse) has also been suspected of this role (Wright, 1971); *B. (B.) beccarii* is an intermediate host in Aden and Saudi Arabia (Wright, 1963a; Arfaa, 1976), with *B. (B.) cernicus* being responsible for transmission in Mauritius. *B. (B.) scalaris* has a wide distribution in Central and Eastern Africa but its status as an intermediate host is unknown. *B. (B.) senegalensis* is found in the Gambia, Senegal and Mauritania (Mandahl-Barth, 1973), but is an intermediate host of *S. haematobium* in the Gambia (Smithers, 1956).

The truncatus/tropicus *complex*

B. truncatus and *B. tropicus* were formerly considered to be members of two different species-groups: members of the *truncatus* group, and in particular *B. (B.) truncatus truncatus* (Audouin), are present in the Near East and Mediterranean countries of Africa, in East, Central, West and parts of southern Africa, being tetraploid species (chromosome number 2n = 72), which transmit, or are able to transmit, particular strains of *S. haematobium*; and the *tropicus* species-group, mainly present in southern Africa, containing diploid species (2n = 36), and generally insusceptible to schistosomes. However, the differences between these species-groups are apparently not as distinct as was formerly thought, Brown and his co-workers (1971) having demonstrated continuous variation in the characters of the radula, and some diploid snails having been found susceptible to *S. haematobium* (Lo *et al.*, 1970; Mandahl-Barth *et al.*, 1976). Tetraploid snails have been found as far south as Malawi (Mandahl-Barth, 1960). The results from morphological, biochemical and cytological studies, therefore, indicate that it is now desirable to refer to a single group of species—the *B. truncatus/tropicus* complex—in which polyploidy has occurred a number of times (Brown, 1980).

As the results of studies (Brown and Wright, 1972; Burch, 1972), at least four species of snails in Ethiopia have been distinguished by differences in numbers of chromosomes which were previously identified as *B. sericinus* (Jickeli) or *B. truncatus sericinus*, and specimens from some areas have been found susceptible to Egyptian *S. haematobium* in the laboratory. *B. truncatus* has been identified from different locations in the Awash valley (Kloos and Lemma, 1974), although *S. haematobium* is transmitted by a member of the *africanus* species-group in the lower Awash. On the Ethiopian plateau, where *B. truncatus* is uncommon, the presence of higher polyploid species probably accounts for the absence of *S. haematobium*, with which they are generally of low compatibility.

B. truncatus, identified by chromosome numbers and egg-proteins, has been found in a wide area of Western Kenya (Brown and Wright, 1974). It has been shown that these snails do not transmit the local strain of *S. haematobium*, which is carried by snails of the *africanus* species-group, but that they are susceptible to an Egyptian strain of the parasite (Southgate and Knowles, 1977). Brown (1976) and Jelnes (1977) have, however, distinguished a different tetraploid species in the Kenya highlands which may be compatible with the local parasite. *B. truncatus*, or related tetraploid populations, are found as far south as Malawi. In south-east Africa, however, the diploid species *B.*

natalensis occurs (Brown *et al.*, 1971) and it has been reported from Nelspruit that snails which resemble *B. truncatus* are susceptible to *S. haematobium*. Successful laboratory infections of diploid snails resembling *B. natalensis* or *B. depressus* are reported (Lo *et al.*, 1970; Mandahl-Barth *et al.*, 1976), although there is no evidence that *S. haematobium* is being transmitted in nature by these snails. In West Africa, *B. truncatus rohlfsi* (Clessin) the principal intermediate host of *S. haematobium* in Volta Lake is widely distributed, but more studies are necessary in relation to *B. rohlfsi* from Nigeria, which apparently differs from Ghanaian specimens in certain characteristics (Brown, 1980).

B. (B.) guernei (Dautzenberg) occurs in the Gambia, where it transmits *S. haematobium*, and in the Senegal/Mali region. It is a poorly known nominal species and further host–parasite compatibility studies are indicated. *B. (B.) coulboisi* (Boirguignat), of which some forms are susceptible to *S. haematobium*, is found in East Africa and the eastern part of Zaire.

The varying susceptibility of local races of bulinid snails to different strains of *S. haematobium* has been recorded by many workers (Wright, 1962b and 1963b; Paperna, 1968). As a result of his experiments, Le Roux (1958) suggested that there are two separate species of parasite, the form transmitted in North Africa by the *truncatus* group of snails being known as *S. haematobium* and that developing in Africa south of the Sahara in the *africanus* species as *S. capense* (Harley, 1864), a view which has been supported by many workers. Other authorities, however, consider that insufficient grounds exist for resurrecting '*S. capense*' to distinguish the South African from the North African strains of the parasite (Nelson *et al.*, 1962). According to Pitchford (1965), a local Nelspruit (South African) snail, identified as a member of the *truncatus* group, was found to be susceptible to the so-called *S. capense* and to *S. mattheei*, being no less susceptible to both these schistosomes than were local *Bulinus (Physopsis)* sp. of the *africanus* group of snails. On the basis of this, and other evidence obtained from the measurement of eggs and anatomical features of the parasites, Pitchford concluded that the name '*S. capense*' should be regarded as synonymous with *S. haematobium*. Wright (1966) commented that there is little interchange of parasites between the groups of bulinids transmitting strains of the *S. haematobium* complex, that the specificity of the forms infecting the *truncatus* and *africanus* groups is very strong, and that in both cases the geographical

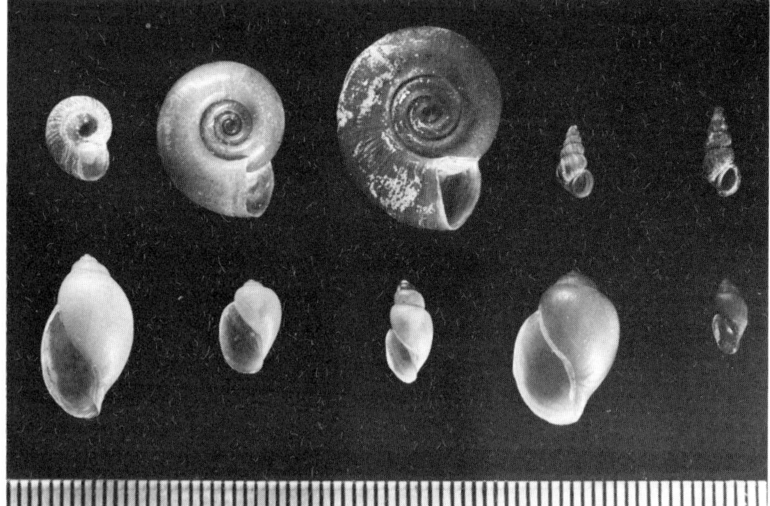

Fig. 2.1 Snail intermediate hosts (scale in mm). Top row, left to right: *B. choanomphala, B. sudanica, B. glabrata, O.h. nosophara, O.h. hupensis.* Bottom row, left to right: *B. (P.) nasutus, B. (B.) rohlfsi, B. (B.) senegalensis, B. (P.) africanus, B. (B.) forskalii.*

range of the snails slightly exceeds that of their schistosome parasites. Wright (1967) further stated that increasing evidence supports the view that we are dealing with a 'composite species of two morphologically similar forms', *S. haematobium sensu stricto* developing only in snails of the *truncatus* and *forskali* species-groups in North Africa, the Middle East, parts of West Africa, Mauritius and the Malagasy Republic, and '*S. capense*' developing in species of the *africanus* complex, generally in Africa south of the Sahara, with a mosaic of both forms in the west.

In order to study the *S. haematobium* problem further, the susceptibility of 11 species of bulinid snails to 4 strains of *S. haematobium* and an Iranian strain of *S. bovis* from different geographic regions was investigated (Webbe and James, 1971a). It was found that *B. globosus* (Nigeria) is highly susceptible to its own strain of parasite, with an infection rate of 71%, whereas *B. truncatus* (Iran), *B. truncatus rohlfsi* (Ghana), *B. africanus ovoideus, B. nasutus productus, B. globosus* (Tanzania) and *B. bavayi* (Malagasy Republic) are completely refractory to this Nigerian strain of *S. haematobium*. It is, however, infective to *B. obtusispira* (Malagasy Republic—30·7%) and to *B. africanus africanus* (South Africa—5·9%). *B. truncatus* (Iran) was found to be susceptible to its own strain of *S. haematobium* (Dezful—43·0%). This strain is also infective to *B. truncatus rohlfsi* (Ghana—4·5%) and to *B. africanus* (South Africa—22·2%), but other species are all refractory to it.

S. haematobium from Alexandria, Egypt, was found to be infective to local *B. truncatus truncatus* (24·3%) and to *B. africanus* (South Africa—12·7%). It was not found to be infective, however, to any of the East African snails nor to *B. globosus* (Nigeria), *B. truncatus* (Iran) or *B. truncatus rohlfsi* (Ghana). It is noteworthy that Iranian, Egyptian and Ghanian bulinids of the *truncatus* species-group were all found to be refractory to strains of *S. haematobium* normally transmitted by snails of the *africanus* species complex. However, both *B. globosus* (Nigeria) and *B. truncatus rohlfsi* (Ghana) have recently been infected with *S. haematobium* isolated from a naturally infected baboon imported from the area of the River Gambia (Fig. 2.1).

Whilst strains of *S. haematobium* which usually develop in bulinid snails of the *truncatus* group may not readily develop in those of the *africanus* group and *vice versa*, it is apparent that exceptions do occur. In Ghana, although a distinction can be made between the strain of *S. haematobium* which is associated with local *B. globosus* and the strain transmitted by *B. truncatus rohlfsi*, the separation is not absolute (Paperna, 1968). In most populations of both *B. globosus* and *B. truncatus rohlfsi* a few snails become infected following exposure to the non-compatible strain of parasite, and a few populations of *B. globosus* even showed a high level of compatibility with the strain normally transmitted by *B. truncatus rohlfsi*, and *vice versa*. Paperna considers that *B. truncatus rohlfsi* appears to be biologically the better adapted host of *S. haematobium*, whereas *B. globosus* is apparently more susceptible to infection and cercarial production is higher, although this snail and the strains of *S. haematobium* transmitted by it usually showed a 'strong tendency to further divergence towards the formation of isolated local host–parasite compatibilities' (Paperna, 1968). Chu and co-workers (1978) have recorded mixing of the two strains of *S. haematobium* near Lake Volta, where the parasite isolated from both individuals and the community developed well in both *B. rohlfsi* and *B. globosus*.

Evidence of the existence of different geographical strains of *S. haematobium* has also been obtained from comparative studies of their characteristics in the hamster (Wright and Bennet, 1967a and 1967b; Webbe and James, 1971b; James and Webbe, 1973 and 1975), while other observations have been made in baboons (Webbe *et al.*, 1974). Pronounced differences in the pathogenicity of strains of *S. haematobium* from various geographical regions have been suggested to account for the apparent severity of human infections recorded in certain endemic areas (Macdonald and Forsyth, 1968) compared with their relatively benign manifestations in others (Walker *et al.*, 1970). Demonstrable differences are apparent between the different geographical strains of *S. haematobium* in the hamster and baboon, but they possess many common characteristics too, and considerable variability has been noted in individual animals both in relation to the growth of parasites and to the number of eggs found in different organs.

While the observed differences in the severity of *S. haematobium* infections from different geographical areas may therefore be attributable, in part, to strain variations of the parasite producing differing intensities of infection, it should not be forgotten that infra-specific variations in the human host, including physiological differences and behavioural patterns, may also profoundly influence the picture.

It is considered that these different strains possess individual characteristics which are probably limited in distribution, and which reflect infra-specific variations of a single complex species, rather than the defined properties of two separate species, *S. haematobium* and '*S. capense*', which have been suggested. *S. haematobium* should be used to describe all strains of the parasite and these strains should be distinguished only by the names of their geographical origins.

INTERMEDIATE HOSTS OF *S. MANSONI*

The genus *Biomphalaria* is widely distributed in Africa south of the Sahara, predominantly above an altitude of approximately 1000 feet, but almost at sea level in parts of North, South and West Africa. It is present in Egypt, Israel and in parts of Arabia, but it does not extend to Iraq. It is found in the southern United States, in the Caribbean Islands and in South America as far south as Chile.

The taxonomic status of the African species has been little changed during the past 20 years and the four species-groups recognised by Mandahl-Barth (1978) continue to be the framework for their classification.

The shell is discoid or lens shaped, being 'ultradextral' and 'biconcave', forming a disc of variable height with a diameter of between 7 mm and 22 mm; 'the number of whorls varies between $3\frac{1}{2}''$ and almost $7'''$; the concavity or umbilicus on the other side of the shell is very wide and shallow in some forms, and in others narrow and deeper; 'the shell is a lighter or darker brownish horn colour, sometimes almost white, in other cases more reddish and very often concealed by a grey or black coating'; curved, transversely arranged growth lines which are sometimes crossed by faint spiral lines comprise the sculpture of the shell (Mandahl-Barth, 1978).

The *pfeifferi* group has several forms and is represented in nearly all parts of Africa south of the Sahara and in Malagasy Republic. Members of this group serve as intermediate hosts of *S. mansoni* in Aden, Yemen and Western Saudi Arabia. It is probably unrealistic, from the medical point of view, to divide *B. pfeifferi* (Krauss) into sub-species since all forms serve as intermediate hosts of *S. mansoni*. *B. pfeifferi rhodesiensis* is, however, an exception as it differs from all the other forms of *B. pfeifferi* (Mandahl-Barth, 1960).

B. rueppelli (Dunker) is regarded as a separate species from *B. pfeifferi* (Wright and Brown, 1962). It is considered that the areas around Lakes Kivu and Tanganyika are centres from which the different forms of *B. pfeifferi* probably spread.

The *choanomphala* group comprises a few forms which are restricted to certain of the great natural lakes. It includes *B. choanomphala choanomphala* (Martens), Lake Victoria; *B. choanomphala elegans* Mandahl-Barth, Lake Albert; *B. smithi* Preston, Lake Edward; and *B. stanleyi* (Smith), Lake Albert.

Certain taxonomic relationships continue to be unresolved, including the question as to whether the more or less *choanomphala*-like *Biomphalaria*, found in a number of lakes in Rwanda, Cameroon and Chad, really belong to the *choanomphala* group or whether they are ecophenotypes of *pfeifferi*.

The *alexandrina* group has a scattered distribution in Africa. *B. alexandrina alexandrina* (Ehrenberg) is present in Egypt and Sudan. The group also includes *B. angulosa* Mandahl-Barth which is distributed in Tanzania, northern Zambia and in eastern South Africa, being closely related to *B. alexandrina*. *B. alexandrina mansoni* (Mandahl-Barth) which is found only in the northern Congo Basin.

The *sudanica* group comprises an East and West African

species, each with sub-species—*B. sudanica sudanica* (Martens), *B. sudanica tanganyicensis* (Smith) and *B. camerunensis camerunensis* (Boettger), *B. camerunensis manzadica* (Mandahl-Barth) respectively. Further taxonomic relationship problems apparently exist in relation to *B. camerunensis, B. salinarium* (Morelet) and *B. pfeifferi*, in Angola.

Although differences in the degree of susceptibility of *Biomphalaria* spp. to infection with *S. mansoni* have been noted, a general compatibility of various strains of *S. mansoni* and *Biomphalaria* is apparent. All African *Biomphalaria* are susceptible to some strains of *S. mansoni* but certain anomalies have been recorded, including certain populations of Egyptian *alexandrina* which are very receptive to infection with the local strain of *S. mansoni*, others less compatible and others virtually impossible to infect. It has been noted, however, that the latter category can be infected with other *mansoni*-strains (Mandahl-Barth, 1978), and that the relationship between the two *mansoni* strains in West Africa, the *pfeifferi*-borne and *camerunensis*-borne, requires further investigation.

In the Western Hemisphere, the genus *Biomphalaria* is represented by some 20 species, of which 15 have been well defined by conchological, anatomical and, in some cases, genetic criteria (PAHO/WHO, 1968). Of these, only *B. glabrata* (Say), *B. straminea* (Dunker) and *B. tenagophila* (Orbigny) have been found naturally infected with *S. mansoni*.

B. amazonica Paraense, *B. helophila* (Orbigny)-syn. *albicans*, and *B. peregrina* (Orbigny)-syn. *chilensis*, have been found susceptible to laboratory infection, but have not been found naturally infected. Other experimental infections have been recorded but the identification of the respective *Biomphalaria* populations requires confirmation.

B. glabrata is found throughout the Caribbean region in Dominican Republic, Vieques, Puerto Rico, St Kitts, Antigua, Dominica, Guadeloupe, Martinique, St Lucia and formerly St Martin (Prentice, personal communication). It is found in Venezuela, in the coastal area of Surinam and French Guiana, and in north-east and south-east Brazil, where there is evidence that it is spreading with consequent increased endemicity of *S. mansoni*. It is considered that *B. glabrata* is the most efficient intermediate host of *S. mansoni* in the Western Hemisphere and, although there is apparently considerable variation in the levels of susceptibility of different populations of the species (Paraense and Correa, 1963), most are highly susceptible to infection giving prolonged daily output of cercariae.

B. straminea is widely distributed, being found in some Caribbean islands (Martinique, Grenada and Trinidad), Costa Rica, Panama, Venezuela, Guyana, Surinam, French Guiana, Brazil, east Peru, east Bolivia, Paraguay and Argentina. It shows considerable ecological adaptation, but it is considered to be a poor host of *S. mansoni*, with very low natural infection rates (Coelho and Barbosa, 1956). It is, however, associated with high human infection rates in north-east Brazil, where it is a more important intermediate host than *B. glabrata* (de Lucena, 1963). *B. straminea* has been found transmitting *S. mansoni* in isolated foci in the Amazonian and central regions of Brazil, but not in any other locations throughout its recorded range (Paraense and Michelson, personal communication).

B. tenagophila is found in Brazil, east Bolivia, Paraguay, Uraguay and Argentina. It serves as an intermediate host of *S. mansoni* in Rio de Janeiro and São Paulo states of Brazil, and its importance has increased during the past 20 years because of the recent adaptation to it of a strain of *S. mansoni* (Paraense and Correa, 1963). Different populations of this species apparently show variable (moderate or low) susceptibility to infection (Paraense and Correa, 1978). Evidence suggests that a closer compatibility exists between *S. mansoni* and its intermediate host in the Western Hemisphere than in Africa (Saoud, 1965a and 1965b) and that *S. mansoni* is not a uniform species but that distinct infra-specific and inter-strain variations occur. Compatibility between parasite and intermediate snail host is largely regulated by genetic factors. *B. glabrata* populations have been categorised according to their infection rates: some were susceptible, others refractory, some were susceptible when juvenile but refractory when adult, and a fourth category was susceptible as juveniles but showed varying degrees of susceptibility as adults. It was found that the juvenile susceptibility status was determined by a complex of four or more genetic factors and factors for lack of susceptibility may, of course, be present even in susceptible snails and *vice versa* (Richards and Meredith, 1972; Richards, 1973, 1975 and 1976). Richards (1977) pointed out that there are probably additional genetic factors for susceptibility in intermediate host snails and for infectivity in parasite strains, and that 'since both snail populations and parasite populations may vary qualitatively in the alleles present and quantitatively in gene frequencies, variations in host–parasite relations when populations from different geographic areas are compared, are to be expected'.

A series of Field Guides to African Freshwater Snails (1973) is available from the WHO Snail Identification Centre, Danish Bilharziasis Laboratory, Charlottenlund, Denmark, as is 'Freshwater snails of Africa' (Brown, 1980). A publication for the identification of snail intermediate hosts in the Americas has also been produced (PAHO/WHO, 1968).

INTERMEDIATE HOSTS OF *S. JAPONICUM*

The oncomelanid shell is small, dextral, conical or sub-conical with four to eight whorls, being 'imperforate' or 'umbilicate' with a corneous or calcareous operculum which is 'concentric' or 'paucispiral'; the height varies from 3 mm to 10 mm and the shell may be smooth, have fine axial growth lines or strong axial ribs (Malek, 1962). *S. japonicum* is transmitted by populations of polytypic *Oncomelania hupensis* (Gredler), of which there are six sub-species: *O.h. hupensis* (Gredler), in Mainland China; *O.h. quadrasi* (Möllendorff) in the Philippines; *O.h. nosophora* (Robson) in Japan; *O.h. lindoensis* (Davis and Carney) in Sulawesi; and *O.h. formosana* (Pilsbry and Hirase) and *O.h. chiui* (Habe and Miyazaki) in Taiwan (Davis, 1978). These taxa are too similar to be regarded as species (Davis, 1968 and 1969; Davis and Carney, 1973). There are races of these sub-species and Davis (1968) recorded that various populations of *O.h. formosana* have distinct electrophoretic patterns and differ in their potential to transmit the Formosan zoophilic strain of *S. japonicum*, such populations being morphologically identical and immunologically indistinguishable. The main differences between the sub-species include shell size and sculpture, electrophoretic and antigenic differences (Davis, 1968), differences in reproductive potential in the same environment (Wagner and Chi, 1959; Van der Schalie and Davis, 1968), differences in susceptibility to different strains of *S. japonicum* (Chiu, 1967; Chi *et al.*, 1971; Davis and Ruff, 1973).

The susceptibility of *Oncomelania* hybrid snails to various geographic strains of *S. japonicum*, hybridisation of *O. hupensis*, and the importance of genetic factors in the transmission of *S. japonicum* were demonstrated (Chi *et al.*, 1971; Davis *et al.*, 1976).

During the past 10 years, *O.h. lindoensis*, which transmits *S. japonicum* in Sulawesi (Celebes), has been discovered and described (Carney *et al.*, 1973; Davis and Carney, 1973) and the snail intermediate host of the Mekong '*japonicum*-like' schistosome was found in '*Lithoglyphopsis*' *aperta* (Temcharoen) (Harinasuta *et al.*, 1972; Sornmani *et al.*, 1973).

As the result of systematic and biological analysis of this snail, the close relationship of '*L.*' *aperta* to the genus *Tricula* was demonstrated and it was suggested that the Mekong schistosome was not *S. japonicum* (Davis *et al.*, 1976). '*L.*' *aperta* has now been shown to be a *Tricula* (Davis, 1979) and the Mekong schistosome has been named *S. mekongi* (Voge *et al.*, 1978; Table 2.2).

Table 2.2   The snail hosts of *S. japonicum* and *S. mekongi*. (After Davis, 1979.)

Sub-class	*Prosobranchia*	
Family	*Pomatiopsidae* Stimpson, 1865	
Sub-family	*Pomatiopsinae* Stimpson, 1865	
Genus	*Oncomelania* Gredler, 1881	
	**O. hupensis* (Gredler, 1881)	
	**O.h. hupensis* (Gredler, 1881)	Mainland China
	**O.h. formosana* (Pilsbry and Hirase, 1905)	Taiwan
	O.h. chiui (Habe and Miyazaki, 1962)	Taiwan
	**O.h. quadrasi* (Möllendorff, 1895)	Philippines
	**O.h. nosophora* (Robson, 1915)	Japan
	**O.h. lindoensis* (Davis and Carney, 1973)	Sulawesi
Sub-family	*Triculinae* Annandale, 1924	
Tribe	*Triculini* Davis, 1978	
Genus	*Tricula* Benson, 1893	Asia
	**T. aperta* (Temcharoen, 1971)	Mekong River Laos, Cambodia

* Indicates hosts transmitting the respective parasite naturally.

T. aperta is endemic in the Mekong River and there are three races of the species—alpha, beta and gamma—which can transmit *S. mekongi*, but only the latter one is considered to be important in transmission (Davis *et al.*, 1976).

ECOLOGY AND BIONOMICS OF INTERMEDIATE HOSTS

The snail intermediate host is an essential link in the schistosome life-cycle and adequate knowledge of its ecology, bionomics and population dynamics is required for a proper understanding of schistosome transmission, or as a basis for the planning and evaluation of measures directed against snails in the control of disease, or both.

There are considerable differences in the susceptibility of different species of snails, and of races of the same species, to different strains of parasites, and in their capacity to serve as intermediate hosts. Effective transmission depends upon the degree of compatibility between the snail host and the local strain of parasite. The degree of susceptibility of the snail host will, of course, influence the production of cercariae and determine the epidemiological pattern. Very few distinct relationships have been established in snail ecology and there is a general lack of precise data (Hubendick, 1958). This is due to the general euryok character of freshwater snails, their wide ecological tolerance and, therefore, lesser adaptation to special conditions than most marine or terrestrial organisms. To a great extent, therefore, various species react similarly to the same environmental influence, their ecological requirements being qualitatively similar but quantitatively different. This is applicable to most aquatic planorbid and bulinid snail intermediate hosts, and it is very difficult to define and evaluate the significance of an individual environmental factor—whether physical, chemical or biological—when all may be mutually affecting one another and their combined effect influencing a particular species or population. A detailed review of abiotic factors influencing the distribution and life-cycle of snail intermediate hosts has recently been produced (Appleton and Stiles, 1976). Although the snail intermediate hosts of *S. japonicum* are amphibious, their responses to differences in physical, chemical and biological factors in water are similar to those of aquatic molluscs, while on land they favour moist and shady conditions.

The habitat

The bulinid and planorbid intermediate hosts are found in many different habitat types, including small ponds (permanent or semi-permanent), marshes and swamps, perennial and seasonal rivers and streams, very large permanent bodies of water such as natural and man-made lakes and habitats such as irrigation channels, drains, dams and rice fields. The bulinid intermediate hosts are generally found in impounded waters, but also in slowly flowing water and in irrigation networks in certain areas, e.g. in Egypt and the Middle East. The planorbid snail hosts are adapted to a wide range of environmental conditions—the general features of the habitat are shallow water in streams with a moderate organic content, little turbidity, a muddy substratum rich in organic matter, submerged or emergent vegetation, rich microflora and moderate light penetration. They are found in freshwater with a pH varying between 5·3 and 9, in tropical forest regions, as well as in arid situations, at low or at high altitudes, and at water temperatures ranging between 18°C and 30°C.

The amphibious *Oncomelania* spp. inhabit floodplains and the many man-made habitats resulting from agricultural development in such areas—drainage channels and roadside ditches, rice fields, and the smaller canals and drains of irrigation works.

Chemical and physical factors

Snails are capable of tolerating different chemical and physical conditions within very wide limits and it is apparently not usually possible to predict colonisation of a particular habitat through chemical analysis of its water content (Webbe and Msangi, 1958; Webbe, 1962a; Sturrock, 1974; Klumpp and Chu, 1977). Interesting results have been obtained, however, by measuring salinity (total concentrations of electrolytes), of which electrical conductivity gives an acceptable estimate. It was found in Puerto Rico that waters having less than 150 mg/l of dissolved solids, represented by a conductivity of approximately 222 micromhos, were free of established colonies of *B. glabrata* (Harry *et al.*, 1957). In the Bukoba area of West Lake Region, Tanzania, no snails were found in waters for which conductivities of 8–19·7 micromhos per cm at 25°C were recorded (McClelland and Jordan, 1962). It is thought that the effect may be due to a low concentration of one or more electrolytes, so that certain species fail to maintain adequate salt balance when the external concentration of a particular ion or ions falls below a particular value. Observations on the distribution of molluscs in relation to water chemistry and the effects of different concentrations of calcium and magnesium upon the natality rates of snails have been made (Schutte and Frank, 1964; Harrison and Shiff, 1966; Harrison *et al.*, 1966; Thomas and Lough, 1974; Thomas *et al.*, 1974).

Low pH may be harmful to molluscs, coagulating the mucus on exposed skin surfaces (Carpenter, 1927), but there may be marked diurnal variations in the reaction of water depending upon the carbon dioxide concentration (Boycott, 1936).

Profound diurnal temperature ranges occur in many of the habitats of snail intermediate hosts, but the existence of micro-habitats having their own microclimates must be considered in this respect. In these conditions higher concentrations of oxygen may be available than those recorded for general water sup-plies—the heart beat and oxygen consumption of snails can be influenced by temperature (Von Brand and Mehlman, 1953; Chernin, 1957). It may be, therefore, that oxygen tension rather than temperature is likely to be the factor of most importance to snails in nature. Its significance as a determining factor in the choice of microhabitat by freshwater snails in relation to *Nympheae* spp. has been recorded (Wright, 1956).

Light

Although increased hydrostatic pressure in deep water may decrease the buoyancy of snail hosts, it does not seem to be a significant factor in most snail habitats. Most of the observations made on the influence of light on host snails are qualitative, but numerous records show that these species are able to survive for several consecutive generations in almost total darkness. It has been suggested by some workers that the effect of sunlight is an indirect one, related to photosynthesis and the availability of food. There is evidence to show that planorbid snails may be negatively phototaxic and that locomotor, feeding and reproduc-tive activities are nocturnal in the case of a variety of aquatic and terrestrial *Pulmonata*. It is also considered that light may be more important than temperature in controlling locomotor activity (Appleton, 1978).

Geology

The distribution of snail intermediate hosts may be influenced by geological factors in many different ways, and this question has been reviewed in relation to snail distribution in the coastal plains of Kenya and Tanzania (McCullough, 1962). It has been shown that in South Africa snails survive in flowing habitats only when rock formations are heterogeneous in hardness (Ap-pleton and Stiles, 1976), thus permitting the development of irregularities in the stream bottom with associated stretches of still water in which snail intermediate hosts can survive. The snail habitat may, of course, be chemically conditioned by ions leached from the related rock formations.

The general topography of an area may influence the distribution of snails. *B. truncatus* does not usually tolerate rapidly flowing water, while *B. alexandrina* is apparently even less able to withstand high rates of flow (Boycott, 1936; Watson, 1950 and 1958). *B. glabrata* is also limited by stream gradient, but in most such cases marginal shallows will occur which are capable of supporting high densities of snails. *O.h. quadrasi* occurs in the Philippines only in very flat regions regardless of the topographical features, including elevation (Pesigan *et al.*, 1958). The relationship betweeen snail ecology and current velocity still requires investigation, but available data indicate that the limiting velocity for most species is probably not less than 30 cm/s (or approximately 1 ft/s). Current velocity is the most important factor influencing the distribution of snails in lotic environments, i.e. river systems (Appleton, 1978).

Density

The maintenance of snail intermediate hosts at high densities may result in reduced growth rates and fecundity, and these effects have been studied in laboratory colonies of *B. glabrata, B. forskali, B. globosus* and *B. angulosa* (Chernin and Michelson, 1957a and 1957b; Wright, 1960; Shiff, 1964a; Sturrock, 1965a). There is evidence that the surface:volume ratio of the water used in these studies may be important, with a relatively large surface reducing the effects of crowding, which suggests that some unstable substances in the water are involved (Berrie, 1970). Growth inhibition has been reported in a natural population of *B. sudanica tanganyicensis* in a small pool in Uganda (Berrie and Visser, 1963; Berrie, 1968). Although the presence of a chemical factor was established, other factors, including 'availability of food and mutual interference in relation to density', may have contributed to the overall picture.

Studies have been made to determine the role of density-dependent factors in relation to numbers of snails. An increased rate of growth and natality of *B. glabrata* resulted in the presence of chemical growth factors of a molecular weight between 500 and 1000, low concentration of ammonia, substances found in snail faeces, and celluloses of snail origin (Thomas, 1973; Thomas *et al.*, 1974; Thomas, Goldsworthy and Aram, 1975;

Thomas, Lough and Lodge, 1975; Thomas *et al.*, 1976). Negative feedback effects were observed through calcium depletion, the presence of concentrations of ammonia above a critical threshold and plant inhibitory factors. Such density-dependent factors are only likely to be effective in impounded waters, since in flowing waters any such inhibiting factors will be diluted and the level of nutrient ions maintained.

Rainfall

Rainfall cycles are among the most important climatic factors that affect the life history of snails and determine seasonal fluctuations in their density. This is particularly so in the Tropics in relation to bulinid snails in areas with temporary and semi-permanent habits (McCullough, 1962; Webbe, 1962a; Shiff, 1964; Webbe, 1965) and intense breeding of planorbid snails has also been reported in areas with seasonal rainfall (Barbosa and Olivier, 1958; Teesdale, 1962; Berrie, 1964; Sturrock, 1973; Fig. 2.2). Rainfall may of course result in sharp reductions in population density where streams and rivers are flushed out (Webbe, 1962b) and in East Africa and the Caribbean a fall in snail density with little or no breeding of planorbid snails occurred during the main periods of rainfall, followed by an upsurge in snail populations with the production of large numbers of young snails during the drier months which follow (Webbe, 1965; Anon, 1971).

Temperature

The distribution and growth of snail populations in a given area depend upon temperature and other incompletely understood factors. Low temperatures in winter reduce breeding or stop it completely in temperate and sub-tropical zones; it is then resumed when temperatures increase, snail population densities becoming maximal. This general pattern is seen in Egypt in relation to *B. truncatus* and *B. alexandrina* (Dazo *et al.*, 1966; Demian and Kamel, 1972) and was also recorded in the case of *O.h. nosophora* in Japan (Ritchie, 1955). High temperatures in summer in the Sudan are responsible for reduced reproduction, *B. truncatus* and *B. pfeifferi* being most abundant in March and April (Malek, 1962), while seasonal temperature changes in Iran are responsible for differences in the local distribution pattern of snails (Najarian, 1961).

A review was made of the distribution of *Biomphalaria* spp. in the coastal regions of East and West Africa (Sturrock, 1965b). It was suggested that temperature limits the distribution of *Biomphalaria*,

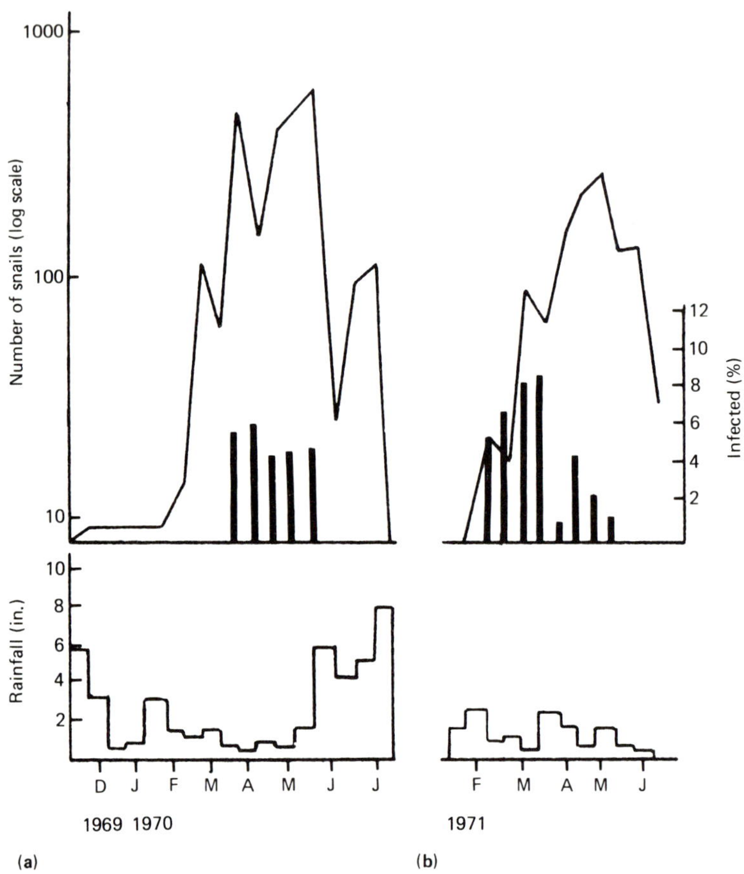

Fig. 2.2 *S. mansoni* transmission data from two stream studies in St Lucia showing the seasonal fluctuation in numbers of snails and cercarial infections obtained by routine sampling fortnightly. (a) Cul de sac Valley, 1970; (b) Richefond Valley, 1971. (After Sturrock, 1973.)

since there appears to be a belt roughly parallel with the Equator and extending some 10–15° north and south of it, depending upon local climatic conditions, within which *Biomphalaria* spp. cannot tolerate the high surface temperatures found at sea level, *S. mansoni* transmission apparently being absent below the 1000 ft (305 m) contour. To the north and south of this belt, coastal temperatures are generally lower and *Biomphalaria* spp. are present at lower altitudes. Life-tables were compiled for *B. pfeifferi* maintained at 19°C, 25°C and 30°C, respectively (Sturrock, 1966) and it was found that the optimal temperature for the rapid expansion of a population of this species was close to 25°C. The maximum temperature tolerated by *B. pfeifferi* appeared to be about 32°C, but under field conditions it was considered doubtful whether colonies would survive temperatures much above 28°C. It is considered that high temperatures are a major barrier to colonisation by *B. pfeifferi* of suitable natural habitats in the coastal areas of Tanzania, whereas *B. globosus* is present (Sturrock and Sturrock, 1972), but that in certain circumstances habitats created in irrigation schemes might support *B. pfeifferi* seasonally.

Laboratory and field studies were made on the influence of temperature on the 'intrinsic rate of natural increase' of *B. (P.) globosus* (Shiff, 1964a and 1964b) and the data suggest that *B. (P.) globosus* is able to survive higher temperatures and to respond to temperature changes more easily than does *B. pfeifferi* (Harrison and Shiff, 1966). The distribution of *B. obtusispira* and *B. pfeifferi* in Malagasy (Brygoo, 1967) and the seasonality of snail densities there in relation to temperature have been well shown (Pflüger, 1976), as has the distribution of different bulinid snails and of *B. pfeifferi* in relation to temperature in South Africa (Van Eeden, 1965; Van Eeden and Combrinck, 1966; Brown, 1967).

It has been shown that where the duration of temperatures greater than 27°C is more than 120 h/week, *B. pfeifferi* is absent in habitats (shallow permanent waterbodies) on the coastal plain of north-eastern Zululand (Appleton, 1977). Temperature, according to available evidence (Appleton, 1978), is apparently the abiotic factor of greatest importance in determining the distribution of host snails in lentic environments (i.e. ponds and lakes).

In certain areas where rainfall, water levels and temperatures are relatively constant, there are no pronounced cyclic changes and reproduction may take place throughout the year. It was found that *O.h. quadrasi* showed only very minor changes in density over a two-year period (Pesigan *et al.*, 1958). There is apparently no conclusive evidence for reproductive and population cycles independent of cyclic fluctuation of environmental factors, but irregular population changes independent of seasonal factors may occur (McMullen *et al.*, 1951; Ritchie *et al.*, 1962).

Biological factors

A number of reports have been made of the food utilised by snail intermediate hosts (Webbe and James, 1971c). The pulmonates are essentially browsing animals which feed continuously as they move (Berrie, 1970). Most aquatic habitats contain rich microflora which, together with decaying vegetable matter, provide the principal food of snails. While there may be no preferences for any particular species of microflora, the quantitative composition of the diet is probably important in conditioning the habitat (Malek, 1958). As the result of seasonal fluctuations in the quantity of microflora (consequent upon changes in rainfall and in temperature and on other ecological factors controlled by them), one might expect the density of a snail population to vary. Habitats devoid of higher plant life, but rich in green algae, blue-green algae and

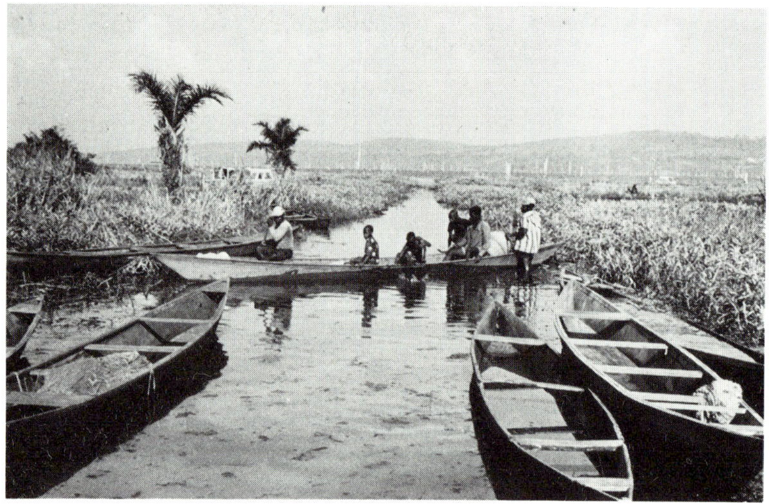

Fig. 2.3 Channel water-contact site on Lake Volta in which focal transmission of *S. haematobium* occurs seasonally in *Bulinus truncatus rohlfsi* associated with *Ceratophyllum* growth.

diatoms have been found to contain thriving snail populations (Webbe, 1962a), but no causal relationship with a particular species of algae or diatom was established. A positive correlation has, however, been found between the presence of green algae and *O.h. quadrasi*, and a negative correlation with blue-green algae (Dazo and Moreno, 1962). The diet of *O.h. nosophora* has also been studied, including the effect of a diatom diet of *Navicula luzonensis* (Davis and Iwamoto, 1969; Davis and Werner, 1970).

There are numerous reports of associations between aquatic snails and different plant species, but these may simply indicate that the plants in question provide a suitable physical environment (Sturrock, 1974). The snails may, of course, be attracted to plants because they offer a major source of food (Jobin and Michelson, 1967; Jobin, 1970). Ecological studies of *B. truncatus rohlfsi* in Volta Lake have shown a correlation between the spread and proliferation of this species and floating masses of vegetation and, in particular, *Ceratophyllum demersum* (Fig. 2.3). It is observed that roots and hollow stems of *Polygonum* provide shelter and protected surfaces for oviposition, and that rotting *Polygonum* serves as an ideal bottom substrate and snail food source (Klumpp and Chu, 1977 and 1978).

There is an apparent association between concentrations of snails and pollution of the habitat and references to certain species being 'sewage snails' and requiring 'fouling of the habitat' are common in literature. In Tanzania it was concluded that the apparent relationship between *Bulinus* and fouling of its habitat was not a direct one, but rather attributable to the attraction of an increased food supply produced by organic waste matter (Maclean *et al.*, 1958). It has been observed, however, that streams receiving the effluent from sewage works are generally free of snails (Malek, 1958).

Aestivation
Aquatic snail intermediate hosts have the capacity to survive out of water for weeks or even months, which has significant consequences in relation to the epidemiology of schistosomiasis and to control measures. Many workers have made observations on the reaction of different molluscan hosts to drying (Webbe and Msangi, 1958; Webbe, 1962a and 1962b; Chu *et al.*, 1967; Richards, 1967; Sturrock, 1970). Infection with schistosomes, however, appears to render snails less tolerant to desiccation and sporocysts and cercariae of *S. mansoni* degenerate on the 20th day in *B. glabrata* subjected to desiccation (Barbosa and Coelho, 1953). Mature *S. mansoni* infections in *B. glabrata* die during aestivation, but snails exposed to miracidia within 25 days of aestivation retain the infection (Barbosa and Coelho, 1955). Immature *S. mansoni* infections have been found in aestivating snails in the field (Barbosa and Olivier, 1958) and *S. haematobium* infection in *B. (P.) nasutus productus* survived drying for 98 days (Webbe, 1962a). It is apparent, therefore, that immature infections of both *S. mansoni* and *S. haematobium* may be carried in

aestivating snails from one wet season to the next, which is of considerable epidemiological significance.

The aquatic snail withdraws the body into the shell when subjected to desiccation and a layer of mucus is produced to cover the opening of the shell, and apertural lamellae may form in aestivating planorbid snails (Richards, 1967). Unlike the amphibious *Oncomelania*, aquatic planorbid and bulinid snails have no operculum, so that the shell cannot be so effectively sealed under dry conditions. Drying apparently affects the amphibious snails much less than aquatic ones, although it does influence their oviposition and eggs are very susceptible to desiccation. Vegetation found in the favoured habitats of *Oncomelania* spp. largely controls an appropriate microhabitat, its temperature and humidity. Desiccation will, of course, ultimately kill all adult and juvenile snails and their ova and it may be used as a method of control in certain circumstances. The capacity of snails to survive in dried mud may also be an important factor in their dissemination and colonisation of new habitats through the agency of animals, birds and even vegetation.

SNAIL LIFE-CYCLES

The aquatic snail intermediate hosts of schistosomes are hermaphroditic and capable of self-fertilisation, but cross-fertilisation is usual. Ova are laid in water over an appreciable range of temperature—for *B. pfeifferi* and *B. globosus*, 20°–30°C—and in nature oviposition probably goes on throughout the year, with a considerable increase in the number of young snails being observed at the beginning of the rainy season in West Africa (Vogel, 1932; Gordon *et al.*, 1934).

Ova of *B. pfeifferi*, when freshly laid, appear as a yellowish transparent gelatinous mass, oval or more-or-less circular in outline. The egg masses vary in size (5–10 mm in diameter), and may contain 6–28 ova. At an aquarium temperature of 26°–28°C, 9–10 days elapsed from deposition of spawn to the hatching of free-living snails in the case of *B. pfeifferi*; a growth-rate of 0.5 mm per week was maintained for about six weeks and thereafter a slower rate; maximum size was attained probably within six months and maturity was observed at about three months (Gordon *et al.*, 1934). Recent life-history data for this species have been obtained (Sturrock, 1966; Shiff and Garnett, 1967); also for *B. sudanica tanganycensis* (Webbe, 1962b), *B. angulosa* (Sturrock, 1965b) and *B. glabrata* (Sturrock and Sturrock, 1970). In appearance, the egg mass of *B. (P.) nasutus productus* is oval in shape, its length varies from 4 mm to 8 mm, and it contains 5–22 ova. Twenty-one egg masses laid by young snails approximately two months old contained an average of 14·5 ova per mass. The numbers of ova per mass apparently varied with the age of the parent snail. Ova hatch 10 to 11 days after oviposition and young snails grow about 0·8 mm per week until they are 7–8 mm (maximum height of shell), and approximately two months old, at which time most snails are mature. The rate of growth then progressively diminishes and combined laboratory and field data indicate that this species attains its full size (20·5 mm maximum recorded height of shell) not less than 12 months after hatching, and probably only after one or even two periods of aestivation (Webbe, 1962a).

Numerous studies have underlined the enormous reproductive potential of snail intermediate hosts and several have shown an apparent correlation between the onset of rains and increased reproductive activity in populations of snails. It may be that the stimulus is provided by an associated drop in water temperature, but the addition of nutrients, the dilution of substances in solution, changes in the size of the habitat, and perhaps associated changes in food supply, could be involved. Snail size and time of year are correlated with the development of the reproductive system in temperate freshwater snails. In the tropical species, egg laying does not always commence when the snails are large enough to reproduce and the delays may be attributable to unfavourable environmental conditions. It is considered that the internal control mechanisms are probably chemical and may involve neurosecretion, which has been shown to influence osmotic regulation (Berrie, 1970).

Apart from the extrinsic factors, which are generally seasonal, the density and age structure of a snail population is therefore also controlled by intrinsically operating factors, such as birth rate, natural mortality and the environmental resistance, which are not constant for a population and will vary with the size and composition of different populations and environmental conditions. Each population of snails, therefore, has an 'intrinsic rate of natural increase', designated 'r', which is a population parameter based upon the survival and fecundity of a species under particular environmental conditions.

The amphibious oncomelanid intermediate hosts of *S. japonicum* are dioecious: *O.h. quadrasi* lays most eggs above the water on a solid substrate, mainly at night; lower temperature, higher humidity and absence of sunlight all contributing to the protection of the female snail during the process of oviposition. *O.h. nosophora*, however, lays more eggs in the water and usually on a muddy substrate. These amphibious snails, when newly hatched, pass through an aquatic phase for a period of two to three weeks, but older snails spend a large proportion of their active life on moist surfaces where they feed on algae and on decaying organic matter. *O.h. quadrasi* apparently feeds more rapidly during the day than at night; the sexes are separate and copulation takes place repeatedly, and at least once every 24 hours. The female is able to lay viable eggs more than three months after isolation from the male (Pesigan *et al.*, 1958)—a similar observation has been made for *O.h. nosophora* (Ritchie, 1955). Eggs are laid singly, the mucous layer being covered by snail faeces and other debris, and hatching takes place some 10–25 days after oviposition. The growth rate of young snails is of course variable (0·25–0·50 mm per week) and becomes slower as maturity is approached which, under favourable conditions is attained in 10–16 weeks. While the life span of oncomelanid snails is variable, observations have shown that some specimens of *O.h. nosophora* in Japan may live for several years, while other data suggest that while the average life span may only be a few months, many snails survive for 12 months or longer. *O.h. quadrasi* in the Philippines lives for 24 to 35 weeks only, with an average longevity of 65·8 days. Mating is minimal in the spring and early summer, and maximal in winter. Aestivation may begin in autumn but egg laying and hatching are continuous throughout the year.

Culturing of *Biomphalaria* and *Oncomelania* for large-scale studies has been described (Anon, 1971). Recent laboratory studies have been made on the growth and fecundity of *O.h. quadrasi* and of *O.h. nosophora* (Iwanaga and Tsuji, 1976; Iwanaga *et al.*, 1977; Anon, 1978).

T. aperta, the snail intermediate host of *S. mekongi*, has been successfully cultivated in a petri dish aquarium provided with mud and algae (Liang and Van der Schalie, 1975). The incubation period of eggs was about 4 weeks; the young grew to maturity in 16–20 weeks and egg laying followed about 6–8 weeks later—the entire cycle taking approximately 6 months. The eggs, each of which had a husk consisting of a thin coating layer of mud, were deposited exclusively at the edge on the wall of the aquarium. The eggs were hemispherical in shape and, together with the husks, measured between 0·37 mm and 0·43 mm in diameter. The newly hatched young snails were 0·24 mm in shell length and full-grown snails were 3·11 mm to 3·36 mm long. It was noted that growth commenced in its logarithmic phase slowly, 11 to 12 weeks after hatching; that 16 to 20 weeks were needed to reach maturity; and that a further 6 to 8 weeks were required to obtain eggs following maturity. The full cycle of growth was completed in about 6 months.

REFERENCES

Anon (1971). *Culturing Biomphalaria and Oncomelania (Gastropoda) for large-scale studies of Schistosomiasis* Biomedical Rep. 19, US Army Medical Research and Development Command, Washington DC.

Anon (1978). *Recent Researches on Schistosomiasis.* Japan International Cooperation Agency.

Appleton, C. C. (1977), *Int. J. Parasit.* **7,** 335.

Appleton, C. C. (1978). *Malac. Rev.* **11,** 1.

Appleton, C. C. and Stiles, G. (1976). *Ann. Trop. Med. Parasit.* **70,** 189.

Arfaa, F. (1976). *Studies on schistosomiasis in Saudi Arabia.* Unpublished report. *WHO/Schisto* **76,** 41. WHO, Geneva.

Barbosa, F. S. and Coelho, M. V. (1953). *Publ. Avuls. Inst. Aggeu Magalhaĕs* **2,** 51.

Barbosa, F. S. and Coelho, M. V. (1955). *Publ. Avuls. Inst. Aggeu Magalhaĕs* **4,** 51.

Barbosa, F. S. and Olivier, L. J. (1958). *Bull. Wld Hlth Org.* **18,** 895.

Berrie, A. D. (1964). *Ann. Trop. Med. Parasit.* **58,** 457.

Berrie, A. D. (1968). *Ann. Trop. Med. Parasit.* **62,** 45.

Berrie, A. D. (1970). *Adv. Parasit.* **8,** 43.

Berrie, A. D. and Visser, S. Z. (1963). *Physiol. Zool.* **36,** 167.

Boycott, A. E. (1936). *J. Anim. Ecol.* **5,** 116.

Brown, D. S. (1967). *Ann. Natal. Mus.* **18,** 477.

Brown, D. S. (1976). *J. Nat. Hist.* **10,** 257.

Brown, D. S. (1980). *Freshwater snails of Africa and their Medical Importance.* Taylor & Francis, London.

Brown, D. S. and Burch, J. B. (1967). *Malcologia* **6,** 189.

Brown, D. S., Oberholzer, G. and Van Eeden, J. A. (1971). *Malacologia* **11,** 141.

Brown, D. S., Schutte, C. H. J., Burch, J. B. and Natarajan, R. (1967). *Malacologia* **6,** 175.

Brown, D. S. and Wright, C. A. (1972). *J. Zool. Lond.* **167,** 97.

Brown, D. S. and Wright, C.A. (1974). *Trans. R. Soc.Trop. Med. Hyg.* **68,** 341.

Brown, D. S. and Wright, C. A. (1978). *J. Nat. Hist.* **12,** 217.

Brygoo, E. R. (1967). *Bull. Soc. Path. Exot.* **60,** 433.

Burch, J. B. (1972). *Malac. Rev.* **5,** 7.

Burch, J. B. and Lindsay, G. K. (1970). *Malac. Rev.* **3,** 1.

Carney, W. P., Hadidjaja, P., Davis, G. M., Clarke, M., Djajasamita, M. and Nalim, S. (1973). *J. Parasit.* **59,** 210.

Carpenter, K. E. (1927). *J. Ecol.* **15,** 33.

Chernin, E. (1957). *Proc. Soc. Exp. Biol. (N.Y.)* **96,** 204.

Chernin, E. and Michelson, E. H. (1957a). *Am. J. Hyg.* **65,** 57.

Chernin, E. and Michelson, E. H. (1957b). *Am. J. Hyg.* **65,** 71.

Chi, L. W., Wagner, E. D. and Wold, N. (1971). *Am. J. Trop. Med. Hyg.* **20,** 89.

Chiu, J. K. (1967). *Malacologia* **6,** 145.

Chu, K. Y., Kpo, H. K. and Klumpp, R. K. (1978). *Bull. Wld Hlth Org.* **56,** 601.

Chu, K. Y., Massoud, J. and Arfaa, F. (1967). *Ann. Trop. Med. Parasit.* **61,** 139.

Coelho, L. R. and Barbosa, F. S. (1956). *Publ. Avuls. Inst. Aggeu. Magalhaẽs* **2,** 159.

Coles, G. C. (1970). *Parasitology* **61,** 19.

Davis, G. M. (1968). *Malacologia* **7,** 17.

Davis, G. M. (1969). In *Proceedings of the Fourth Southeast Asian Seminar on Parasitology and Tropical Medicine, Schistosomiasis and other Snail-Transmitted Helminthiases*, p. 93. Ed. C. Harinasuta. S.E. Asian Minister of Education Council, Bangkok.

Davis, G. M. (1979). *The origin and evolution of the gastropod family Pomatiopsidae, with emphasis on the Mekong River Triculinae.* Monograph of the Academy of Natural Sciences of Philadelphia, **20,** 1–120.

Davis, G. M. and Carney, W. P. (1973). *Proc. Acad. Nat. Sci., Philadelphia* **125,** 1.

Davis, G. M. and Iwamoto, Y. (1969). *Am. J. Trop. Med. Hyg.* **18,** 629.

Davis, G. M., Kitkoon, V. and Temcharoen, P. (1976). *Monograph. Malacologia* **15,** 241.

Davis, G. M. and Lindsay, G. K. (1967). *Malacologia* **5,** 311.

Davis, G. M. and Ruff, M. D. (1973). *Malac. Rev.* **6,** 181.

Davis, G. M. and Werner, J. K. (1970). *Jap. J. Parasit.* **19,** 35.

Dazo, B. C., Hairston, N. G. and Dawood, I. K. (1966). *Bull. Wld Hlth Org.* **35,** 339.

Dazo, B. C. and Moreno, R. G. (1962). *Trans. Am. Micro. Soc.* **81,** 341.

Demian, S. S. and Kamel, E. G. (1972). *Proc. Egyptian Acad. Sci.* **25,** 37.

Gadgil, R. K. and Shah, S. N. (1956). *Indian J. Med. Res.* 577.

Gordon, R. M., Davey, T. H. and Peaston, H. (1934). *Ann. Trop. Med. Parasit.* **28,** 323.

Harinasuta, C., Sornmani, S., Kitkoon, V., Schneider, C. and Pathammavong, O. (1972). *Trans. R. Soc. Trop. Med. Hyg.* **66,** 184.

Harley, J. (1864). *Med. Chir. Trans.* **47,** 55.

Harrison, A. D., Nduku, W. and Hooper, A. S. C. (1966). *Ann. Trop. Med. Parasit.* **60,** 212.

Harrison, A. D. and Shiff, C. J. (1966). *S. Afr. J. Sci.* **62,** 253.

Harry, H. W., Cumbie, B. G. and Martinez de Jesus, J. (1957). *Am. J. Trop. Med. Hyg.* **6,** 313.

Hubendick, B. (1955). *Trans. Zool. Soc. Lond.* **28,** 453.

Hubendick, B. (1958). *Bull. Wld Hlth Org.* **18,** 1072.

Iwanaga, Y., Santos, M. J. and Blas, B. L. (1977). *Hiroshima, J. Med. Sci.* **26,** 5.

Iwanaga, Y. and Tsuji, M. (1976). *S.E. Asian J. Trop. Med. Publ. Hlth* **7,** 223.

James, C. and Webbe, G. (1973). *J. Helminth.* **47,** 49.

James, C. and Webbe, G. (1975). *J. Helminth.* **49,** 191.

Jelnes, J. E. (1977). *Steenstrupia* **4,** 139.

Jobin, W. R. (1970). *Am. J. Trop. Med. Hyg.* **19,** 1038.

Jobin, W. R. and Michelson, E. H. (1967). *Bull. Wld Hlth Org.* **37,** 657.

Kloos, H. and Lemma, A. (1974). *Ethiop. Med. J.* **12,** 157.

Klumpp, R. K. and Chu, K. Y. (1977). *Bull. Wld Hlth Org.* **55,** 715.

Klumpp, R. K. and Chu, K. Y. (1978). *Proc. Int. Conf. Schisto., 1975* **1,** 85.

Le Roux, P. L. (1958). *Trans. R. Soc. Trop. Med. Hyg.* **52,** 12.

Liang, Y. S. and Van der Schalie, H. (1975). *J. Parasit.* **61,** 915.

Lo, C. T., Burch, J. B. and Schutte, C. H. (1970). *Malac. Rev.* **3,** 121.

Lucena, D. T. de (1963). *Revta Bras. Malar, Doenc. Trop.* **15,** 13.

Macdonald, G. and Forsyth, D. M. (1968). *Trans. R. Soc. Trop. Med. Hyg.* **62,** 766.

McClelland, W. F. J. and Jordan, P. (1962). *Ann. Trop. Med. Parasit.* **56,** 396.

McCullough, F. S. (1962). *Trop. Geogr. Med.* **24,** 199.

Maclean, G., Webbe, G. and Msangi, A. S. (1958). *E. Afr. Med. J.* **35,** 7.

McMullen, D. B., Komiya, S. and Endo-Itabashi, T. (1951). *Am. J. Hyg.* **54,** 402.

Malek, E. A. (1958). *Bull. Wld Hlth Org.* **18,** 785.

Malek, E. A. (1962'. *Laboratory Guide and Notes for Medical Malacology*, p. 66. Burgess Publishing Co., Minneapolis.

Mandahl-Barth, G. (1958). *Intermediate Hosts of Schistosoma: African Biomphalaria and Bulinus.* WHO Monograph Series No. 37, WHO, Geneva.

Mandahl-Barth, G. (1960). *Bull. Wld Hlth Org.* **22,** 565.

Mandahl-Barth, G. (1965). *Bull. Wld Hlth Org.* **33,** 33.

Mandahl-Barth, G. (1973). *Proc. Malac. Soc. Lond.* **40,** 277.

Mandahl-Barth, G. (1978). *Schisto/WP* **78,** 5. WHO, Geneva.

Mandahl-Barth, G., Frandsen, R. and Jelnes, J. E. (1976). *Trans. R. Soc. Trop. Med. Hyg.* **70,** 88.

Najarian, H. H. (1961). *Bull. Wld Hlth Org.* **25,** 435.

Nelson, G. S., Teesdale, C. and Highton, R. B. (1962). In *Bilharziasis: A Ciba Foundation Symposium*, p. 127. Eds. G. E. W. Wolstenholme and M. O'Connor. Churchill, London.

PAHO/WHO (1968). *An Introductory Guide for Intermediate Hosts of Schistosomiasis in the Americas.* WHO, Washington DC.

Paperna, I. (1968). *Ann. Trop. Med. Parasit.* **62,** 13.

Paraense, W. L. and Correa, L. R. (1963). *Revt. Int. Med. Trop. S. Paulo* **5,** 15.

Paraense, W. L. and Correa, L. R. (1978). *J. Parasit.* **64,** 822.

Pesigan, T. P., Hairston, N. G., Jauregui, J. J., Garcia, E. G., Santos, A. T., Santos, B. C. and Besa, A. A. (1958). *Bull. Wld Hlth Org.* **18,** 481.

Pflüger, W. (1976). *Arch. Inst. Pasteur Madagascar* **45,** 79.

Pitchford, R. J. (1965). *Bull. Wld Hlth Org.* **32,** 105.

Ritchie, L. S. (1955). *Am. J. Trop. Med. Hyg.* **4,** 426.

Ritchie, L. S., Radke, M. G. and Ferguson, F. F. (1962). *Bull. Wld Hlth Org.* **27,** 171.

Richards, C. S. (1967). *Am. J. Trop. Med. Hyg.* **16,** 797.

Richards, C. S. (1973). *Am. J. Trop. Med. Hyg.* **22,** 748.

Richards, C. S. (1975). *Parasitology* **70,** 231.

Richards, C. S. (1976). *Bull. Wld Hlth Org.* **54,** 706.

Richards, C. S. (1977). *Expl Parasit.* **42,** 165.

Richards, C. S. and Meredith, J. W. Jr. (1972). *Am. J. Trop. Med. Hyg.* **21,** 425.

Saladin, B., Degremont, A. and Weiss, N. (1976). *Acta Trop.* **33,** 376.

Saoud, M. F. A. (1965a). *J. Helminth.* **39,** 101.

Saoud, M. F. A. (1965b). *J. Helminth.* **39,** 363.

Schutte, C. H. J. and Frank, G. H. (1964). *Bull. Wld Hlth Org.* **30,** 389.

Shiff, C. J. (1964a). *Ann. Trop. Med. Parasit.* **58,** 94.

Shiff, C. J. (1964b). *Ann. Trop. Med. Parasit.* **58,** 106.

Shiff, C. J. and Garnett, B. (1967). *Archiv. für. Hydrobiol.* **62,** 429.

Smithers, S. R. (1956). *Trans. R. Soc. Trop. Med. Hyg.* **50,** 354.

Sornmani, S., Kitkoon, V., Schneider, C., Harinasuta, C. and Pathammavong, O. (1973). *S.E. Asian J. Trop. Med. Publ. Hlth* **4,** 218.

Southgate, V. R. and Knowles, R. J. (1975). *Trans. R. Soc. Trop. Med. Hyg.* **69,** 356.

Southgate, V. R. and Knowles, R. J. (1977). *Trans. R. Soc. Trop. Med. Hyg.* **71,** 82.

Southgate, V. R., Van Wyk, J. A. and Wright, C. A. (1976). *Ztschr. Parasitkde* **49,** 145.

Sturrock, R. F. (1965a). *Bull. Wld Hlth Org.* **32,** 225.

Sturrock, R. F. (1965b). *Ann. Trop. Med. Parasit.* **59,** 1.

Sturrock, R. F. (1966). *Ann. Trop. Med. Parasit.* **60,** 100.

Sturrock, R. F. (1970). *Int. J. Parasit.* **3,** 175.

Sturrock, R. F. (1973). *Int. J. Parasit.* **3,** 165.

Sturrock, R. F. (1974). *Carib. J. Sci.* **14,** 149.

Sturrock, R. F. and Sturrock, B. M. (1970). *Ann. Trop. Med. Parasit.* **64,** 349.

Sturrock, R. F. and Sturrock, B. M. (1972). *Ann. Trop. Med. Parasit.* **66,** 385.

Teesdale, C. (1962). *Bull. Wld Hlth Org.* **27,** 759.

Thomas, J. D. (1973). *Adv. Parasit.* **11,** 307.

Thomas, J. D., Benjamin, M., Lough, A. and Aram, R. H. (1974). *J. Anim. Ecol.* **43,** 839.

Thomas, J. D., Goldsworthy, G. J. and Aram, R. H. (1975). *J. Anim. Ecol.* **44,** 1.

Thomas, J. D. and Lough, A. (1974). *J. Anim. Ecol.* **43,** 861.

Thomas, J. D., Lough, A. S. and Lodge, R. W. (1975). *J. Appl. Ecol.* **12,** 421.

Thomas, J. D., Powles, M. and Lodge, R. (1976). *Biol. Bull.* **151,** 386.

Van der Schalie, H. and Davis, G. M. (1968). *Malacologia* **6,** 321.

Van Eeden, J. A. (1965). *Tyskr. Natuurw.* **5,** 152.

Van Eeden, J. A. and Combrinck, C. (1966). *Zoologica Africana* **2,** 95.

Voge, M., Bruckner, D. and Bruce, J. (1978). *J. Parasit.* **64,** 577.

Vogel, H. (1932). *Arch. Schiffa., Tropenhyg.* **36,** 108.

Von Brand, T. and Mehlman, B. (1953). *Biol. Bull., Wood's Hole* **104,** 301.

Wagner, E. D. and Chi, L. W. (1959). *Am. J. Trop. Med. Hyg.* **8,** 195.

Walker, A. R. P., Walker, B. T. and Richardson, B. D. (1970). *Am. J. Trop. Med. Hyg.* **19,** 792.

Watson, J. M. (1950). *J. Roy. Fac. Med. Iraq* **14,** 148.

Watson, J. M. (1958). *Bull. Wld Hlth Org.* **18,** 833.

Webbe, G. (1962a). *Bull. Wld Hlth Org.* **27,** 59.
Webbe, G. (1962b). In *Bilharziasis: A Ciba Foundation Symposium*, p. 7. Eds G. E. W. Wolstenholme and M. O'Connor. Churchill, London.
Webbe, G. (1965). *Bull. Wld Hlth Org.* **33,** 147.
Webbe, G. and James, C. (1971a). *J. Helminth.* **45,** 403.
Webbe, G. and James, C. (1971b). *J. Helminth.* **45,** 271.
Webbe, G. and James, C. (1971c). *Symp. Br. Soc. Parasit.* **9,** 77.
Webbe, G., James, C. and Nelson, G. S. (1974). *Ann. Trop. Med. Parasit.* **68,** 187.
Webbe, G. and Msangi, A. S. (1958). *Ann. Trop. Med. Parasit.* **52,** 302.
Wright, C. A. (1956). *Ann. Trop. Med. Parasit.* **50,** 346.
Wright, C. A. (1960). *Ann. Trop. Med. Parasit.* **54,** 224.
Wright, C. A. (1961). *Trans. R. Soc. Trop. Med. Hyg.* **55,** 225.
Wright, C. A. (1962a). *Bull. Zool. Nom.* **19,** 39.
Wright, C. A. (1962b). In *Bilharziasis: A Ciba Foundation Symposium*, p. 103. Eds G. E. W. Wolstenholme and M. O'Connor. Churchill, London.
Wright, C. A. (1963a). *Trans. R. Soc. Trop. Med. Hyg.* **57,** 142.
Wright, C. A. (1963b). *Bull. Br. Mus. Nat. Hist. Zool.* **10,** 447.
Wright, C. A. (1966). *J. Helminth.* **40,** 403.
Wright, C. A. (1967). In *Bilharziasis:* p. 3. Ed. F. K. Mostofi. Springer-Verlag, Berlin, Heidelberg, New York.
Wright, C. A. (1971). *Phil. Trans. Roy. Soc. Lond. B.* **260,** 299.
Wright, C. A. (1974). *Biochemical and Immunological Taxonomy of Animals*, p. 351. Ed. C. A. Wright. Academic Press, London, New York.
Wright, C. A. (1977). In *Medicine in a Tropical Environment*, p. 291. Ed. J. N. S. Gear. Balkema, Cape Town.
Wright, C. A. and Bennet, M. S. (1967a). *Trans. R. Soc. Trop. Med. Hyg.* **61,** 221.
Wright, C. A. and Bennet, M. S. (1967b). *Trans. R. Soc. Trop. Med. Hyg.* **61,** 228.
Wright, C. A. and Brown, D. S. (1962). *Bull. Brit. Mus. (Nat. Hist.) Zool.* **8,** 287.
Wright, C. A. and Rollinson, D. (1979). *Parasitology* **79,** 95.
Wright, C. A., Southgate, V. R. and Knowles, R. J. (1972). *Trans. R. Soc. Trop. Med. Hyg.* **66,** 26.

3 The Life-Cycle of the Parasites

Gerald Webbe

THE LIFE-CYCLE

The life-cycle is complex, involving alternating parasitic and free-living stages: the egg, miracidium, first-stage (mother) sporocyst, second-stage (daughter) sporocyst, cercaria, schistosomulum, and adult schistosome (see Fig. 1.1).

The yellowish eggs are non-operculate and have a spine. The embryo (miracidium) develops inside the egg over a period of 6 days. If the egg remains in the tissues, it lives for another 15 days, during which time it secretes histiolytic antigenic material, and dies approximately 21 days after oviposition, releasing products of autolysis. The eggshell is destroyed over a period of weeks or months depending upon whether or not calcification has taken place (Warren, 1973). Ova passing through the bladder or intestinal wall (probably less than 50% of total egg production) contain embryos which are usually visibly motile and ready to hatch when the eggs are voided. In a suitable environment in which the urine or faeces are diluted by freshwater, and generally under the influence of warmth (10–30°C) and light, the miracidia become active and emerge from the eggshell through slits caused in part by osmotic effects and in part by the activity of the larvae (Fig. 3.1).

THE MIRACIDIUM

The miracidia of the human schistosomes differ in size (*S. mansoni* 0·160 mm in length, 0·062 mm in breadth) but are similar in their behaviour and morphology. Essential morphological features include an apical papilla (tenebratorium), epidermal plates arranged in four tiers and covered with cilia of

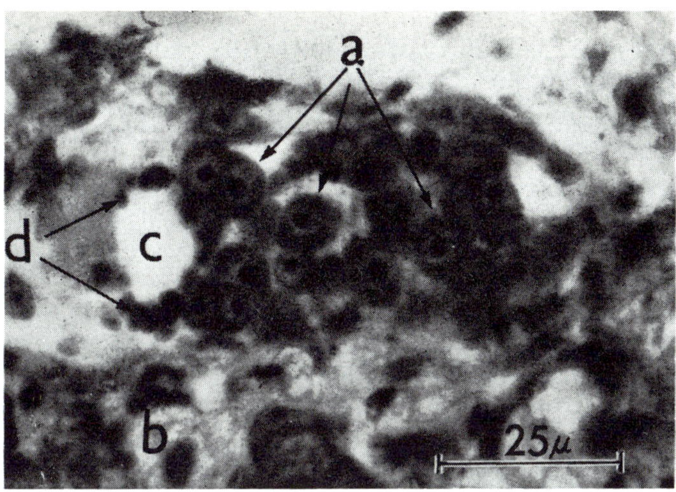

Fig. 3.1(a) Young mother sporocyst in foot of snail, 48 h. a, growing germinal cells; b, host tissue; c, penetration gland; d, somatic cells. (Giemsa stain sectioned 6 μ.)

equal length (which enable the organism to swim rapidly in straight lines), a subepithelium lined by a continuous row of arched cells, a primitive gut, a pair of cephalic penetration glands which are unicellular and periodic acid-Schiff staining, each opening antero-laterally by a duct at the base of the tenebratorium, a neural mass, two pairs of flame cells and germinal cells (Faust and Russell, 1964; Pan, 1965; Schutte, 1974a).

Miracidia swim actively (approximately 2 mm per second) and exhibit behaviour patterns similar to those of the molluscan intermediate host (Smyth, 1966). The miracidia of *S. mansoni* and *S. japonicum* are usually positively phototactic and negatively geotactic, while those of *S. haematobium* are negatively phototactic and apparently unable to distinguish low light intensities from darkness—however, they show strong positive geotaxis (Prah and James, 1977). There is evidence that the behaviour of miracidia is related to the ecology of their snail intermediate hosts, and adaptive behaviour patterns have been discussed in relation to irrigation canals (Wright, 1962), bottom-living *B. choanomphala* in Lake Victoria (Webbe, 1962; Prentice *et al.*, 1970) and an Iraqi strain of *S. haematobium* (Wajdi, 1972).

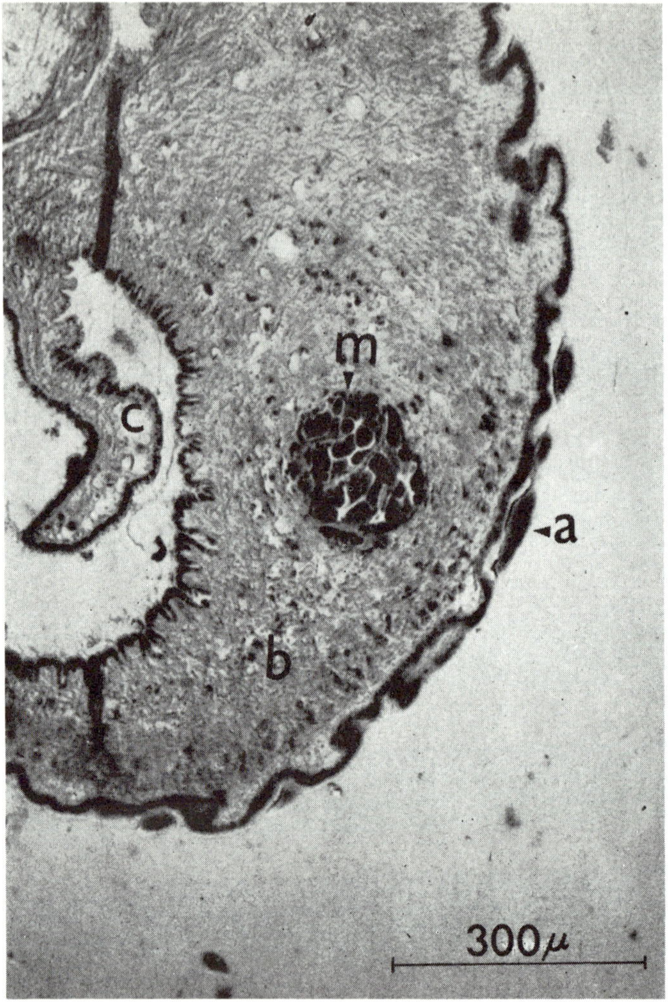

Fig. 3.1(b) Section of foot showing mother sporocyst (m) 10 days post-infection. a, foot epithelium; b, host connective tissue and mucous gland cells; c, mantle collar. (Giemsa stain sectioned 6 μ.)

Infection of snails

The behaviour of miracidia after hatching has been studied (Wright, 1958 and 1965; Chernin and Dunavan, 1962; Etges and Decker, 1963). Miracidia remain infective to their snail inter-mediate hosts for some 8–12 hours, swimming randomly in long sweeping lines in a 'scanning phase' of host location and increasing their turning rate sharply when stimulated by chemical substances emitted by snails and other organisms, until contact is made. The mechanism by which the molluscan hosts of schistosomes are located by miracidia continues to be investigated. Host location appears to be the result of characteristic ciliary locomotion of miracidia, conditioned by their orientation to different physical stimuli (light, gravity, contact etc.), until a chemical substance—the so-called 'miraxone', used to describe

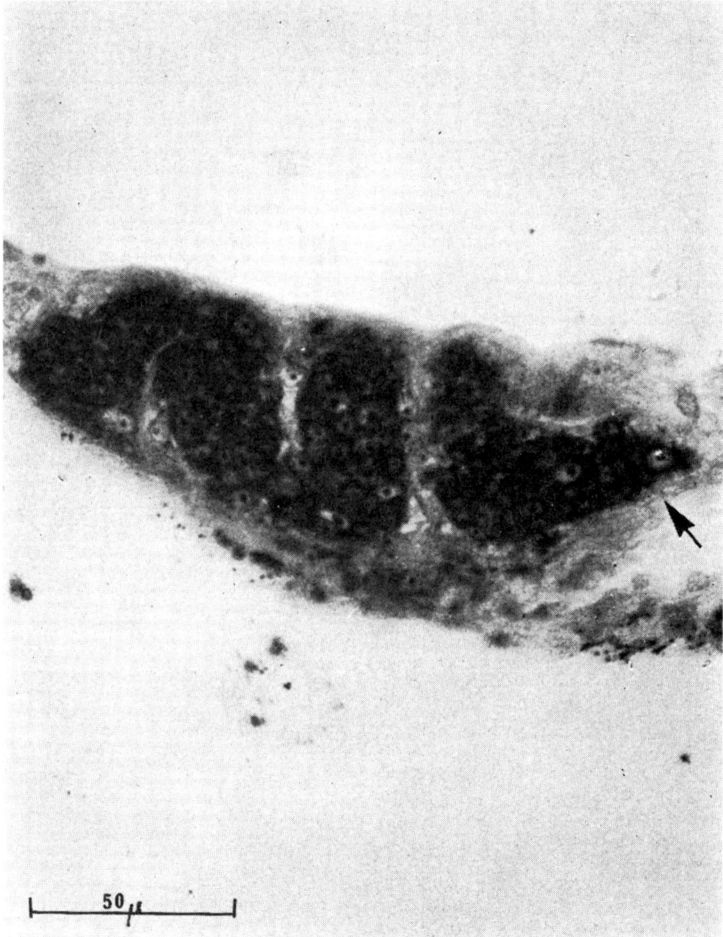

Fig. 3.1(c) Migrating daughter sporocyst in section of mantle, 19 days post-infection. Arrow indicates the cone-shaped muscular anterior portion. (Giemsa stain sectioned 6 μ.)

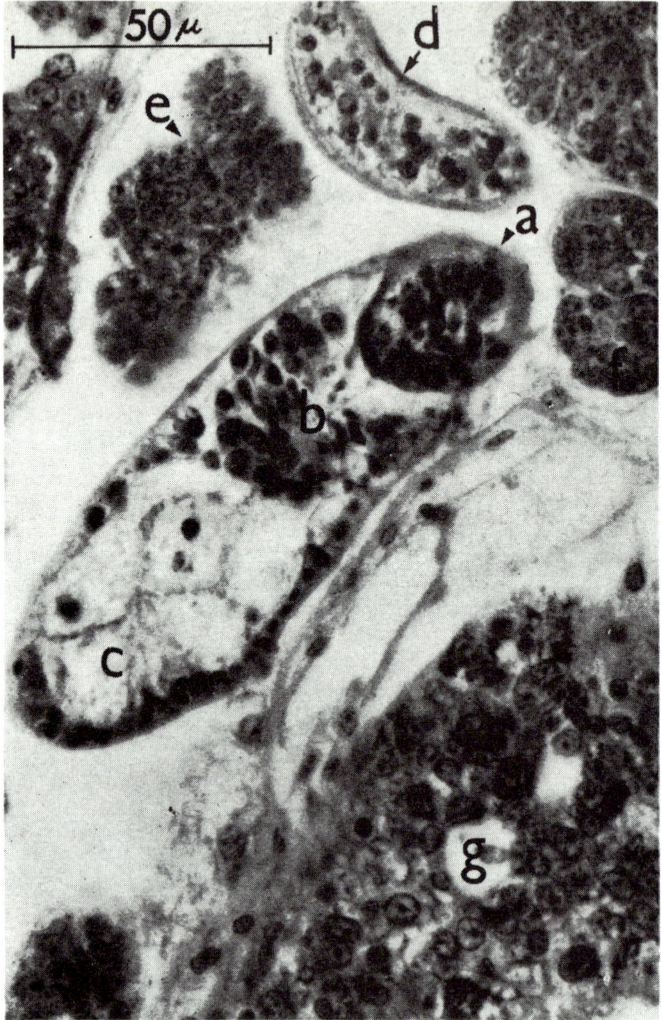

Fig. 3.1(d) Section of liver tissue containing nearly mature cercaria within a daughter sporocyst, 70 days post-infection. a, oral sucker; b, neural mass; c, penetration glands; d, exhausted sporocyst containing interstitial and germinal cells; e, regenerating daughter sporocyst; f, cercarial germ ball; g, liver tissue. (Iron haematoxylin stain sectioned 6 μ.)

the undefined complex of substances emitted by host snails which produce this effect (Chernin, 1970)—stimulates them to exhibit excited locomotor behaviour (Etges *et al.*, 1975). Evidence of the effects of pH, salinity and turbidity on miracidial infectivity in the *S. mansoni–B. glabrata* complex and of the stimulatory effect of divalent inorganic cations has been produced (Short and Saladin, 1973; Sturrock and Upatham, 1973). The available evidence suggests that the 'miraxone' is a complex of soluble substances, emitted by snails and other aquatic organisms, which may include the neurogenic product serotonin.

The activity of schistosome miracidia in water conditioned by host snails has been established by different techniques (Chernin, 1970; Shiff and Kriel, 1970; Mason and Fripp, 1976). Fatty acids and/or amino acids have been shown to stimulate schistosome miracidia (MacInnis, 1965), and these were found in the materials released by *B. glabrata*, forming an active component of 'snail-conditioned' water (MacInnis *et al.*, 1974). The miracidia of *S. mansoni* have been shown to respond to 'snail-conditioned' water even in the absence of a concentration gradient (Mason and Fripp, 1976), which supports the suggestion that 'active spaces' may be more significant in host location than chemotactic responses to a chemical diffusion gradient (Miller, 1976). Further experiments have been conducted to identify chemicals known to be released from snails which stimulate *S. mansoni* miracidial movements in the absence of a concentration gradient and ammonia was shown to induce miracidia to increase their klinokinetic (turning) movements, thus restricting their dispersion (Mason and Fripp, 1976 and 1977).

In addition to penetrating intermediate snail hosts, miracidia will penetrate a variety of natural and synthetic agents, and it is clear that the stimulus is non-specific. Under field conditions, the depth of water is probably not an important barrier to snail location by miracidia of *S. mansoni*, but certain submerged margins probably represent sites where miracidia–snail contact is most likely to occur. Factors which influence the infection of snails by miracidia include: the age of snails and miracidia; the number of miracidia per snail; dispersion of snails and miracidia; the temperature of the exposure and the temperature of the habitat or microhabitat in which the snails live during the prepatent period; the length of contact time; water turbulence, flow and ultraviolet light (Webbe, 1967).

The influence of temperature upon the penetration of *Biomphalaria spp.* by *S. mansoni* miracidia has been investigated. The infection rate in snails increases with increasing temperature, up to the thermal death point of snails (Stirewalt, 1954; Purnell, 1966a).

The number of miracidia to which a group of snails is exposed apparently influences the proportion of snails which become infected. If particular species of *Biomphalaria* or *Bulinus* are exposed to sufficient miracidia of a compatible strain, 100% infection will be achieved, and failure to achieve this level of infection has been attributed to deficient infectivity of the miracidia rather than to innate resistance on the part of the snails (Etges, 1963; Chu, Massoud and Sabbaghian, 1966a). There is, however, clear evidence that various degrees of innate resistance to infection occur among different races of the same species of snail.

The evidence suggests that *S. haematobium* miracidia are less able to locate their hosts than are *S. mansoni* miracidia, and that dispersion of their snail hosts results in greater fluctuations in infection rates than is the case with *S. mansoni* (Jordan and Webbe, 1969).

In studies of host location of *S. haematobium* in a natural pond during the summer and winter, it was found that in summer miracidia–snail contacts were most frequent on the bottom or at the surface in the shade—contacts did not occur in the open water; in winter there was a decline in the number of contacts occurring along the bottom, while there was an increase in those among snails confined at the surface, both in the shade and light. The normal negative response to light was apparently reversed when temperatures dropped to 18°C or 13°C. Under normal conditions, with prevailing stimuli of light and temperature, miracidia seemed to scan the surface nearest to which they hatched, and become aggregated in particular parts of the habitat (Shiff, 1974).

Highly susceptible races of snails show no variation in infectability at different ages, but there is evidence that such variation does exist in other cases (Chu, Sabbaghian and Massoud, 1966; Berrie, 1970). Schistosome miracidia have a pronounced scanning capacity and, although a decline in infection rate was observed with a decrease in miracidial density, the infection rates in both *B. pfeifferi* and *B. globosus* were found to be more than 50% at 0·4–0·8 miracidia/l; in both species of snail, infection rates of 36–44% were obtained when host snails were situated at a distance of 5 m from the miracidial source, and equally high infection rates (39–40%) occurred in snails placed in flowing water at a velocity of 12–15 cm/s (James and Prah, 1978).

Flowing water is clearly of considerable significance in the epidemiology of schistosomiasis, since infective miracidia can be distributed over appreciable distances, thereby increasing their scanning capacity and potential contact with snail intermediate hosts. Infected *Biomphalaria* spp. have been collected from water courses in some parts of which flow rates as high as 122–176 cm/s were recorded in the rainy season (Webbe, 1965). In an experimental flowing water system, water velocity was shown to influence miracidia in the infection of *B. sudanica tanganyicensis*— the numbers of miracidia used ranged from less than 1 to 50 per snail and these were tested at water velocities from 0·15 m/s to 1·07 m/s. High infection rates were obtained in all the tests carried out, but it was recognised that the recorded rates of flow in the experimental channel employed were probably much higher than those within the relatively sheltered conditions of the snail cages used (Webbe, 1966a). Other observations have shown that infections generally occur at flow rates of 10 cm/s and below (Shiff, 1968; Upatham, 1973). Further, it has been shown that a water velocity exceeding 0·33 m/s at shell height produces a hydrodynamic drag force sufficient to dislodge *B. glabrata* (Jobin and Ippen, 1964), and evidence suggests that snails may be successfully infected at any water velocity which they can withstand—although most infections probably occur in the relatively sheltered conditions of the microhabitats provided along the margins of streams, in pools or within vegetation.

Penetration of the miracidium occurs when the larva becomes attached to the body surface of the snail by a secretion from the apical gland cells. Penetration is initiated by the papilla, the boring movements of the miracidium probably being assisted by lytic enzymes secreted from the 'gut' (Wajdi, 1963, 1966 and 1972).

Development in the intermediate host and effects of infection

When penetration is complete, the ciliated surface of the larva disappears and within a few days development into a mother sporocyst takes place near to the point of penetration. This development takes place only if the appropriate species of snail has been entered, otherwise the miracidium is destroyed by phagocytic action. A classical study of the host–parasite relationship and tissue responses in *B. glabrata* infected with *S.*

mansoni (Pan, 1963 and 1965) shows that only a small proportion of the miracidia that enter the snail host develop to mature mother sporocysts and these, usually localised in the head–foot of snails, only rarely provoke 'non-specific minimal focal proliferative tissue reactions'. These reactions usually occur within the first 48 hours after infection. The muscle layers of the miracidium degenerate 48 hours after penetration, and the cephalic penetration glands also disappear during this period. The mother sporocyst at 96 hours is an elongated sac, almost filled with germinal cells and small centrally placed vacuoles. At 8 days it appears to have grown considerably into a 'non-motile convoluted tube coiled into a globular shape'; germ balls are budded off from the epithelial lining and these develop into daughter sporocysts which are opaque and have a spine-covered anterior end. They migrate to other parts of the snail's body, primarily through loose connective tissue to the digestive gland (liver or ovotestis). In the connective tissue of the liver, further production of germ balls takes place and ultimately the final larval form of the cercaria is produced. Thus, from a single miracidium, due to a process of asexual multiplication within both mother and daughter sporocysts, thousands of cercariae are produced—all of the same sex. Regeneration of a daughter sporocyst may take place following the exhaustion of cercarial production, and is 'accomplished by growth of mesenchymatous tissue to fill the empty spaces, and later by replacement of the mesenchymatous tissue with germinal balls' (Pan, 1965).

Pathological changes produced by *S. mansoni* in a susceptible strain of *B. glabrata* include a 'marked generalised proliferative tissue reaction which is incited by cercariae trapped and dying in the loose vascular connective tissue and which appears some one or two weeks after cercariae begin emergence from snails'. A high mortality of snails is noted at this time. The daughter sporocysts which mature in the liver apparently provoke a reaction which is intermediate between the focal and generalised type of tissue response; 'extensive infiltration of hypertrophic amoebocytes around the daughter sporocysts in the liver usually appears after the generalised tissue reaction has commenced; fibroblasts in loose connective tissue transform readily into hypertrophic, phagocytic amoebocytes which are the most important cellular element in the generalised tissue reaction' (Pan, 1965).

Other detailed studies of intra-molluscan larval development have been made (Meuleman, 1972; Schutte, 1974b; Etges *et al.*, 1975). Tissue extracts prepared from infected *B. glabrata* contain substances capable of immobilising the miracidia of *S. mansoni* (Michelson, 1963 and 1964), extracts from uninfected snails immobilised up to 22% of the miracidia, and a much higher degree of activity was found in most snails with an infection more than 9 days old. Evidence suggests that a developing infection produces some type of immunity to re-infection in snails. It takes about 9 days to develop and is then only partial—bisexual infections and evidence of repeated successful miracidial invasions having been shown in *B. glabrata* and *B. truncatus* (Berrie, 1970).

Production of mature cercariae from the time of miracidial penetration takes approximately 4–5 weeks for *S. mansoni*, 5–6 weeks for *S. haematobium*, and 7 weeks or even longer for *S. japonicum*. The length of the prepatent period may vary according to temperature, the age of the snail and the number of miracidia infecting it (Chu, Massoud and Sabbaghian, 1966a, 1966b, 1966c; Chu, Sabbaghian and Massound, 1966).

Studies of the influence of *S. mansoni* infection on the growth rate and reproduction of *B. pfeifferi* indicate that, in snails of all ages, infection causes a shortened life span but a temporary acceleration in the growth rate which is proportional to the intensity of infection (as judged by cercarial output) of individual snails. Snails which are infected before maturity lay some eggs throughout life, but complete sterility results when snails are infected after maturity. Amongst those that exhibit self-cure, egg laying returns to normal. Eggs laid by infected snails have a higher sterility and a lower hatching rate than eggs of uninfected snails (Sturrock, 1966). Similar results were noted in *B. glabrata* infected with *S. mansoni* (Pan, 1963 and 1965), but *S. haematobium* in *B. truncatus* caused only reduced egg production (Najarian, 1961).

While the infection is usually terminated by the death of the snail (McClelland, 1965), many *Biomphalaria* spp. apparently survive infections, as does *B. nasutus productus* infected with *S. haematobium* (Sturrock, 1967), and *B. truncatus* infected with *S. haematobium* (Webbe and James, 1972). Production of cercariae of *S. mansoni* in *B. glabrata* and *B. pfeifferi* and of *S. haematobium* in *B. truncatus* may persist for 8 months and these snails may become spontaneously cured and can then be subsequently re-infected (Pan, 1965; Pitchford and Visser, 1965; Chu, Massoud and Sabbaghian, 1966a).

The development of *S. japonicum* in *O.h. quadrasi*, the susceptibility of the snail to infection and the mortality rates of infected snails have been fully described (Hunter *et al.*, 1947). From field data, it appears that more female *O.h. quadrasi* are infected with *S. japonicum* than males, and suggestions to explain the disparity in infection rates have been made (Pesigan *et al.*, 1958). Since the miracidium has no clear preference for either sex, and since studies showed no great dissimilarity of habitats between male and female snails, males may be more resistant to penetration by the miracidia than females, or miracidia may not develop to cercariae as well in males as in females, or both. Fewer eggs were laid by infected snails with similarly poor hatchability rates, as compared with non-infected snails, the effect being more severe among younger specimens. Spontaneous cure of *S. japonicum* in *O.h. quadrasi* is apparently negligible, if it occurs at all.

CERCARIAE

When mature, cercariae escape from the daughter sporocyst and emerge from the snail; this is a free-swimming stage, adapted for host invasion. All cercariae developing from one miracidium are of the same sex. The furcocercariae of the *Schistosomatidae* generally swim with the tail pushed forward so that it pulls the body along. They may, however, swim head first, but this depends upon the angle between the furca. Cercariae are often observed sinking through the water with the entire body elongated but inactive; they may also hang head downwards, with the furca extended during a resting phase, but intermittent swimming activity may be observed so that only a small proportion of quite a large collection of cercariae may be actually swimming. On the surface film or on the bottom of a containing vessel, they may perform a looping movement, also referred to as 'measuring worm movement' (Smyth, 1966). In a test tube, the cercariae of *S. mansoni* are predominantly near the surface of the water, whereas *S. haematobium* cercariae form an inverted pyramid extending some way down the test tube. The cercariae of *S. japonicum* are markedly adhesive.

The cercariae of the principal human schistosomes are alike, being furcocercous (brevifurcate) and lacking eye spots or pharynx. They are small and less than 1 mm long; they have a muscular, eversible oral sucker which occupies about one-third of the body and a smaller ventral sucker (acetabulum). The entire trilaminate tegument is covered with minute spines and hairs which are concentrated along the anterior sixth of the body and its posterior margin and also on the acetabulum. The digestive system has a mouth situated sub-terminally in the centre of the oral sucker, an oesophagus and a pair of short, dorsally placed caeca. The nervous system, which lies ventral to the gut, consists of a mass of nerve fibres behind the oral sucker, from which three pairs of nerves lead. The excretory system consists of three pairs of flame cells, collecting tubules and a posterior excretory bladder, and one pair of protonephridia in the tail, the tubules of which open at the tips of the furca (Dawes, 1946; Smyth, 1962).

There are six pairs of 'cephalic glands'; two pairs are pre-acetabular—one pair being escape glands to facilitate the emergence of the cercariae from the snail (Smyth, 1966)—and four pairs are post-acetabular glands occupying the posterior two-thirds of the body. The contents of these glands empty through ducts opening at the edge of the oral sucker. The primary function of the pre-acetabular secretion is probably enzymatic, while the secretion of the post-acetabular glands is believed to be mainly adhesive in function and deposited as the cercariae move over the skin during exploration and in the early phase of penetration. The pre-acetabular glands contain alkaline alizarin-staining material, while the post-acetabular glands contain 'finely granular periodic acid-Schiff staining contents', of which small quantities are secreted each time the oral sucker is attached to a surface (Stirewalt, 1959; Stirewalt and Kruidenier, 1961). These secretions swell in water to provide a sticky mucus for attachment of the oral and ventral suckers as the cercariae begin to penetrate.

Production of cercariae

Light is the principle stimulus causing the release of the cercariae of both *S. haematobium* and *S. mansoni*, usually at temperatures between 10°C and 30°C and possibly higher; cercariae are shed in small numbers in the dark, but periodic peaks of output apparently occur because of an 'innate rhythm' (McClelland, 1965). In the laboratory, the patterns of cercarial output of *S. haematobium* and *S. mansoni* are constant but different; when *B. nasutus* and *B. sudanica* are exposed to light and heat continuously from 0830 to 1730 or 1830 hours, there is one peak during the day—for *S. mansoni* after two hours (with almost the whole day's output emerging within five hours), and for *S. haematobium* after four hours (with nearly all the day's output *being produced over a six-hour period).* More *S. haematobium* cercariae emerge than do *S. mansoni* (McClelland, 1967). High temperatures appear to have a supplementary effect of causing greater output than illumination, but within the range given above, temperature appears to be of secondary importance.

In the field, the pattern of output of *S. mansoni* cercariae from *B. glabrata* corresponded to the curves for temperature and intensity of illumination; from 0900 hours onwards, large numbers of cercariae are produced and this output rises to a peak at 1500 hours, then drops, a few cercariae emerging between 1900 and 2100 hours, the maximum temperature recorded being 37·5°C (Barbosa *et al.*, 1954). Other work in Brazil, in which mice were exposed in a pond, confirmed this picture but revealed the continued presence of cercariae during the night (Pellegrino and de Maria, 1966). These findings are in accord with those of other workers and with the pattern of recovery of cercariae from natural waters in Puerto Rico (Rowan, 1958). Under tropical conditions, when temperatures are high, daytime illumination is probably sufficient to stimulate the emergence of *S. mansoni* cercariae (McClelland, 1965); in Puerto Rico it has been noted that the recovery of cercariae from a pond was the same on dull as on clear days (Maldonado, 1959). In Tanzania, in a natural water course, the peak *S. mansoni* cercarial shedding occurred between 1000 and 1400 hours (Webbe and Jordan, 1966). In South Africa, similar but slightly later peaks for *S. mansoni* and *S. haematobium*, an early (0700–1100 hours) diurnal pattern for *S. bovis*, equal day and night cercarial densities of *S. mattheei*, and a nocturnal shedding pattern (peak at 2100 hours) for *S. rodhaini* have been demonstrated (Pitchford and Visser, 1966). The pattern for *S. rodhaini* is probably an adaptation to the rodent hosts, which are mainly nocturnal.

Cercariae of *S. japonicum* are most abundant in the field during the early part of the night. Estimates of cercarial densities taken at four-hour intervals between 1100 hours and 2300 hours showed that peak densities were found at 2300 hours and a minimum concentration was recorded at 1500 hours. Prolonged exposure to light is necessary, so that cercariae are most abundant in the field during the early part of the night (Pesigan *et al.*, 1958).

Number of cercariae produced

The number of cercariae produced by a snail varies from day to day and is related to the susceptibility of the snail to infection. Few cercariae are produced when a snail first begins to shed, but the number increases to a peak, after which it falls to a relatively constant level which is maintained usually until a short time before the death of the snail, or until spontaneous cure occurs (McClelland, 1965; Chu, Sabbaghian and Massoud, 1966). Among equally susceptible snails, the size of the host is probably the most important factor determining the output of cercariae, with large snails shedding more than small ones. The output from *B. glabrata* is high—1000–3000 per day and 100 000 during the course of an infection are frequently observed. African *Biomphalaria* spp. shed about 500 cercariae per day or less and rarely exceed 1500 per day (Gordon *et al.*, 1934; Sturrock, 1965; McClelland, 1967; Chu and Dawood, 1970; Sturrock and Sturrock, 1970; Klumpp and Chu, 1977). Similar numbers of cercariae are shed by the larger bulinid snails and only a small proportion exceed 2000 per day (McClelland, 1965 and 1967; Chu, Sabbaghian and Massoud, 1966; Berrie, 1970), but individual snails have been found to shed much higher numbers (Webbe and James, 1972).

It has been reported that *B. nasutus productus* with unisexual infections shed significantly fewer cercariae than those with bisexual infections (McClelland, 1965), and that *B. truncatus* which were exposed to two or more miracidia produced twice as many cercariae as those exposed to a single miracidium (Chu, Sabbaghian and Massoud, 1966). It was also observed, however, that *B. glabrata* exposed to one miracidium shed more cercariae than snails exposed to two, and as many as snails exposed to four miracidia (Sturrock and Sturrock, 1970). Similar results were obtained in the case of *B. globosus* exposed to one, three and seven miracidia, respectively (Webbe and James, 1972). Further, it has been shown that in *O.h. quadrasi* the mean daily output of cercariae from snails into which one miracidium has penetrated is nearly twice as high as that from snails into which two to five miracidia have penetrated. The difference is believed to be due to overcrowding of sporocysts, leading to poorer development of cercariae (Pesigan *et al.*, 1958). Other evidence supports the view that the development of sporocysts restricts the penetration of additional miracidia, thus affecting host regulation of parasite numbers. However, the number of parasites and the extent of their development required to produce the effect have not been ascertained.

The snail hosts of *S. japonicum* are much smaller than most of the hosts of other schistosome species. When infected *O.h. quadrasi* were permitted to shed naturally, the mean number of cercariae produced was 15 per day but, under particular conditions, as many as 160 could be obtained. Cercarial output is not apparently continuous in this species, and snails which have been infected for some time frequently shed no cercariae for many days (Pesigan *et al.*, 1958). *O.h. nosophora* from Japan apparently produces several times as many cercariae as *O.h. quadrasi*.

Double infections of *Bulinus* and *Biomphalaria* occur in nature, different species of these genera serving as intermediate hosts of a number of trematodes including echinostomes (Berrie, 1970). Such infections may influence the output of schistosome cercariae, and larval antagonism caused by concomitant echinostome redial infections has been considered as a biological control mechanism (Lim and Heyneman, 1972). It is doubtful, however, whether such a mechanism will significantly alter schistosome infection rates in nature and affect cercarial output to a degree which would influence transmission.

Behaviour of cercariae

While cercariae are influenced by the effect of light, gravity, agitation and touch, and these factors apparently increase the probability of infection of a definitive host, the nature of the habitat and the behaviour of the definitive host chiefly condition the importance of these stimuli. The swimming activity of cercariae may apparently be induced either by reduced light intensity or by mechanical stimuli, the latter producing only activating stimuli which are not affected by simultaneous light stimuli. There is no evidence that chemotaxis is involved in the location of the host by cercariae, but they may exhibit positive thigmotaxis and most species show negative geotaxis. When cercariae reach a surface, they continue to swim to the film and back a short distance from it, but usually they remain just under the surface. The duration of swimming beneath the surface is apparently closely related to the length of free life of the cercariae which has already elapsed, and after a period of time at the surface, they fall passively to the bottom (Smyth, 1966).

Cercariae are relatively short-lived (up to 48 h), non-feeding organisms which have large glycogen reserves. The length of life of a cercaria is dependent upon these glycogen reserves, and any extrinsic factors, such as turbulence or temperature, which may stimulate use of them will therefore reduce viability.

It has been suggested that cercariae become fatigued in fast-flowing, turbulent water (Radke *et al.*, 1961). In East Africa during the rains, high velocities (1·8 m/s; 5·8 ft/s) were recorded in some sections of a natural water course, which may have accounted for the low infection rates and low worm loads recorded from mice exposed in the stream, despite the high snail–cercarial rates found. The almost complete absence of flow in the stream at other times (less than 6 cm/s—0·2 ft/s—during June, July and August), with minimal contact of cercariae and mouse, might have accounted for similar low infection rates and worm loads in exposed animals, even though very high cercarial infection rates were recorded. These anomolous results were, in part, explained by data from an experimental flowing water system designed to study the effect of water velocity on the infection of animals exposed to *S. mansoni* cercariae under controlled conditions. Maximum worm burdens were obtained at a velocity of about 30 cm/s (1 ft/s) and were found to be correspondingly lower at both slower and faster water flows (Webbe, 1966b). Velocity may be important in mixing cercariae in the water and in effecting contact with an exposed host.

Laboratory studies have shown that most cercariae are infective to vertebrate hosts at temperatures normally encountered in the field. The percentage recovery of adult worms from laboratory infected mice increases curvilinearly to a peak at 24°C and then decreases symmetrically (Purnell, 1966a). The survival of *S. mansoni* cercariae decreases with age but is independent of maintenance temperatures from 12–27°C, but above 27°C there is an accelerated rise in mortality of the older cercariae (Purnell, 1966b). In hamsters, the worm load from 100 cercariae decreases significantly both with increase in maintenance temperature in the range 12–33°C and with increase in the age of the cercariae. Cercariae apparently move more rapidly at high temperatures, but they age quickly and soon die. At high temperatures some cercariae which manage to penetrate may not mature if they have used up reserves of glycogen by vigorous movement. At temperatures of 20–24°C, most species of cercariae probably exhaust their glycogen resources within 8 to 12 h.

Addition of glucose to the water can considerably increase the survival period, suggesting that cercariae can apparently utilise substrates for energy purposes but not for synthetic purposes (Smyth, 1966).

The number of *S. mansoni* cercariae which die during penetration of mouse abdominal skin steadily increases with the age of the cercariae. An initial mortality level of about 30% is observed for 2-hour-old cercariae, which rises to 50% at 8 hours and 85% at 24 hours. Losses in the skin also increase with the age of the host up to about 28–35 days (Ghandour and Webbe, 1973). Ultraviolet radiation has a damaging effect on the cercariae of *S. mansoni* and *S. haematobium*. Radiation of cercariae for intervals as short as 5–20 s markedly increased their mortality during penetration of host skin and inhibited migration of schistosomula in the lungs beyond 3–4 days post-infection (Ghandour and Webbe, 1975a). It was found that gamma-radiation (6000r) inhibited the migration and maturation to the adult stage of *S. mansoni* schistosomula; penetration of irradiated cercariae into host skin, however, proceeded normally and the first site of damage was in the lungs (Ghandour and Webbe, 1975b). It is considered that the cercaricidal action of solar u.v. radiation in natural water bodies might reduce the numbers of cercariae in surface waters, but is likely to have little effect at depths greater than 15 cm, since radiation only penetrates the top layers of still, clear water and is quickly absorbed in turbid conditions (Prah and James, 1977).

After emergence from the snail host, the fate of cercariae has not been well studied. Although very large numbers are produced, consideration should be given to their 'density–volume relationship' in natural habitats, and to the possible deleterious effects of chemicals and physical factors in different environments (McClelland, 1965). Using sentinel rodents, exposures were made to *S. mansoni* cercariae in a large volume of water and a factorial design was used to investigate the effects of cercarial concentration and length of exposure on infection rates and worm burdens (Upatham and Sturrock, 1973). Statistical analysis showed that both infection rates and mean worm burdens were related to the two main factors, but the relationship was complicated in each case by curvilinear effects and by a significant interaction between the main factors. The results of these experiments suggest that exposures of less than 1 minute carry little risk of infection at low cercarial concentrations, that repeated exposures will probably not increase the risk substantially and it will only rise if the cercarial concentration increases. There is apparently a greater risk of infection with a low worm burden for activities involving prolonged exposures to low cercarial concentrations, while prolonged exposures to high concentrations carry the greater risk of high infection rates and worm burdens.

Studies on infectivity, population dynamics, dispersion and host-finding capacity of schistosome cercariae under laboratory and field conditions have been based either on cercariometry or direct microscopic observations of free-swimming or penetrating cercariae, or on the ratio of the number of mature worms recovered at autopsy of infected laboratory hosts to the number of available larvae at their exposures. A new radioisotope assay system has been developed (Christensen and Frandsen, 1977) which may overcome some of the problems inherent in other methods—in that precise determination of tissue-bound radio-activity is possible—and may permit of further studies of host-finding capacity relative to physical, chemical and biological characteristics of the aquatic environment.

THE SCHISTOSOMULUM

Cercariae penetrate the skin of the definitive host with the assistance of lytic substances from the penetration glands. The process of penetration is quite rapid and many cercariae penetrate the stratum corneum within a few minutes, the larva changing in appearance to become a schistosomulum. The schistosomulum is tailless, worm-like in appearance and has shed the cercarial glycocalyx, being adapted to serum and saline but unable to survive in water for even a brief period. It does not form the pericercarial sero-envelope in antiserum. After penetration, the trilaminate tegument of the cercaria is replaced by the seven-layered membrane of the schistosomulum and adult worm, which consists of two closely opposed lipid bilayers (Hockley and McLaren, 1973; Stirewalt, 1974; Hockley et al., 1975).

The passage through the subcutaneous tissue is usually affected within 48 hours, and peripheral lymphatic or venous vessels are then penetrated, from which transportation to the right heart and the lungs is accomplished. In mice, schistosomula can be found in the lungs after 4 days and they attain a peak concentration at this site in 5–7 days. A small proportion only apparently feed in the lungs and no real growth takes place there. After 8 days, a few schistosomula are found in the portal

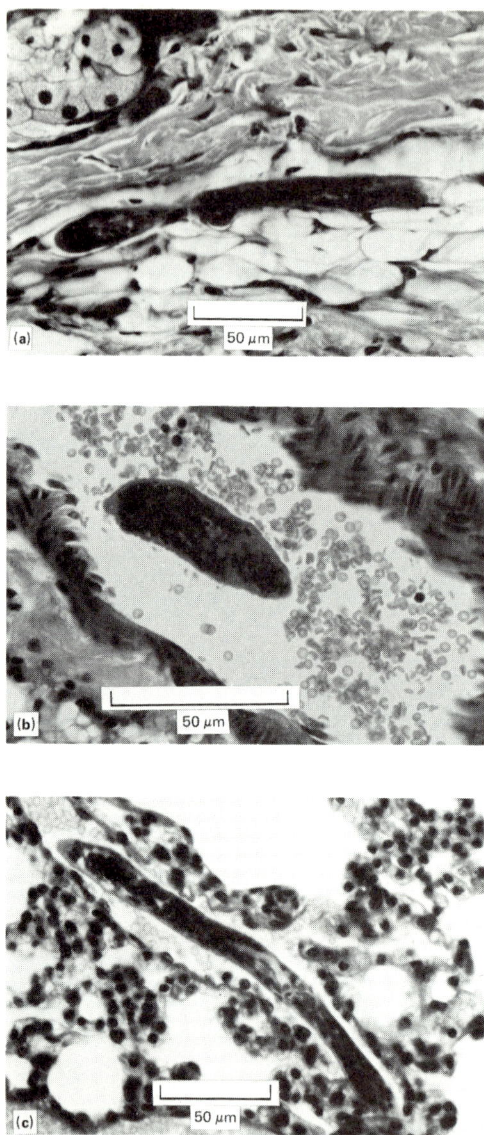

Fig. 3.2 Schistosomula (*S. mansoni*) seen intravascularly in tissues of the mouse without any apparent cellular reaction. All sections stained H & E. (Photographs by courtesy of Dr M. Nilsson.)
(a) Within a dermal blood vessel 3 days post-infection.
(b) Non-elongated form within pulmonary blood vessel 7 days post-infection.
(c) Elongated form within pulmonary blood vessel 7 days post-infection.

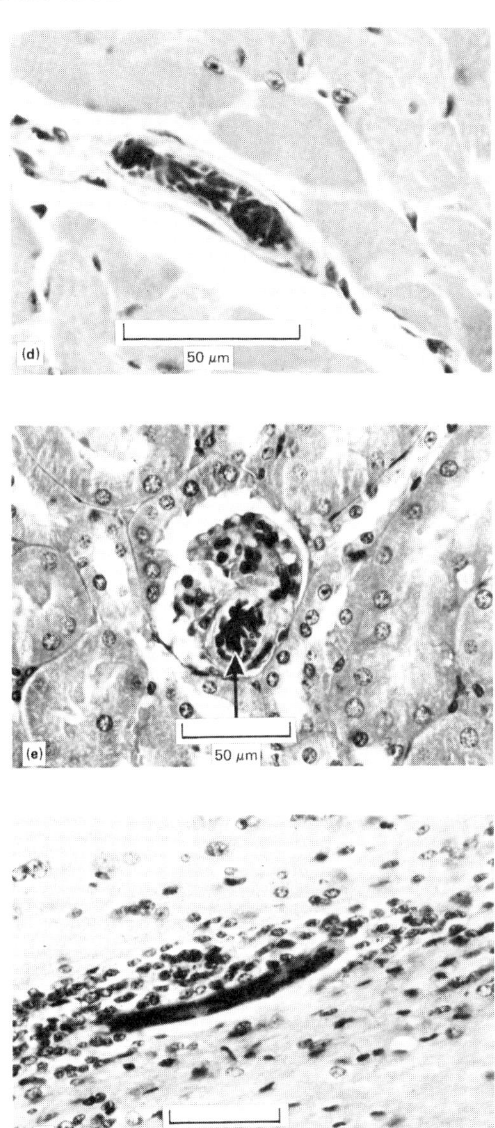

(d) Within a diaphragmatic blood vessel 11 days post-infection.
(e) Within a capillary tuft of a renal glomerulus 15 days post-infection (schistosomulum arrowed).
(f) Within a blood vessel in a nerve cell of the olfactory bulb 15 days post-infection.

vessels of the liver, where active mitosis and growth take place. Paired worms may be found in the mesenteric and portal veins after about 26 days. When the worms are sexually mature, growth slows markedly but still continues. *S. haematobium* schistosomula remain in the skin of the hamster for at least 3 days; some leave this site by day 4 and most by day 5. A similar experiment with *S. mansoni* cercariae showed that the schistosomula stay in the skin for 2 days and begin to migrate on day 3. *S. haematobium* schistosomula can be recovered from the lungs in small numbers from day 5 onwards—peak recoveries of about 20% of the cercariae applied occurring on day 8, compared with day 5 for *S. mansoni* (Smith *et al.*, 1975). *S. haematobium* worms were first found in the mesenteric veins of the hamster on day 29, but males did not pair with females until day 31—normal eggs being produced from day 65 onwards and in the faeces on day 70 (Smith *et al.*, 1976).

The route of migration of the schistosomulum of *S. mansoni* has been studied and certain evidence shows that, following penetration, worms remain in mouse skin for a mean period of 88 h (S.D. ± 23 h), that worms leave the skin mainly by the blood vascular system and are quickly carried passively to the lungs, and that within the lungs there is a 'growth period' of at least 72 h (Miller, 1976; Miller and Wilson, 1978). Between 3 and 6 days after infection, the maximum extension of worms recovered from the lungs more than doubles and this is the probable explanation of the 'growth phase' (Miller, 1976), postulated as lasting up to 72 h after arrival in the lungs (Wilson *et al.*, 1978). It was previously suggested that worms migrate from the lungs to the liver via the pleural cavity, diaphragm and liver capsule (Wilks, 1967), but from some recent work (Miller, 1976) it is concluded that the route of migration is entirely 'intravascular'. It is suggested that worms exit from the lungs via the pulmonary veins and pass through the heart to the systemic circulation, and that an individual worm may make several circuits of the pulmonary/systemic circulation before entering a blood vessel which leads to the hepatic portal system.

Other evidence, however, clearly indicates that the lymphatic system is involved in the migration routes of schistosomula. Recovery of a schistosomulum of *S. japonicum* has been made from a lymph node in a dog (Miyagawa, 1913). Studies of the degree of cell division of schistosomula of *S. mansoni* in the mouse, using radioactive thymidine and inhibition of dividing cells in metaphase with colchicine, also clearly show that no 'real growth' in terms of 'cell division' takes place in the lungs and that there is even a time lag before growth commences in the liver—also that the lymphatics are definitely used in the migration of schistosomula (Nilsson, personal communication).

Most sexually mature worms leave the liver when they have mated and, according to the species, then migrate to the mesenteric veins or to the veins of the vesical plexus, where egg laying begins. The period between successful cercarial penetration and the appearance of eggs in the urine or stools of the definitive host may be 30–40 days, but it is often much longer. There is available evidence that the presence of male worms is essential for the full maturation of the females, and it has been reported that females of one species are aided by males of another species both in maturation and transport from the liver to the mesenteric vessels.

Transformation and cryopreservation of schistosomula

A study of the transformation of cercariae to schistosomula has been carried out and a quantitative comparison made of transformation techniques and of infectivity by different infection routes of the organisms produced (James and Taylor, 1976). At perfusion, the largest numbers of adult worms were recovered from mice injected intramuscularly with organisms produced by the syringe technique (mechanical disruption by passage through a syringe and 21-gauge needle) and control mice given cercariae percutaneously. Other comparisons of transformation techniques included: incubation of cercariae in an isotonic medium; penetration of isolated skin; stimulation with crude egg lecithin; whorling of cercariae with a vortex mixer; syringe transformation followed by incubation.

Following storage at $-196°C$, successful recovery of infective schistosomula of *S. mansoni* has been reported (James and Farrant, 1977). The technique involves a two-step cooling procedure—slow cooling ($0.65°C$ min^{-1}) to an intermediate temperature of $-28°C$, followed by rapid cooling into liquid nitrogen ($10\,000°C$ min^{-1}). It was found that rewarming ($10\,000°C$ min^{-1}) and rapid dilution to remove the cryoprotectant (17.5% methanol) produced motile organisms, some of which develop to adult worms in mice following intramuscular injection.

Immunisation against schistosomes by the administration of living, radiation-attenuated schistosomula will only be feasible if a satisfactory procedure for their storage is developed (Taylor *et al.*, 1977).* It has now been shown that normal cryopreserved schistosomula give rise to adult worm infections which can stimulate concomitant resistance to re-infection; and further, that cryopreserved irradiated schistosomula are as effective in conferring protection in mice as fresh irradiated schistosomula. Partially motile but non-infective frozen schistosomula failed to stimulate protection, indicating the importance of a period of survival within the host (Bickle and James, 1978).

The three major schistosomes which infect man have been cultured *in vitro* with varying degrees of success. *S. mansoni* can be cultured in a simple system *in vitro* from the cercarial stage to adults which mate, but the female does not form ova (Clegg, 1965). The culture of *S. haematobium* has also been described (Smith *et al.*, 1976), and while males formed some spermatozoa, pairing did not take place and females did not complete sexual maturation. It was found that the use of one culture system for both *S. mansoni* and *S. haematobium* has considerable potential value for studying cross-immunity between the species (Smith and Webbe, 1974).

ADULT WORMS

The body orifices of adult worms include a mouth that perforates the oral sucker, a gonopore which is slightly posterior to the ventral sucker, and a posterodorsal excretory pore. The integument in many species is covered with spines, tubercles, and/or hairs. Unlike the tegument of some other parasites, that of the schistosome is a living tissue rather than a dead protective sheath—it comprises 5–7 layers and the outermost of these are continuously being regenerated.

Circular and longitudinal muscles together with a network of mesenchymal cells surround the internal organs, including the digestive system which consists of a short oesophagus leading to the intestine that divides in front of the ventral sucker and reunites behind the gonads as a blind, posterior gut caecum. The

---

* *See also* Taylor, M. G. (1980) in 18th Sympos. Brit. Sc. Parasit Oxford: Blackwell Scientific Publ. 115–40.

gut contents, particularly in females, are usually black and contain pigment (haematin) derived from ingested blood. The excretory–water balance system is made up of flame cells, collecting tubules with an excretory bladder and a terminal pore. In the male, the testes are arranged in one or two rows above the ventral sucker. In the female, a single pyramidal ovary lies in the mid-body line, anterior to the seminal vesicle and posterior to the ootype from which the single, straight uterus leads to the gonopore.

Biology

Adult worms may live for 20–30 years, but the mean length of life span is much shorter (3–8 years). Each worm pair produces 300 to more than 3000 eggs per day. The adults worms do not have a functional Kreb's cycle, but utilise glucose at a rate equal to approximately one-fifth of their dry body weight per hour, via the Embden–Meyerhof pathway, and excreting fatty acids such as lactic, acetic and propionic acids. There is apparently a functional citric acid cycle in the egg, but it is not known whether glycolysis or oxidative metabolism is of greater importance to energy formation in the egg. It appears that oxidation is complete in the free-living stages (miracidia and cercariae) that are not present in an energy-rich environment. The worms ingest red blood cells and possess a protease that breaks down globulin and haemaglobin, releasing tyrosine. A haematin-like pigment is regurgitated by the adult worms and this is taken up by reticuloendothelial cells in the liver and spleen.

As is the case with most helminths, the adult schistosomes do not multiply in the definitive host and, in terms of host–parasite populations, this means that 'the infection process produces, or tends to produce, an over-dispersed distribution of parasites within the host population', in which most individuals carry very few parasites and a small proportion are heavily parasitised (Crofton, 1971a and 1971b). Thus, unlike bacteria or protozoa, the distribution of the schistosomes in definitive host populations does not follow the normal Poisson or bell-shaped curve, but fits a truncated, negative binomial model. It is considered that, in the case of schistosomiasis, ecological data and egg counts in man indicate that this precept is followed and that, even if the proportion of those with infections of high intensity is low, morbidity may be considerable (Warren, 1973).

Metabolism and drug action*

The surface proteins of cercariae and schistosomula are qualitatively similar, apart from one protein band which is lost on penetration. The schistosomular coat, however, lacks the large amounts of glycolipid found in the surface coat of adult worms (Kusel, 1972). Oxidative phosphorylation is still important in the energy formation of the schistosomulum which excretes lactic acid as well as uses oxygen. Little is known about the biochemistry of the developing worms, but the ratio of lactate production under air and nitrogen is comparable in 3-week-old and adult worms, suggesting a similar importance of glycolysis and oxidative phosphorylation in energy formation (Coles, 1973a). It is commonly observed that drugs which affect adult worms are not usually effective against juvenile stages and worms in the third and fourth weeks appear to be particularly resistant to most available schistosomicides, but how far this is due to the worm metabolism changing and how much it is related to the different positions of the parasite within the host is not yet known (Coles, 1973b).

The schistosomes are, of course, unisexual and there are differences in biochemistry between males and females. There is a difference in drug response—male worms are more susceptible to hycanthone and oxamniquine, but females are more susceptible to niridazole and antimony. The former may kill worms because of its effect on glycogen breakdown; following treatment, there is a fall in worm glycogen and decreased inactivation of schistosome phosphorylase by phosphorylase phosphatase. Antimony compounds are believed to be toxic to schistosomes because of their inhibition of phosphofructokinase (PFK). Hycanthone interchelates with DNA, and it is believed that it probably acts in this way on schistosomes. Metrifonate, an organophosphorous ester, and its metabolite, dichlorvos, are inhibitors of cholinesterase and acetycholinesterase and the effect is quantitatively the same for *S. mansoni* and *S. haematobium* (Coles, 1973b). Differences in drug responses between species may be much greater than between strains of the same species. Although the mechanisms of drug uptake are clearly of considerable importance, they remain almost completely unknown. The uptake of a drug may result in a rapid or delayed migration of worms from the mesenteric veins to the liver and/or from the

* Van den Bossche, H. (1980) *Biochem. Pharma.*, **29,** 1981.

vesical plexus to the lungs (James *et al.*, 1972; James and Webbe, 1974). The use of certain drugs at sublethal doses causes a reversible shift of worms to the liver, but the death of most worms is apparently due to their becoming trapped and subsequently phagocytosed. It is thought that this is probably due to the surface coat of the worm being damaged or 'recognised' by the host (Standen, 1962). Worms may also be attacked by leucocytes while they are still alive (Striebel, 1969).

The integument of the worm is an important site of many types of nutrient transfer, much of which will probably be active transport; the gut is another source of nutrients for the worms (Fripp, 1967; Senft, 1969; Coles, 1973b). Knowledge of nutrient uptake mechanisms, as well as those of drug uptake, is wanting and more information is required about metabolic pathways in schistosomes—such as the citric acid cycle, the pentose phosphate pathway, the importance of fatty acid elongation, and amino acid metabolism—before structurally related drug formulations can be considered (Coles, 1973b).

REFERENCES

Barbosa, F. S., Coelho, M. de V. and Dobbin, J. E. Jr. (1954). *Publ. Avuls. Inst. Aggeu Magalhães.* **3,** 79.
Berrie, A. D. (1970). *Adv. Parasit.* **8,** 43.
Bickle, Q. D. and James, E. R. (1978). *Trans. R. Soc. Trop. Med. Hyg.* **72,** 677.
Chernin, E. (1970). *J. Parasit.* **56,** 287.
Chernin, E. and Dunavan, C. A. (1962). *Am. J. Trop. Med. Hyg.* **11,** 455.
Christensen, N. and Frandsen, F. (1977). *J. Helminth.* **51,** 105.
Chu, K. Y. and Dawood, I. K. (1970). *Bull. Wld Hlth Org.* **42,** 575.
Chu, K. Y., Massoud, J. and Sabbaghian, H. (1966a). *Bull. Wld Hlth Org.* **34,** 113.
Chu, K. Y., Massoud, J. and Sabbaghian, H. (1966b). *Bull. Wld Hlth Org.* **34,** 131.
Chu, K. Y., Massoud, J. and Sabbaghian, H. (1966c). *Bull. Wld Hlth Org.* **34,** 135.
Chu, K. Y., Sabbaghian, H. and Massoud, J. (1966). *Bull. Wld Hlth Org.* **34,** 121.
Clegg, J. A. (1965). *Expl Parasit.* **16,** 133.
Coles, G. C. (1973a). *Int. J. Parasit.* **3,** 783.
Coles, G. C. (1973b). *Int. J. Biochem.* **4,** 319.
Crofton, H. D. (1971a). *Parasitology* **62,** 179.
Crofton, H. D. (1971b). *Parasitology* **63,** 343.
Dawes, B. (1946). *The Trematoda.* Cambridge University Press, Cambridge.
Etges, F. J. (1963). *J. Parasit.* **49** (Suppl.), 26.
Etges, F. J., Carter, O. S. and Webbe, G. (1975). *Ann. N.Y. Acad. Sci.* **266,** 480.
Etges, F. J. and Decker, C. L. (1963). *J. Parasit.* **57,** 217.

Faust, E. C. and Russell, P. F. (1964). *Craig and Faust's Clinical Parasitology*, 7th edn, p. 534. H. Kimpton, London.

Fripp, P. J. (1967). *Comp. Biochem. Physiol.* **23,** 893.

Gordon, R. M., Davey, T. H. and Peason, H. (1934). *Ann. Trop. Med. Parasit.* **28,** 323.

Hockley, D. J. and McLaren, D. J. (1973). *Int. J. Parasit.* **3,** 13.

Hockley, D. J., McLaren, D. J., Ward, B. J. and Nermut, M. V. (1975). *Tissue and Cell.* **7,** 485.

Hunter, G. W., Bennett, H. J., Ingalls, J. W. and Greene, E. (1947). *Am. J. Trop. Med. Hyg.* **27,** 597.

Ghandour, A. and Webbe, G. (1973). *Int. J. Parasit.* **3,** 789.

Ghandour, A. and Webbe, G. (1975a). *J. Helminth.* **49,** 153.

Ghandour, A. and Webbe, G. (1975b). *J. Helminth.* **49,** 161.

James, C. and Prah, S. K. (1978). *J. Helminth.* **52,** 221.

James, C., Preston, J. and Webbe, G. (1972). *Ann. Trop. Med. Parasit.* **66,** 467.

James, C. and Webbe, G. (1974). *Trans. R. Soc. Trop. Med. Hyg.* **68,** 413.

James, E. R. and Farrant, J. (1977). *Trans. R. Soc. Trop. Med. Hyg.* **71,** 498.

James, E. R. and Taylor, M. G. (1976). *J. Helminth.* **50,** 223.

Jobin, W. R. and Ippen, A. T. (1964). *Science, N.Y.* **145,** 1324.

Jordan, P. and Webbe, G. (1969). *Human Schistosomiasis*, p. 212. Heinemann Medical Books, London.

Klumpp, R. K. and Chu, K. Y. (1977). *Bull. Wld Hlth Org.* **55,** 715.

Kusel, J. R. (1972). *Parasitology* **65,** 55.

Lim, H. K. and Heyneman, D. (1972). *Adv. Parasit.* **10,** 191.

McClelland, W. F. J. (1965). *Bull. Wld Hlth Org.* **33,** 270.

McClelland, W. F. J. (1967). *Expl Parasit.* **20,** 205.

MacInnis, A. J. (1965). *J. Parasit.* **51,** 731.

MacInnis, A. J., Bethel, W. M. and Cornford, E. M. (1974). *Nature (Lond.)* **248,** 361.

Maldonado, J. F. (1959). *Bol. Assoc. Med. P. Rico* **51,** 36.

Mason, P. R. and Fripp, P. J. (1976). *J. Parasit.* **62,** 721.

Mason, P. R. and Fripp, P. J. (1977). *Ztschr. Parasitenk.* **53,** 287.

Meuleman, E. A. (1972). *Neth. J. Zool.* **22,** 355.

Michelson, E. H. (1963). *Ann. N.Y. Acad. Sci.* **113,** 486.

Michelson, E. H. (1964). *Am. J. Trop. Med. Hyg.* **13,** 36.

Miller, P. (1976). PhD Thesis. University of York.

Miller, P. and Wilson, R. A. (1978). *Parasitology* **77,** 281.

Miyagawa, Y. (1913). *Zbl. Bakt.* **69,** 132.

Najarian, J. J. (1961). *Tex. Rep. Biol. Med.* **19,** 327.

Pan, C. (1963). *Ann. N.Y. Acad. Sci.* **113,** 475.

Pan, C. (1965). *Am. J. Trop. Med. Hyg.* **14,** 931.

Pellegrino, J. and de Maria, M. (1966). *Am. J. Trop. Med. Hyg.* **15,** 333.

Pesigan, T. P., Hairston, N. G., Jauregui, J. J., Garcia, E. G., Santos, A. T., Santos, B. C. and Besa, A. A. (1958). *Bull. Wld Hlth Org.* **18,** 481.

Pitchford, R. J. and Visser, P. S. (1965). *Bull. Wld Hlth Org.* **132,** 83.

Pitchford, R. J. and Visser, P. S. (1966). *S. Afr. Med. J.* **40,** 1.

Prah, S. K. and James, C. (1977). *J. Helminth.* **51,** 73.

Prentice, M. A., Panesar, T. S. and Coles, G. C. (1970). *Ann. Trop. Med. Parasit.* **64,** 339.

Purnell, R. E. (1966a). *Ann. Trop. Med. Parasit.* **60,** 90.

Purnell, R. E. (1966b). *Ann. Trop. Med. Parasit.* **60,** 182.
Radke, M. G., Ritchie, L. S. and Rowan, W. B. (1961). *Expl Parasit.* **11,** 323.
Rowan, W. B. (1958). *Am. J. Trop. Med. Hyg.* **7,** 374.
Schutte, C. H. J. (1974a). *S. Afr. J. Sci.* **70,** 299.
Schutte, C. H. J. (1974b). *S. Afr. J. Sci.* **70,** 327.
Senft, A. W. (1969). *Ann. N.Y. Acad. Sci.* **160,** 571.
Shiff, C. J. (1968). *J. Parasit.* **54,** 1133.
Shiff, C. J. (1974). *J. Parasit.* **60,** 578.
Shiff, C. J. and Kriel, R. L. (1970). *J. Parasit.* **56,** 281.
Short, R. B. and Saladin, K. (1973). *J. Parasit., Progr. Abst.* **64,** 1.
Smith, M., Clegg, J. A., Kusel, J. R. and Webbe, G. (1975). *Experimentia* **31,** 595.
Smith, M., Clegg, J. A. and Webbe, G. (1976). *Ann. Trop. Med. Parasit.* **70,** 101.
Smith, M. and Webbe, G. (1974). *Trans. R. Soc. Trop. Med. Hyg.* **68,** 70.
Smyth, J. D. (1962). *Introduction to Animal Parasitology.* English University Press, London.
Smyth, J. D. (1966). *The Physiology of Trematodes, University Reviews in Biology,* pp. 96, 105, 106, 107, 110, 115, 135. Oliver and Boyd, Edinburgh, London.
Standen, O. D. (1962). *Ciba Foundation Symposium on Bilharziasis,* p. 266. Eds G. E. W. Wolstenholme and M. O'Connor. Churchill, London.
Stirewalt, M. A. (1954). *Expl Parasit.* **3,** 504.
Stirewalt, M. A. (1959). *Expl Parasit.* **8,** 199.
Stirewalt, M. A. (1974). *Adv. Parasit.* **12,** 115.
Stirewalt, M. A. and Kruidenier, F. J. (1961). *Expl Parasit.* **11,** 191.
Striebel, H. P. (1969). *Ann. N.Y. Acad. Sci.* **160,** 491.
Sturrock, B. M. (1966). *Ann. Trop. Med. Parasit.* **60,** 187.
Sturrock, B. M. (1967). *Ann. Trop. Med. Parasit.* **61,** 321.
Sturrock, B. M. and Sturrock, R. F. (1970). *Ann. Trop. Med. Parasit.* **64,** 357.
Sturrock, R. F. (1965). *Ann. Trop. Med. Parasit.* **59,** 1.
Sturrock, R. F. and Upatham, E. S. (1973). *Int. J. Parasit.* **3,** 35.
Taylor, M. G., James, E. R., Bickle, Q. D., Doenhoff, M. J. and Nelson, G. S. (1977). *INSERM.* **72,** 291.
Upatham, E. S. (1973). *Int. J. Parasit.* **3,** 289.
Upatham, E. S. and Sturrock, R. F. (1973). *J. Parasit.* **59,** 448.
Wajdi, N. (1963). *Studies on the larval development of schistosomes.* PhD Thesis, University of London.
Wajdi, N. (1966). *Trans. R. Soc. Trop. Med. Hyg.* **60,** 774.
Wajdi, N. (1972). *Bull. Wld Hlth Org.* **46,** 115.
Warren, K. S. (1973). *Helm. Abstr.* **42,** 591.
Webbe, G. (1962). *Ciba Foundation Symposium on Bilharziasis,* p. 7. Eds G. E. W. Wolstenholme and M. O'Connor. Churchill, London.
Webbe, G. (1965). *Bull. Wld Hlth Org.* **33,** 155.
Webbe, G. (1966a). *Ann. Trop. Med. Parasit.* **60,** 85.
Webbe, G. (1966b). *Ann. Trop. Med. Parasit.* **60,** 78.
Webbe, G. (1967). *Ann. Soc. Belg. Méd. Trop.* **47,** 97.
Webbe, G. and James, C. (1972). *J. Helminth.* **46,** 185.
Webbe, G. and Jordan, P. (1966). *Trans. R. Soc. Trop. Med. Hyg.* **60,** 279.
Wilks, N. E. (1967). *Am. J. Trop. Med. Hyg.* **16,** 599.
Wilson, R. A., Draskau, T., Miller, P. and Lawson, J. R. (1978). *Parasitology* **77,** 57.

Wright, C. A. (1958). *Ann. Trop. Med. Parasit.* **53,** 288.
Wright, C. A. (1962). *Ciba Foundation Symposium on Bilharziasis,* p. 103.
  Eds G. E. W. Wolstenholme and M. O'Connor. Churchill, London.
Wright, C. A. (1965). *Proc. 1st Inst. Congr. Parasit., Rome.* Pergamon Press,
  Oxford.

4 Infection with *S. haematobium*

Herbert M. Gilles

In endemic areas, *S. haematobium* is the commonest cause of haematuria. Evidence is now available which indicates a correlation between the intensity of *S. haematobium* infection and the clinicopathological effects of the disease. However, in endemic areas with light or moderate infections, the degree of morbidity is often difficult to determine.

The target organs are in the urinary tract—the bladder, ureters and kidney—but ectopic deposition of eggs can occur in any part of the body, resulting in specific localised lesions.

PATHOLOGY

The main histopathological features of the disease have been described in detail (Edington and Gilles, 1976).

The bladder

Many lesions occur in the bladder. Although the mechanism of egg deposition is not clear, it seems likely that the female worm deposits her eggs in terminal blood vessels in the submucosa of the bladder (Fig. 4.1), and that the miracidia in the mature eggs secrete a histolytic substance which acts on the bladder wall to such an extent that, when the bladder contracts, eggs are forced through the tissues into the lumen of the organ (Barlow, 1949; Kloetzel, 1969). In the early stages the bladder may only be hyperaemic, with or without petechial haemorrhages (Fig. 4.2). Ova retained in the epithelium or in the vesical tissues, most usually in the subepithelial layer, cause the formation of pseudo-tubercles and the bladder may be studded by these small, yellow seed-like bodies surrounded by a zone of hyperaemia, later resembling white sago grains. They are most frequently present

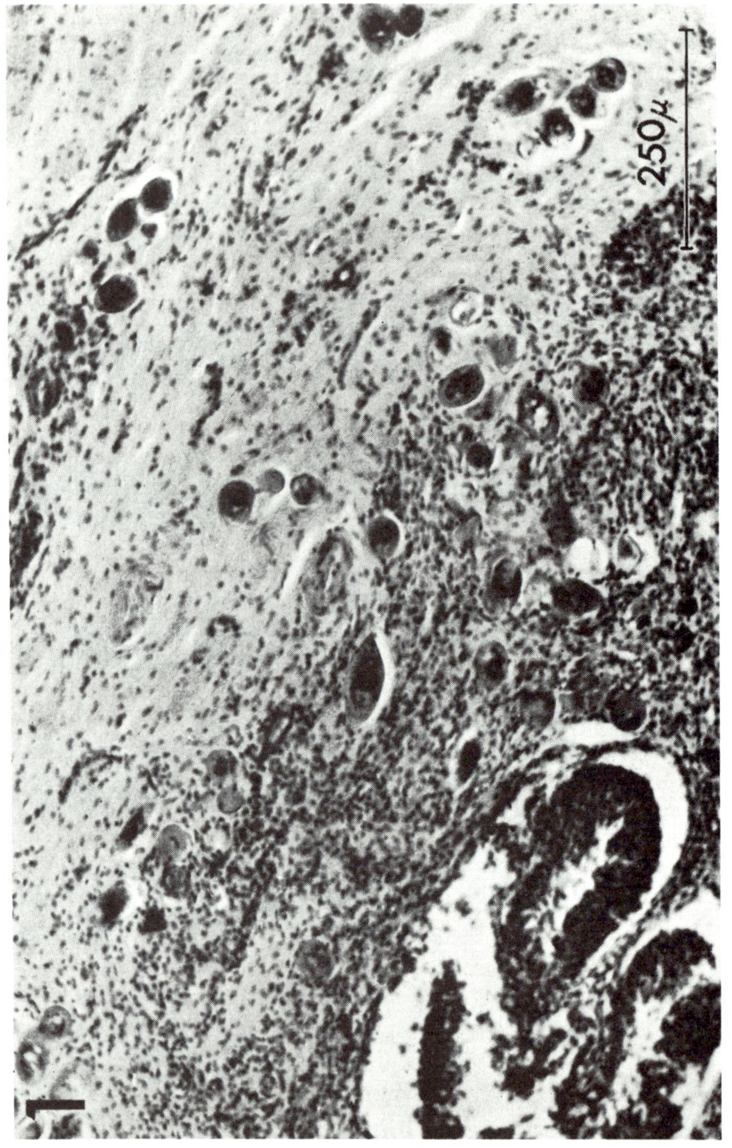

Fig. 4.1 Section of bladder showing *S. haematobium* eggs in submucosa, some eggs in 'nests' showing partial calcification. (Material from the Department of Helminthology, London School of Hygiene and Tropical Medicine.)

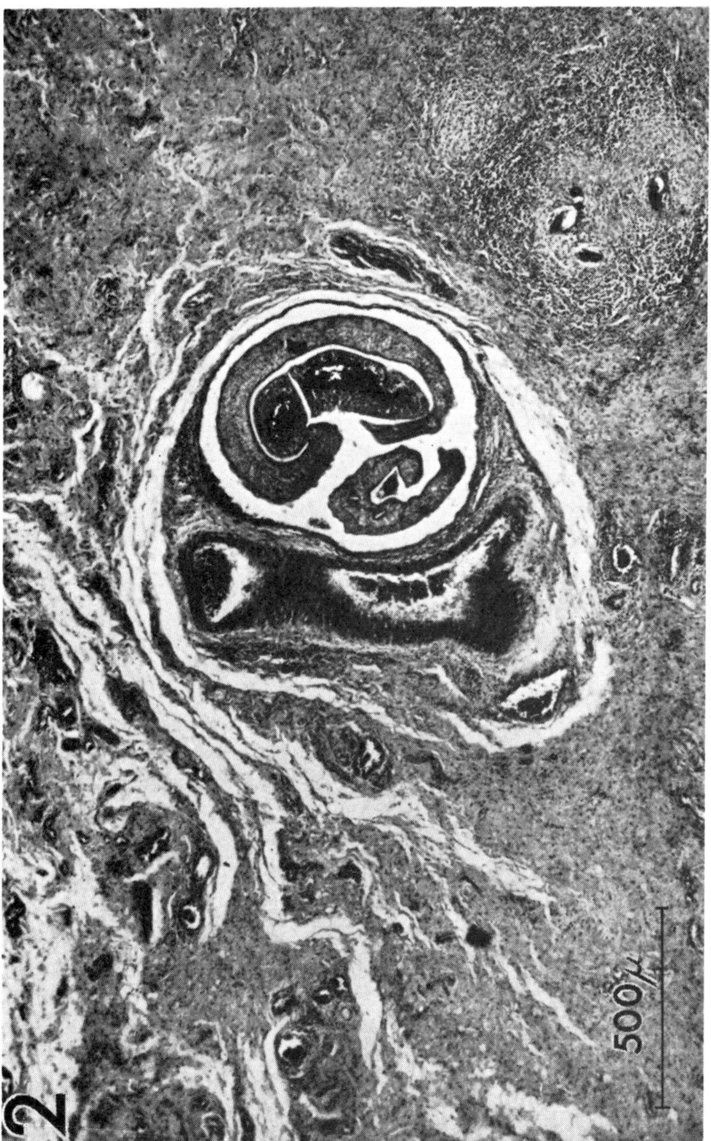

Fig. 4.2 Section of bladder showing adult male and female worms of *S. haematobium* in a venule and *S. haematobium* eggs. Note the absence of tissue reaction around the adults. (Material from the Department of Helminthology, London School of Hygiene and Tropical Medicine.)

in the areas of the trigone, with the base and lateral walls next most commonly affected. Adult schistosomes are frequently present in the neighbouring vesical veins. Nodular or polypoid lesions may be formed by coalescence of the tubercles, hyperplasia of the mucosa, and early fibrosis and hypertrophy of muscle. In the early stages these are hyperaemic and mulberry like. These active, proliferating papillomatous or granulomatous lesions are responsible for the bladder-filling defects seen radiologically in the early stages (Gelfand and Gilles, 1966). Later, the ova become calcified; atrophy of the mucosa with underlying fibrosis of the connective tissue occurs and the lesions shrink and are represented by white, fibrous plaques on the mucosal surface (Fig. 4.3). With less severe proliferation, the bladder mucosa may eventually present a flat, ground-glass appearance due to widespread atrophy of the epithelium with underlying fibrosis. In addition to the mulberry-like multiple granulomatous polyps described, a fibro-calcific type also commonly occurs. This is a small, usually solitary lesion with the raised surface resembling microscopically the sandy patch. The central core of dense fibrous tissue contains dilated capillaries and calcified ova. The epithelium is denuded. A third type of polyp (the villous) is less common and has thickened, club-shaped fronds covered with hyperplastic epithelium. These polyps rarely resemble the classical polyp with its delicate fronds covered by transitional epithelium.

However, the most common lesion in vesical schistosomiasis is the so-called 'sandy patch'. This is a late lesion and is most often seen in the trigone area in which the mucosa is roughened, raised and greyish-golden-brown in colour. The overlying epithelium may be irregularly thickened or atrophic and areas of squamous metaplasia have been described. In the submucosa and muscularis, pseudotubercles and foreign-body granulomas may be seen surrounding ova in various stages of disintegration or calcification, but the predominant feature is fibrosis, with calcified ova scattered in variable numbers in the dense collagenous tissue. In many instances, the cellular reaction disappears or scanty lymphocytes and plasma cells may be present.

The epithelium of the bladder may undergo a number of changes, varying from marked hyperplasia to atrophy. Foci of leukoplakia may be present. At the edges of nodules or polyps, the mucous membrane is folded, forming shallow pits or pseudoglands, the lumina of which may become occluded by hypertrophy of the epithelium, with the formation of broad epithelial

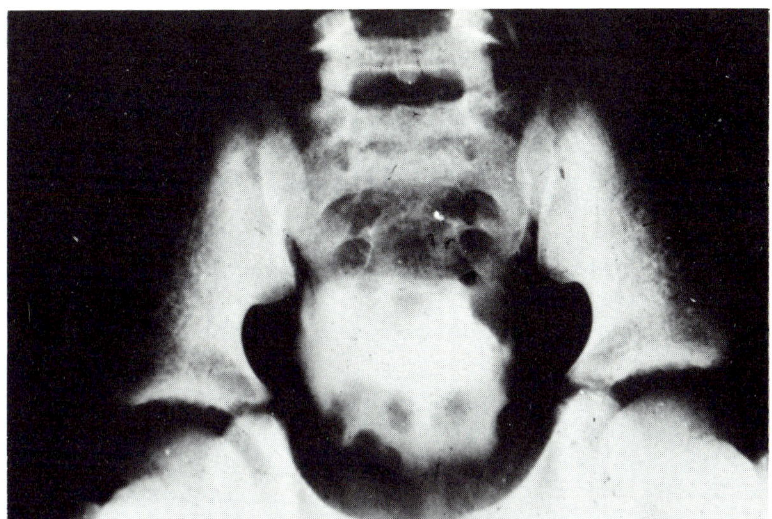

Fig. 4.3 Bladder-filling defects seen in the early stages of *S. haematobium* infection. These lesions are reversible with medical treatment in the majority of cases.

pegs which may become detached from the surface, giving the appearance of isolated islets of epithelium in the submucosa— the so-called Brunn's nests. These downgrowths may become vesicular and lined by tall columnar epithelium (cystitis glandularis) and, in the presence of a lymphocytic infiltration, may resemble cystitis cystica.

It must be emphasised that in vesical schistosomiasis, all types of lesions may be seen in one bladder and all areas in the bladder wall may undergo fibrosis and calcification—in others, focal muscular hypertrophy and diverticula may be found. With fibrosis of the bladder, the trigone and bladder neck are pulled forward anteriorly with consequent bladder-neck obstruction, a late complication which is seen frequently in Egypt, with all the consequent effects of urinary retention, including multiple sinuses in the scrotum and perineum (Atala *et al.*, 1969). In a detailed study of bladder-neck obstruction in Egypt, it was shown that in many cases the fibrotic obstruction occurred in the posterior urethra and that urethroscopy was the most satisfactory method of definitive diagnosis.

The ureters

The lower thirds of the ureters are frequently bilaterally affected, as they have a common blood supply with the bladder. In addition, there may be secondary changes induced by the bladder lesions. In the early stages in up to 20% of children in endemic areas, uretero-vesical incompetence with reflux and, in a lesser proportion, hydronephrosis can be demonstrated. It is probable that these changes are due to oedema and congestion, perhaps with pseudotubercle formation in the region of the vesical portion of the ureter, with consequent distortion. Pseudo-tubercles, with all the consequential changes described in the bladder, may occur in the ureteric wall. Mucoid degeneration of Brunn's nests may occur just as in the bladder, with the formation of ureteritis glandularis, including polyps and ureteritis cystica. Stricture and/or dilatation of the ureter eventually result. Fibrosis of the bladder may also result in stenosis of the ureteric orifices. It has been stated that in 70% of patients the ureters are affected. Linear calcification in the ureter wall may occur, usually at the lower end, and is said to be pathognomonic. On the other hand, punctate spots of calcification may be seen (ureteritis calcinosa), the calcification arising in the contents of ureteritis cystica. Occasionally, also calcification may arise in a polyp (Maged and Soliman, 1968). Lymphoedema of the penis and scrotum has been reported, and urethritis cystica of the posterior portion of the urethra has been described in Egypt (Zaher and El Deeb, 1969).

The kidney

Lesions directly due to the parasite are not commonly seen in the kidney, but occasionally ova are found in the renal parenchyma or in the submucous tissue of the calyces and renal pelvis. Interstitial nephritis has been described in a few patients. Rarely, adult worms may enter the interlocular veins and after their death cause an acute eosinophilic necrotising lesion (Arean, 1966). Calcification of the renal capsule has been reported in one case; ova were noted histologically, but the renal parenchyma was not affected (Atala and Zaher, 1969).

Hydronephrosis, pyonephrosis, and acute pyelonephritis due to vesical and ureteric lesions are, however, not uncommon and may cause death (Edington, 1957).

Classical comparative studies on the pathological effects of *S. haematobium* infection in Ibadan and Egypt have been carried out (Edington *et al.*, 1970; von Lichtenberg *et al.*, 1971; Smith *et al.*,

1974 and 1975; Cheever *et al.*, 1977) and the salient pathological features of *S. haematobium* infection have been described from the Sudan (Hasan *et al.*, 1977). Techniques used for the recovery of worms and eggs at necropsy have been evaluated (Kamel *et al.*, 1977).

CLINICAL FEATURES

The earliest symptom is severe itching at the sites of skin penetration—'cercarial dermatitis'—which lasts two to three days and is accompanied sometimes by the appearance of small red papules (Barlow and Meleney, 1949). The early stages of *S. haematobium* infection, i.e. **the stages of invasion and maturation**, are rarely seen in indigenous people living in endemic areas.

About eight weeks later, an allergic reaction appears which may include pyrexia, headache, generalised pains and anorexia. There may also be nausea, vomiting, diarrhoea, cough and localised signs such as hepatic tenderness and splenomegaly. An accompanying blood eosinophilia, which may be as high as 80% will suggest an helminthic infection, and even at this early stage, ova may be found in the urine (Walt, 1954). This toxaemic stage is once again rare in indigenous people of endemic areas. Whether it is due to differences in host response (Gelfand, 1967), genetic experience of the parasite (Elsdon-Dew, 1966), or is merely undiagnosed because of the non-specificity of the illness coupled with the paucity of medical care in many rural areas, is difficult to ascertain.

The stage of **established infection** occurs 10–12 weeks after cercarial penetration and is usually manifested by haematuria and egg extrusion. The haematuria is often transitory, and although specimens of urine passed one day may be heavily loaded with blood, those passed the following day may be free from it. Frank haematuria may continue at intervals for a number of years in untreated cases, steadily declining in severity. Microscopic blood will be present between episodes in most cases, together with eggs of the parasite, but these also are excreted in diminishing numbers over the years (see Chapter 10). The blood lost in the urine is rarely sufficient to cause anaemia *per se.* In patients with mild to moderately severe infections, the loss has been calculated, using ^{59}Fe and chemical methods, to be up to 6 ml per day (Gerritsen *et al.*, 1953; El-Bishlawi, 1973). Red blood cells seem to adhere to the ova and release their haemoglobin (Campbell and Dickinson, 1968; Cheever *et al.*, 1977). Loss of protein in *S. haematobium* eggs (Richard *et al.*, 1966) as well as an increased excretion of amino acids have been reported. Protein loss in urine in *S. haematobium* appears, however, to make little contribution to the severity of protein energy malnutrition, except perhaps in extreme cases (Norden and Gelfand, 1973).

The bladder

The symptoms of irritability of the bladder manifest themselves with dysuria, and a steady increase in frequency and urgency of micturition. When schistosomal ulceration occurs, it is usually accompanied by suprapubic or perineal pain (Dimmette *et al.*, 1955). Two clinicopathological entities have been reported:

(i) sloughing of polypoid patches in early active disease; and

(ii) chronic ulceration occurring at sites of very heavy *S. haematobium* egg burdens (Smith, Kelada and Khalil, 1977).

Polypoid lesions of the bladder may persist as polyps into later inactive stages of the disease if the antecedent active infection is heavy (Smith, Torky *et al.*, 1977).

Vesical fibrosis with contraction of the bladder and calcification of eggs retained in the tissues occurs in chronic infections. In some cases, however, probably owing to a reduced blood supply, the bladder wall may become atrophic, leading to a greater bladder capacity than normal (Honey and Gelfand, 1960); but this effect may be the result of involvement of the neck of the bladder, leading to obstruction and back pressure (Makar, 1967), though bladder neck involvement is not recognised by all urologists. Calcification is common in children and young adults. When schistosome ova die in the bladder mucosa, they undergo degenerative changes and, if they are not broken down by giant cells and other phagocytes, become calcified (Buchanan and Gelfand, 1970). In none of the cases examined was there any evidence that the bladder tissue, as opposed to the ova, had undergone calcification (Barlow and Meleney, 1949). X-ray evidence of bladder calcification then would indicate that the patient had a heavy bilharzial infection. Calcified ova could be seen adjacent to the urothelium and in some instances breaking through it. The significance of this is that a patient could have a 'calcified' bladder but, in time, most if not all of the calcified ova could be discharged and the bladder wall could then return to relative normality. This would be in keeping with the evidence that advanced lesions of the disease may resolve spontaneously (Powell, 1967; see Chapter 10). It has been estimated that as few as 100 000 eggs per cm^2 might be detected in a clinical radiograph (Cheever *et al.*, 1975). There is a general correlation between the severity of calcification noted radiologically, the extent of sandy deposits noted grossly, and the number of eggs counted after digestion of the bladder (Fig. 4.4).

The ureters

Ureteric involvement is common in *S. haematobium* infection (Gelfand, 1948; von Lichtenberg *et al.*, 1971; Smith *et al.*, 1975). The lesions are commonly bilateral but may be unilateral, and the left ureter is more commonly affected than the right (Makar, 1968). Severe infections produce sandy patches, polyps, ureteritis cystica, ureteritis glandularis and ulcers. Ureteric stenosis occurs, the commonest site for stricture being the intravesical portion of the ureter. Stenosis of the lower ureter comes next in frequency and it occurs least often in the upper half of the ureter (Fig. 4.5).

Hydro-ureter develops secondary to ureteric stenosis. With distal stenosis, the ureter not only dilates but becomes lengthened and tortuous. Hydro-ureter may develop in the absence of stenosis from functional inco-ordination or aperistalsis. There is a great anatomical variability of schistosomal hydro-ureter (Sayegh, 1950; Chapman, 1966). Lower urinary tract infection, pyelonephritis and urolithiasis are sequelae. A clinicopathological study of schistosomal obstructive uropathy in 155 Egyptian patients treated surgically has been reported (Smith, Kelada *et al.*, 1977).

The kidneys and renal function

Pyonephrosis and hydronephrosis (Fig. 4.5) develop secondarily to schistosomal obstructive lesions. Pyelonephritis occurs more frequently among cases of schistosomal obstructive uropathy than in control series (Elwi *et al.*, 1974; Smith *et al.*, 1974).

An association between *S. haematobium* and the nephrotic syndrome has been suggested (Gelfand, 1963; Sabbour *et al.*, 1973; Ezzat *et al.*, 1974), but the epidemiological and pathological evidence for this association remains to be conclusively demonstrated (Sadigursky *et al.*, 1976).

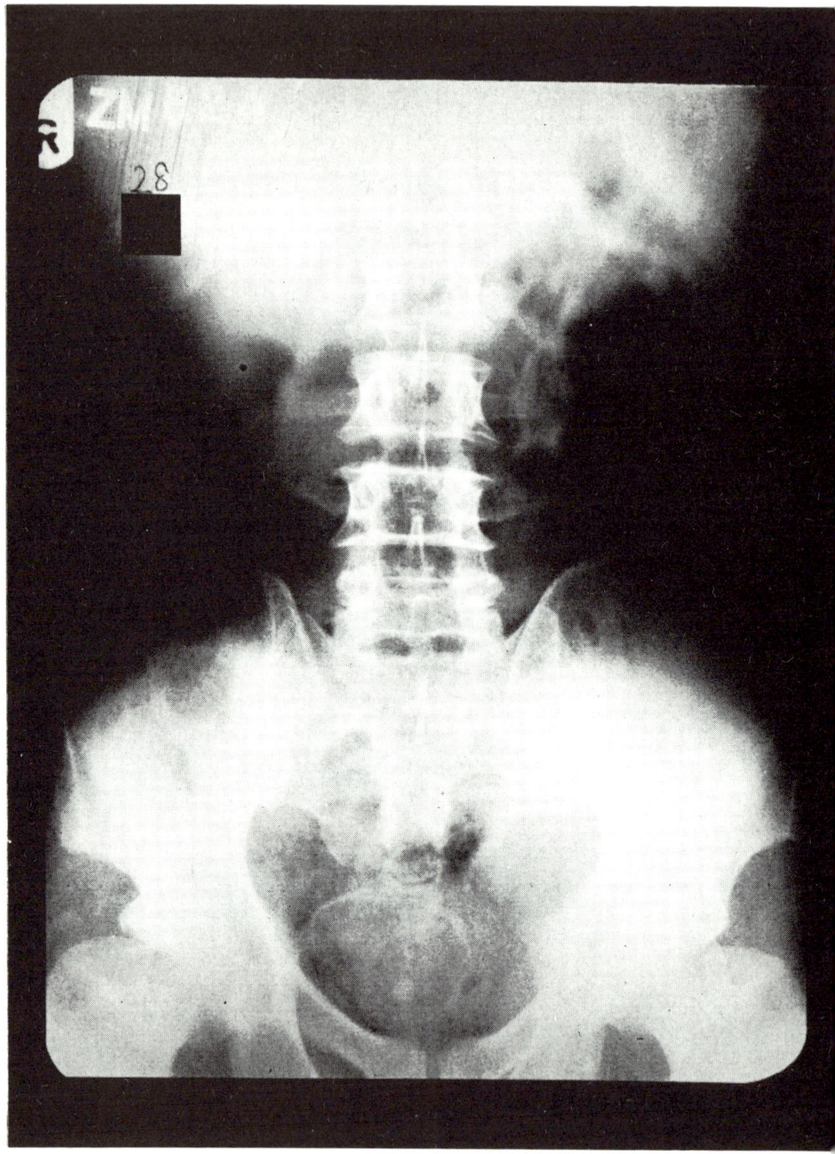

Fig. 4.4 Plain x-ray of the abdomen in a male, approximately 50 years old, showing calcification of the bladder. (X-ray by courtesy of Dr D. M. Forsyth.)

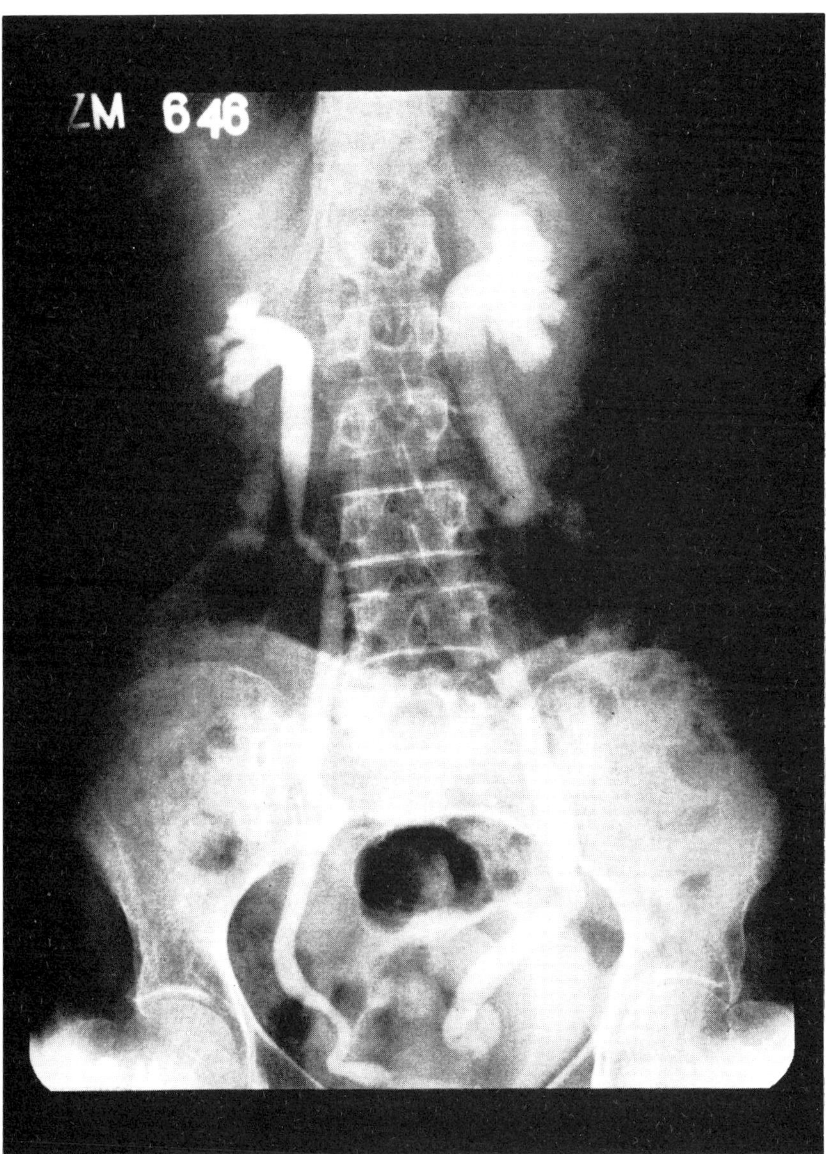

Fig. 4.5 IVP in a female over the age of 45 years, showing bilateral hydronephrosis and deformity of both ureters. (X-ray by courtesy of Dr D. M. Forsyth.)

Hypertension was not related to *S. haematobium* infection, either in East Africa or in Nigeria (Forsyth and Bradley, 1966; Pugh *et al.*, 1979). A minimal increase was reported from South Africa (Gelfand, 1964), and in the Gambia the infection may sometimes result in hypertension, though no clear-cut association was established (Wilkins, 1977).

Hospitalised patients with *S. haematobium* infection and obstructive uropathy had a reduction in maximal urinary concentrating ability, while phenolsulphonphthalein excretion was frequently abnormal. Additional evidence for renal disease could be inferred from the presence of proteinuria and urine casts (Lehman *et al.*, 1970).

β-glucuronidase activity in the urine was significantly greater in persons with *S. haematobium* infection than in controls (Norden and Gelfand, 1972), and impaired renal function was demonstrated using ^{131}I hippuran; subsequent improvement followed therapy (Oyediran *et al.*, 1975).

Day-to-day changes in creatinine concentration correlated with changes in egg count, which were in proportion, smaller (Wilkins, 1977) and both creatinine clearance and blood urea were within normal values in mild to moderately infected patients in northern Nigeria (Pugh *et al.*, 1980). In the Gambia, the levels of proteinuria and haematuria were related to the intensity of infection. The effect of treating all the subjects who had 30 mg/100 ml or more of protein and at least a trace of haematuria would have been very similar to treating all those with an egg count of 200 ova/100 ml or more (Wilkins *et al.*, 1979; Pugh *et al.*, 1980).

Impairment of total hydrogen ion excretion (TH+) was mainly associated with bacteriuria, but the effects of unilateral or bilateral obstruction and bacteriuria on urine osmolality were additive. These abnormalities were usually corrected after therapy (Young *et al.*, 1979).

Bacteriuria

Bacteriuria is often present in hospital patients with *S. haematobium* infection in Egypt (Abdallah, 1946; Shokeir *et al.*, 1972; Lehman *et al.*, 1973), and in a field study in the Gambia 6·6% of males under 25 were found to have bacteriuria. A 5·1% prevalence was found in schoolboys aged 5–16 years in Egypt (Laughlin *et al.*, 1978). This rate is more than 10 times greater than that found in comparable surveys in areas non-endemic for urinary schistosomiasis. Reports from sub-Saharan Africa conflict with these findings (Pi-Sunyer *et al.*, 1965; Forsyth and Bradley, 1966; Dukes *et al.*, 1967; Pugh and Gilles, 1979; Pugh *et al.*, 1980), perhaps because of a different intensity and pattern of infection. The pus cells frequently reported in the urine of patients have been shown to be eosinophils derived from the inflammatory lesions around ova in the bladder wall (Powell *et al.*, 1965), and their numbers are unrelated to bacteriuria but are related to the rate of *S. haematobium* egg excretion (Dukes *et al.*, 1967).

In Egypt, it has been shown that *S. haematobium* infection predisposes to the patient becoming a chronic carrier of *Salmonella typhi* and *S. paratyphi* after acute infection and it has been suggested that, in patients with *S. haematobium*, the main site of *Salmonella* infection is the urinary tract and that the clinical picture resembles that of other urinary tract infections. Response to chloramphenicol is more rapid in these cases than in the patients who do not suffer from schistosomiasis (Hathout *et al.*, 1966 and 1967; Farid *et al.*, 1972).

Calculi

Calculi have been described in relation to haematobium infection in the urethra, bladder, ureter and kidney and are found in up to 25% of infected persons in Egypt, although they are rare in most other parts of Africa. The centre of these calculi consists of oxalate, with an outer uric acid layer frequently incorporating schistosome ova. Where the primary causative environmental factors for stone formation exist, *S. haematobium* infection and urinary stasis are most probably potent contributory factors (Ghorab, 1962; Straffon and Higgins, 1970).

RADIOLOGICAL CHANGES

The main urinary tract lesions caused by *S. haematobium* include nodular egg granulomas of the bladder and ureters (seen as single or multiple filling defects on radiography), unilateral and bilateral hydro-ureter and hydronephrosis (schistosomal obstructive uropathy), calcification of the bladder and ureters, and finally radiographic non-functioning kidneys (Forsyth, 1969; Young *et al.*, 1973a; Umerah, 1977).

Radiographic studies have now shown conclusively that, following treatment and possibly even spontaneously, some of these lesions are reversible. The disappearance of bladder granuloma following treatment of schistosomiasis with subsequent relief of obstruction and resolution of hydro-ureter and hydronephrosis has now been fully confirmed. This is particularly evident in young patients in whom fibrosis of the ureteric lesions with subsequent development of irreversible stenosis has not had time to develop (Lucas *et al.*, 1966; Farid *et al.*, 1967 and 1970; Lehman *et al.*, 1973). Longitudinal studies have also demonstrated that bladder calcification will in general either decrease markedly or completely disappear (Forsyth and Hughes, 1973; Young *et al.*, 1973b; Ezzat *et al.*, 1974). An excellent review of the reversibility of lesions in schistosomiasis is given by Farid and his co-workers (1967). It appears that the renogram is a more sensitive test for evaluating the efficacy of treatment in patients with schistosomal obstructive uropathy than urography (Young *et al.*, 1978) (Fig. 4.6).

CARCINOMA OF THE BLADDER (see also Bland, 1979)

Since a causal relationship between *S. haematobium* and cancer of the bladder was claimed (Ferguson, 1911), evidence confirming and contradicting this has been found in Egypt, where the occurrence of bladder cancer is much greater than in European countries (Makar, 1955). Striking figures have also been given from Mozambique (Prates and Torres, 1965), where bladder cancer in all age groups is very much more common than in North America and Nigeria (Edington, 1967; Fig 4.7).

Using the technique of exfoliative cytology for diagnosing cancer of the bladder, evidence in support of a correlation with *S. haematobium* was obtained in a village survey in Egypt where 2·5% of males over the age of 6 years who had *S. haematobium* were diagnosed as having cancer, compared with 0·3% of those not excreting eggs. Amongst the females, the cancer rates were 1·1% and 0·2% respectively (Dimmette *et al.*, 1955). Using the same technique in a random sample of male out-patients in an Egyptian hospital, 5 of 526 with *S. haematobium* had cancer, compared with none of the 475 patients who were not excreting eggs (Halawani and Tamani, 1955).

Autopsy studies in Egypt (Mohamed, 1954a) and Iraq

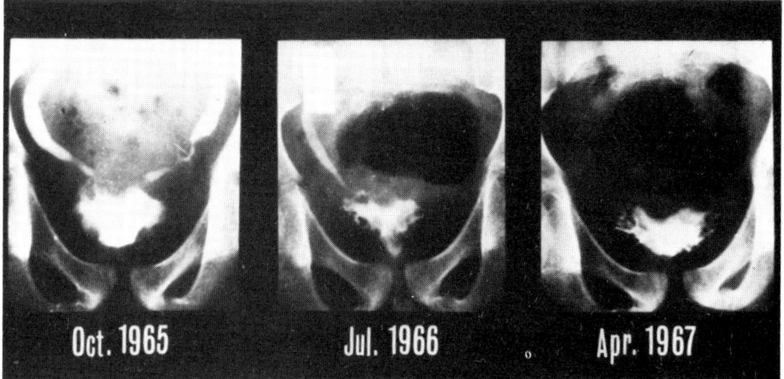

Fig. 4.6   Bilateral dilatation of the ureters in a Nigerian child aged 14 years. Note the normal appearance of the ureters two years (approximately) after a course of treatment with niridazole.

(Shamma, 1955) supported the correlation between *S. haematobium* and cancer, but this was not confirmed (El-Gazayerli and Khalil, 1959). In a study amongst new admissions to a hospital in Egypt (Mustacchi and Shimken, 1958), of 300 males over the age of 15 years excreting *S. haematobium* ova, 8·3% were found to have cancer, compared with 1·5% of those not excreting eggs, and recent studies from the Sudan and Zambia show an association between the two (Malik *et al.*, 1975; Bhagwandeen, 1976).

In other parts of Africa, however, the picture appears to be very different. In East Africa, no cases of bladder cancer were detected in extensive surveys using plain and intravenous pyelograms (IVP), x-ray examination of the urinary tract (Forsyth and Bradley, 1966), and in Nigeria the age-specific rates per 100 000 per year for bladder cancer are no higher than the figures from the US (Edington, 1967). In South Africa, bladder cancer is no more common than in countries where *S. haematobium* is not endemic (Powell *et al.*, 1968), but a higher incidence of calcified bladders and rectal biopsies positive for *S. haematobium* eggs were, however, found in patients with carcinoma of the bladder when compared with patients matched for sex and age in Cape Town, and it was considered that heavy infestation with *S. haematobium* leads to bladder cancer (Gelfand, 1967; Gelfand *et al.*, 1967).

It thus appears that while *S. haematobium* is apparently associated with bladder cancer in some areas, there is less evidence for such an association in other parts of Africa, and some workers believe the available evidence for such a relationship is

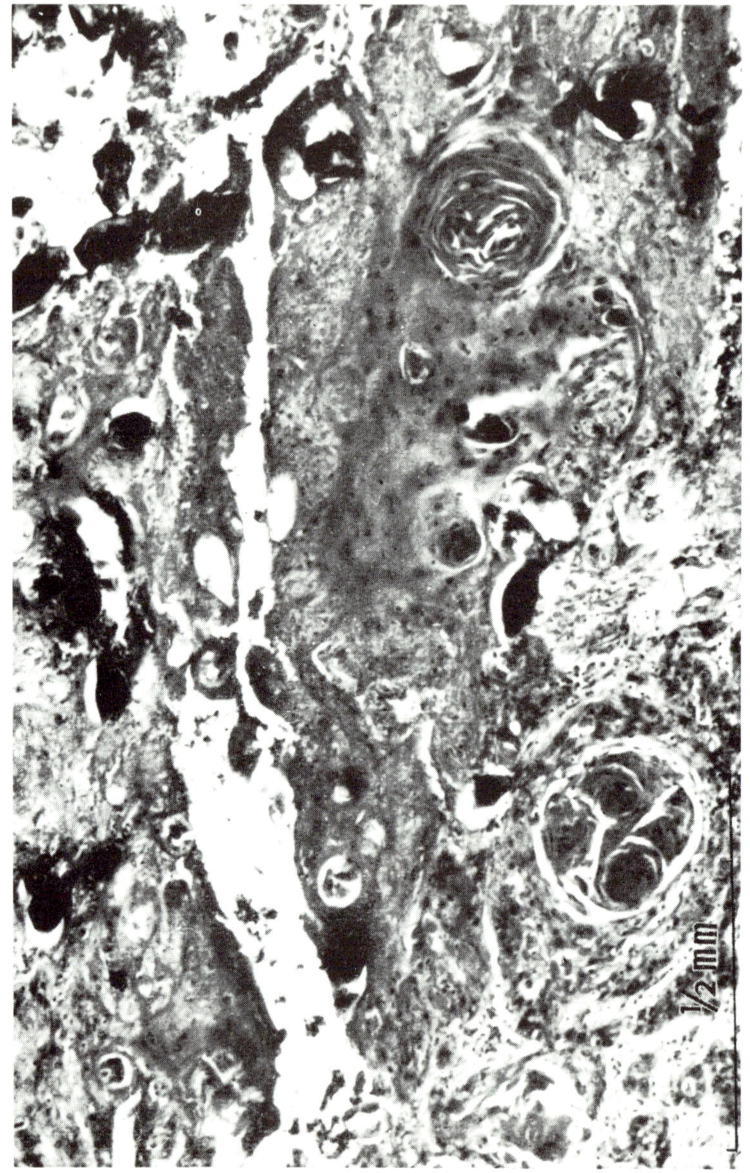

Fig. 4.7 Section of *S. haematobium*-infected bladder in association with neoplasm, showing horny cell nests and calcified ova. (Material from the Department of Helminthology, London School of Hygiene and Tropical Medicine.)

weak (Attah and Nkposong, 1976). However, most investigators would not agree (Docquier, 1976; Ghoneim *et al.*, 1976; Zahran *et al.*, 1976); and Case having analysed various relevant reports (see Fripp, 1965a), concluded 'that at a practical level there can be little doubt that *S. haematobium* infection is a cause of bladder cancer. This is so in all areas which could be studied and it would be wise to consider it to be so wherever *S. haematobium* is found unless and until adequate surveys show otherwise'.

The theories that have been put forward to account for the malignant changes have been discussed by Mohamed (1954b). It has been suggested that in the presence of secondary infection of a schistosomal cystitis, the urine is alkaline and the mucosa is thus subjected to chronic irritation. It has also been suggested that during contraction of the bladder the deeper layers of the mucosa rub against the calcified eggs in the submucosa. A miracidial toxin has also been proposed, which might act on the mucosa, so that when eggs are trapped in the tissue, a high concentration of the toxin accumulates locally.

More recently, attempts have been made to detect carcinogenic substances in the urine. The enzyme β-glucuronidase is excreted in the urine of workers in analine-dye and benzidine manufacturing plants. The enzyme is also excreted by persons with an active *S. haematobium* infection when the diurnal pattern of egg excretion is accompanied by a similar pattern of enzyme excretion (Fripp, 1961).

The enzyme has been shown to be present in miracidia and also in the adult worms and cercariae. In the presence of dietary or other exogenous carcinogenic substances, the increased urinary β-glucuronidase may hydrolyse inactive carcinogenic glucuronide present in the urine, leading to an increase in the concentration of active carcinogen which may affect the epithelial cells leading to tumour formation (Fripp, 1965b).

It is of interest to note in this respect that no unusual amino acid or indole excretion pattern was found in *S. haematobium*-infected children in an area in Tanzania where cancer of the bladder is rarely seen (Fripp, 1965b), but that in Egypt raised urinary levels of metabolites of tryptophan, serotonin and the carcinogen 3-hydroxyanthrilic acid, were found in the urine of infected patients, and in those with cancer of the bladder, levels about eight times normal were found (Abul-Fadl and Khalafallah, 1961; Khalafallah and Abul-Fadl, 1964).

In Uganda, in an area where plantains form the basic diet, high urinary levels of serotonin metabolites and particularly 5-hydroxyindolylacetic acid were found, and bladder cancer in these areas is not uncommon, although *S. haematobium* is not widespread.

Differences in the indoles excreted by *S. haematobium* patients in Lourenço Marques and Johannesburg have also been reported and considered to be due to dietary factors (Trout *et al.*, 1962—quoted by Fripp, 1965b).

Whether dietary factors are involved in causing cancer is, as yet, uncertain, but investigations into this aspect of the problem and other carcinogenic substances which may be ingested (derived possibly from different types of cooking pots) would seem worthy of further investigation. Typically, schistosomal bladder cancer is squamous celled—40% to 75% of cases in different series (Bhagwandeen, 1976; Tannenbaum, 1976).

From a study of the site of origin of 91 schistosomal bladder cancers, it appears that few arise in the trigone region (2), and the superior apical area (9), while the posterior and anterior areas (28 and 24) accounted for the majority, though in many cases (28) the site of origin was described as 'diffuse multiple' (Ishak *et al.*, 1967).

The malignant growth occurs more in younger persons than does the non-schistosomal bladder cancer, and has been diagnosed in children. Males are generally more frequently affected than females (Kamel and Attar, 1962).

The activity of urinary α-esterases as a screening test for bilharzial bladder cancer has been recommended (El-Sewedy *et al.*, 1978).

ECTOPIC LESIONS

Ectopic migration of *S. haematobium* worms and oviposition can occur anywhere in the body, resulting in a variety of lesions (Edington *et al.*, 1975).

Reproductive organs

The female genital tract—the cervix, vulva and vagina, ovaries and Fallopian tubes—is frequently found to harbour *S. haematobium* ova (Gelfand *et al.*, 1971). The ova may be found in cervical and vaginal smears but there is no evidence of a predisposition to malignancy in these cases, although they may occur in association with carcinomatous change (Badawy, 1962; Berry, 1966).

Eggs have also been recovered from the placenta and the uterus (Sutherland *et al.*, 1965; Adeleye and Odjegba, 1975). Healing of vesicovaginal fistulae is adversely affected in patients with urinary bilharziasis (Bland and Gelfand, 1970).

The ova rarely give rise to symptoms but, in view of the widespread involvement of the female genital tract, it might be expected that ectopic pregnancies would result. There is, however, little documented support for this view, although it is held by some workers in endemic areas. Again, while the claim that infertility may be due to schistosomiasis has not been substantiated, in hyperendemic areas some medical workers believe that the treatment of a co-existing schistosomal infection is frequently followed by conception.

Ova have been found at autopsy in the vas deferens, prostate, tunica vaginalis, scrotal skin, pampiniform plexus and epididymis (Gelfand *et al.*, 1970; Kazzaz and Salmo, 1974). Although involvement of the testes appears to be rare, fibrous tumour formations have been reported in the epididymis and cord in West Africans (Camain, 1952). Bilateral infarction of the testes of schistosomal origin (the species was not identified) was also reported (Joshi, 1962).

Gastrointestinal tract and liver

It is not uncommon to find *S. haematobium* eggs in the rectal mucosa on biopsy, but generally there are no intestinal symptoms associated with this infection, although granulomas in the large intestines leading to acute obstruction have been reported (Gelfand and Hammer, 1966) and involvement of the appendix may cause inflammation. In many regions of Africa, especially the Nile Delta and Zimbabwe, mixed infections with *S. haematobium* and *S. mansoni* are extremely common and it may be difficult to determine the pathology due to each parasite as the eggs are often too distorted in section for identification.

Owing to the location of adult worms in the vesical plexus rather than in the portal venous system, fewer eggs get swept to the liver than in *S. mansoni* infections. However, eggs are found on digesting liver tissue, and granulomas may be seen on histological examination. The tissue reaction is much less severe than in *S. mansoni* and serious liver damage is generally not associated with *S. haematobium* (Higginson and de Meillon, 1955), though results of cephalin cholesterol flocculation and thymol turbidity tests suggest that some liver involvement does occur (Shamma and Al-Azzawi, 1964). The electrophoretic pattern of serum shows an increased gamma-globulin and in some cases decreased albumin (Shamma and Azzo, 1966). In a pure *S. haematobium* area of upper Egypt, hepatic enlargement was more common in infected persons than in controls (Allam *et al.*, 1974), but in 400 consecutive autopsies in Cairo there was no relation between the presence and intensity of *S. haematobium* infection to Symmers' clay pipestem fibrosis of the liver (Kamel *et al.*, 1978).

Lungs

Lungs may become involved at different stages of *S. haematobium* infection.

In the acute stage, the schistosomula complete a part of their development in the lungs and, in experimental infections in mice, this stage has been shown to be associated with temporary pulmonary haemorrhages (Olivier, 1952). At this time there may be little symptomatology to direct attention to the lungs apart, possibly, from a slight cough, and miliary lesions in the lungs have been reported (Ritchken and Gelfand, 1954).

Following treatment, the adult worms may move to the lungs under the influence of a schistosomicidal drug (Forsyth, 1965). Proof of this in humans and animals is needed, but the normal laboratory animals are unlikely to be of much use since *S. haematobium* adults are found in the portal rather than in the systemic venous system. Transient changes in the x-ray appearance of the lungs following treatment of *S. haematobium* have been reported (Erfan and Deeb, 1949; El Gholmy, 1956), as have reactionary pneumonitis and pleurisy (Abou-Senna, 1965), but the pathology associated with these changes is unknown. A fatal case of acute focal verminous pneumonia following therapy must be considered unusual (Kenawy and Girges, 1940), as must the report of septicaemia thought to have resulted from lung changes associated with an embolised adult worm in a medium-sized interlobular artery (Payet and Camain, 1952). Adult worms were found in the lungs in 10 of 282 autopsies on patients with schistosomiasis and in only one of these were the worms dead (Shaw and Ghareeb, 1938).

The fate of adult worms after treatment and their movements are perhaps worthy of more investigation. Mass treatment with drugs is becoming possible and, while the parasitological results may be encouraging, the possibility of adult worms being moved to an abnormal situation in the body cannot be overlooked. The long-term results of this in relation to potential chronic lung disease due to embolisation of arterioles is unknown, but it has been suggested that 'if the worm has been accompanied by a sexual partner egg laying *in situ* may be resumed and ova will be voided in the sputum. Unaccompanied, the schistosome is doomed to celebate impotency . . .' (Forsyth, 1965). Living worms are comparatively harmless, but dead ones can cause a focal pneumonitis which heals with connective tissue surrounding the calcified remains of the adult worm.

The role of adult worms in pulmonary disease is questionable, but there is considerable evidence, particularly from Egypt, of lung changes which may be associated with cor pulmonale arising as a result of damage by eggs.

The pulmonary changes due to *S. haematobium* may lead to cor pulmonale (Shaw and Ghareeb, 1938; Jawahiry and Karpas, 1953) which may occur in adolescence (Payet *et al.*, 1953). Cor pulmonale may, however, develop from other causes in the presence of a *S. haematobium* infection and it has been pointed out that only by performing a lung biopsy can schistosomal pulmonary arteriolitis be diagnosed, and care should be taken in labelling a case as of shistosomal origin even if eggs are found in the urine or stool (Gelfand, 1957).

Schistosomal lesions have been noted in the myocardium but these are generally rare (Al-Zahawi and Shukri, 1956; Gelfand *et al.*, 1959).

Central nervous system

Involvement has been reported by many workers. Differentiation of the species of parasite in such cases may be difficult, but *S. haematobium* and *S. mansoni* generally affect the spinal cord while *S. japonicum* has a predilection for the brain (Marcial-Rojas and Fiol, 1963; Odeku *et al.*, 1968; Ruberti and Chopra, 1976; Dar, 1977; Lechtenberg and Vaida, 1977; Siddorn, 1977; see also Chapter 6).

Cutaneous manifestations

These have been recorded by many workers; the lesions are frequently in the genital and perigenital regions, but have also been noted elsewhere (Cahill and Mofty, 1964; Macdonald, 1976).

EXPERIMENTAL STUDIES

S. haematobium is not a uniform species. There is a variety of geographical strains which have been characterised by their different snail hosts and their pathogenesis in mice and hamsters (Wright and Knowles, 1972; James and Webbe, 1973).

Observations have been made on the clinical and pathological features of *S. haematobium* infections in chimpanzees, vervet monkeys, opossums, baboons, gibbons and hamsters (Obuyu, 1970; Sadun *et al.*, 1970; Kuntz, 1972; Webbe *et al.*, 1974; Kuntz *et al.*, 1975; Hicks *et al.*, 1977). Many of the changes found simulate those seen in man.

REFERENCES

Abdallah, A. (1946). *J. Egypt. Med. Ass.* **29,** 33.
Abou-Senna, H. O. (1965). *Med. Parasit. and Parasit. Dis.* **34,** 420.
Abul-Fadl, M. A. M. and Khalafallah, A. S. (1961). *Br. J. Cancer* **15,** 479.
Adeleye, J. A. and Odjegba, A. (1975). *Trop. Georgr. Med.* **27,** 206.
Allam, F. A., Hassanien, F. and Hamman, H. M. (1974). *J. Egypt. Publ. Hlth Ass.* **49,** 97.
Al-Zahawi, S. and Shukri, N. (1956). *Trans. R. Soc. Trop. Med. Hyg.* **50,** 166.
Arean, V. M. (1966). *Path. Arch.* **1,** 68.
Atala, A. and Zaher, M. F. (1969). *J. Urol.* **101,** 125.
Atala, A., Zaher, M. F. and Ragu, I. (1969). *J. Urol.* **101,** 183.
Attah, E. B. and Nkposong, E. O. (1976). *Trop. Geogr. Med.* **28,** 268.
Badawy, A. H. (1962). *Br. Med. J.* **1,** 369.
Barlow, C. H. (1949). *J. Parasit.* **35,** 205.
Barlow, C. H. and Meleney, H. E. (1949). *Am. J. Trop. Med.* **29,** 79.
Berry, A. (1966). *J. Path. Bact.* **91,** 325.
Bhagwandeen, S. B. (1976). *S. Afr. Med. J.* **50,** 1616.
Bland, K. G. (1979). *Acta Trop.* **36,** 203.
Bland, K. G. and Gelfand, M. (1970). *Trans. R. Soc. Trop. Med. Hyg.* **64,** 588.
Buchanan, W. M. and Gelfand, M. (1970). *Trans. R. Soc. Trop. Med. Hyg.* **64,** 593.
Cahill, K. M. and Mofty, A. M. (1964). *Am. J. Trop. Med. Hyg.* **13,** 80.
Camain, R. (1952). *Bull. Med. de L'Afrique-Occidentale Francaise* **9,** 265.

Campbell, E. J. M. and Dickinson, C. J. (1968). *Clinical Physiology*, 3rd edn. Blackwell Scientific Publications, Oxford.

Chapman, D. S. (1966). *Br. J. Surg.* **53,** 544.

Cheever, A. W., Kamel, I. A., Elwi, A. M., Mosimann, J. E. and Danner, R. (1977). *Am. J. Trop. Med. Hyg.* **26,** 702.

Cheever, A. W., Young, S. W. and Shehata, A. (1975). *Trans. R. Soc. Trop. Med. Hyg.* **69,** 410.

Dar, J. (1977). *Surg. Neurol.* **8,** 416.

Dimmette, R. M., Sproat, H. F. and Klimt, C. R. (1955). *Am. J. Clin. Path.* **25,** 1032.

Docquier, J. (1976). *Acta Urologica Belgica* **44,** 41.

Dukes, D. C., McDougall, B. R. D., Orne-Gliemann, R. H. and Davidson, L. (1967). *Br. Med. J.* **1,** 537.

Edington, G. M. (1957). *W. Afr. Med. J.* **6,** (N.S.) 45.

Edington, G. M. (1967). *Bilharziasis*, p. 128. Ed. F. K. Mostofi. Springer-Verlag, Berlin, Heidelberg, New York.

Edington, G. M. and Gilles, H. M. (1976). *Pathology in the Tropics*, 2nd edn. Edward Arnold, London.

Edington, G. M., Lichtenberg, F. von, Nwabuebo, I., Taylor, J. R. and Smith, J. H. (1970). *Am. J. Trop. Med. Hyg.* **19,** 982.

Edington, G. M., Nwabuebo, I. and Junaid, T. A. (1975). *Trans. R. Soc. Trop. Med. Hyg.* **69,** 153.

El-Bishlawi, O. (1973). *Trans. R. Soc. Trop. Med. Hyg.* **67,** 307.

El-Gazayerli, M. and Khalil, H. A. (1959). *Alexandria Med. J.* **5,** 31.

El Gholmy, A. (1956). *Gaz. Egypt. Paediat. Ass.* **4,** 275.

El-Sewedy, S. M., Arafa, A., Abdel-Aal, G. and Mostafa, M. H. (1978). *Trans. R. Soc. Trop. Med. Hyg.* **72,** 525.

Elsdon-Dew, R. (1966). *S. Afr. J. Sci.* **62,** 242.

Elwi, A. M., Nada, G., Safouh, M. and Issa, H. (1974). *J. Egypt. Publ. Hlth Ass.* **49,** 27.

Erfan, M. and Deeb, A. A. (1949). *Br. J. Radiol.* **22,** 638.

Ezzat, E., Osman, R. A., Ahmet, K. Y. and Soothill, J. F. (1974). *Trans. R. Soc. Trop. Med. Hyg.* **68,** 315.

Farid, Z., Bassily, S., Abdel-Wahab, M. F., Lehman, J. S., Hassan, A. and Kent, D. C. (1970). *Trans. R. Soc. Trop. Med. Hyg.* **64,** 122.

Farid, Z., Bassily, S., McConnell, E., Schulert, A., Sabour, M. and Abdel-Wahab, M. F. (1967). *Lancet* **ii,** 1110.

Farid, Z., Higashi, G. I., Bassily, S., Young, S. W. and Sparks, H. A. (1972). *Am. J. Trop. Med. Hyg.* **21,** 578.

Ferguson, A. R. (1911). *J. Path. Bact.* **16,** 76.

Forsyth, D. M. (1965). *Lancet* **ii,** 354.

Forsyth, D. M. (1969). *Bull. Wld Hlth Org.* **40,** 771.

Forsyth, D. M. and Bradley, D. (1966). *Bull. Wld Hlth Org.* **34,** 715.

Forsyth, D. M. and Hughes, M. (1973). *Trans. R. Soc. Trop. Med. Hyg.* **67,** 671.

Fripp, P. J. (1961). *Ann. Trop. Med. Parasit.* **55,** 328.

Fripp, P. J. (1965a). *Proceedings 1st Int. Congr. Parasit., Rome.* Pergamon Press, Oxford.

Fripp, P. J. (1965b). *Br. J. Cancer* **19,** 292.

Gelfand, M. (1948). *Br. Med. J.* **1,** 1228.

Gelfand, M. (1957). *Trans. R. Soc. Trop. Med. Hyg.* **51,** 533.

Gelfand, M. (1963). *Trans. R. Soc. Trop. Med. Hyg.* **57,** 191.

Gelfand, M. (1964). *Cent. Afr. J. Med.* **10,** 1.

Gelfand, M. (1967). *Bilharziasis*, p. 104. Ed. F. K. Mostofi. Springer-Verlag, Berlin, Heidelberg, New York.

Gelfand, M., Alves, W. and Woods, R. W. (1959). *Trans. R. Soc. Trop. Med. Hyg.* **53,** 282.

Gelfand, M. and Gilles, H. M. (1966). *J. Trop. Med. Hyg.* **69,** 4.

Gelfand, M. and Hammer, B. (1966). *Trans. R. Soc. Trop. Med. Hyg.* **60,** 231.

Gelfand, M., Ross, C. M. D., Blair, D. M., Castle, W. M. and Weber, M. C. (1970). *Am. J. Trop. Med. Hyg.* **19,** 779.

Gelfand, M., Ross, C. M. D., Blair, D. M. and Weber, M. C. (1971). *Am. J. Trop. Med. Hyg.* **20,** 846.

Gelfand, M., Weinberg, R. W. and Castle, W. (1967). *Lancet* **i,** 1249.

Gerritsen, T., Walker, A. R. P., de Meillon, B. and Jeo, R. M. (1953). *Trans. R. Soc. Trop. Med. Hyg.* **47,** 134.

Ghoneim, M. A., El-Bolkainy, M. N., Mansour, M. A., El-Hamady, S. M., Ashamallah, A. G. and Soliman, El-Sayed H. (1976). *Urology* **8,** 547.

Ghorab, M. M. A. (1962). *Br. J. Urol.* **34,** 33.

Halawani, A. and Tamani, M. (1955). *J. Egypt. Med. Ass.* **38,** 455.

Hasan, A. M. El, Satir, A. A., Ahmed, M. A. and Omer, A. (1977). *Trop. Geogr. Med.* **29,** 56.

Hathout, S. E., El-Gaffar, Y. A. and Awny, A. Y. (1967). *Am. J. Trop. Med. Hyg.* **16,** 462.

Hathout, S. E., El-Gaffar, Y. A., Awny, A. Y. and Hassan, K. (1966). *Am. J. Trop. Med. Hyg.* **15,** 156.

Hicks, R. M., James, C., Webbe, G. and Nelson, G. S. (1977). *Trans. R. Soc. Trop. Med. Hyg.* **71,** 288.

Higginson, J. and de Meillon, B. (1955). *Arch. Path.* **60,** 341.

Honey, R. M. and Gelfand, M. (1960). *The Urological Aspects of Bilharziasis in Rhodesia*. E. and S. Livingstone, Edinburgh and London.

Ishak, K. G., Le Golvan, P. C. and El-Sebai, I. (1967). *Bilharziasis*, p. 58. Ed. F. K. Mostofi. Springer-Verlag, Berlin, Heidelberg, New York.

James, C. and Webbe, G. (1973). *J. Helminth.* **47,** 49.

Jawahiry, K. I. and Karpas, C. M. (1953). *Am. Rev. Resp. Dis.* **88,** 517.

Joshi, R. A. (1962). *Am. J. Trop. Med. Hyg.* **11,** 357.

Kamel, M. and Attar, F. (1962). *J. Egypt. Med. Ass.* **45,** 1146.

Kamel, I. A., Cheever, A. W., Elwi, A. M., Mosimann, J. E. and Danner, R. (1977). *Am. J. Trop. Med. Hyg.* **26,** 696.

Kamel, I. A., Elwi, A. M., Cheever, A. W., Mosimann, J. E. and Danner, R. (1978). *Am. J. Trop. Med. Hyg.* **27,** 931.

Kazzaz, B. A. and Salmo, N. A. M. (1974). *Trop. Geogr. Med.* **26,** 333.

Kenawy, M. R. and Girges, B. (1940). *Prov. Kasr-el-Aimy-Cliss Soc.* **8,** 156.

Khalafallah, A. S. and Abul-Fadl, M. A. M. (1964). *Br. J. Cancer* **18,** 592.

Kloetzel, K. (1969). *Trans. R. Soc. Trop. Med. Hyg.* **63,** 459.

Kuntz, R. E. (1972). *Bull. Wld Hlth Org.* **45,** 1.

Kuntz, R. E., Cheever, A. W., Myers, B. J., Young, S. W. and Moore, J. A. (1975). *Trans. R. Soc. Trop. Med. Hyg.* **69,** 494.

Laughlin, L. W., Farid, Z., Mansour, N., Edman, D. C. and Higashi, G. I. (1978). *Am. J. Trop. Med. Hyg.* **27,** 916.

Lechtenberg, R. and Vaida, G. A. (1977). *Neurology* **27,** 55.

Lehman, J. S. Jr., Farid, Z., Bassily, S. and Kent, D. C. (1970). *Am. J. Trop. Med. Hyg.* **19,** 1001.

Lehman, J. S. Jr., Farid, Z., Smith, J. H., Bassily, S. and El-Masry, N. A. (1973). *Trans. R. Soc. Trop. Med. Hyg.* **67,** 384.

Lichtenberg, F. von, Edington, G. M., Nwabuebo, I., Taylor, J. R. and Smith, J. H. (1971). *Am. J. Trop. Med. Hyg.* **20,** 244.

Lucas, A. O., Adeniyi Jones, C. C., Cockshott, W. P. and Gilles, H. M. (1966). *Lancet* **i,** 631.

Macdonald, D. M. (1976). *Br. Med. J.* **2,** 619.

Maged, A. and Soliman, L. A. M. (1968). *J. Urol.* **99,** 30.

Mahmoud, A. (1966). *Trans. R. Soc. Trop. Med. Hyg.* **60,** 766.

Makar, N. (1955). *Urological aspects of bilharziasis in Egypt.* Cairo Societe Orientale de Publicite Press.

Makar, N. (1967). *Bilharziasis*, p. 45. Ed. F. K. Mostofi. Springer-Verlag, Berlin, Heidelberg, New York.

Makar, N. (1968). *Br. J. Surg.* **36,** 148.

Malik, M. O. A., Veress, B., Daoud, E. H. and El Hassan, A. M. (1975). *J. Trop. Med. Hyg.* **78,** 219.

Marcial-Rojas, R. A. and Fiol. R. E. (1963). *Ann. Intern. Med.* **59,** 215.

Mohamed, A. S. (1954a). *J. Egypt. Med. Ass.* **37,** 987.

Mohamed, A. S. (1954b). *J. Egypt. Med. Ass.* **37,** 1066.

Mustacchi, P. O. and Shimken, M. B. (1958). *J. Nat. Cancer Inst.* **20,** 825.

Norden, D. A. and Gelfand, M. (1972). *Trans. R. Soc. Trop. Med. Hyg.* **66,** 864.

Norden, D. A. and Gelfand, M. (1973). *Trans. R. Soc. Trop. Med. Hyg.* **67,** 607.

Obuyu, C. K. A. (1970). *Ann. Trop. Med. Parasit.* **64,** 395.

Odeku, E. L., Lucas, A. O. and Richard, D. R. (1968). *J. Neurosurgery* **4,** 417.

Olivier, L. (1952). *Am. J. Hyg.* **55,** 22.

Oyediran, A. B. O. O., Abayomi, I. O., Akinkugbe, O. O., Bohrer, S. P. and Lucas, A. O. (1975). *Am. J. Trop. Med. Hyg.* **24,** 274.

Payet, M., Berte, E., Camain, R. and Pene, P. (1953). *Bull. Soc. Path. Exot.* **46,** 688.

Payet, M. and Camain, R. (1952). *Bull. Soc. Path. Exot.* **45,** 680.

Pi-Sunyer, F. X., Gilles, H. M. and Wilson, A. M. (1965). *Ann. Trop. Med. Parasit.* **59,** 304.

Powell, S. J. (1967). *S. Afr. Med. J.* **41,** 991.

Powell, S. J., Englebrecht, H. E. and Welchman, J. M. (1968). *Trans. R. Soc. Trop. Med. Hyg.* **62,** 231.

Powell, S. J., Maddison, S. E. and Elsdon-Dew, R. (1965). *S. Afr. Med. J.* **39,** 165.

Prates, M. D. and Torres, F. O. (1965). *J. Nat. Cancer Inst.* **35,** 729.

Pugh, R. N. H. and Gilles, H. M. (1979). *Ann. Trop. Med. Parasit.* **73,** 191.

Pugh, R. N. H., Bell, D. R. and Gilles, H. M. (1980). *Ann. Trop. Med. Parasit.* **74,** 597.

Pugh, R. N. H., Gilles, H. M. and Sanderson, J. E. (1979). *Ann. Trop. Med. Parasit.* **73,** 293.

Richard, J., Moreau, J. P. and Dodin, A. (1966). *Arch. Inst. Pasteur Madagascar* **35,** 164.

Ritchken, J. and Gelfand, M. (1954). *Br. Med. J.* **1,** 1419.

Ruberti, R. F. and Chopra, S. A. (1976). *Med. Afr. Noire* **23,** 77.

Sabbour, M. S., El-Said, W. and Abou-Gabal, I. (1973). *Bull. Wld Hlth Org.* **47,** 2932.

Sadigursky, M., Andrade, Z. A., Danner, R., Cheever, A. W., Kamel, I. A. and Elwi, A. M. (1976). *Trans. R. Soc. Trop. Med. Hyg.* **70,** 322.

Sadun, E. H., Lichtenberg, F. von, Cheever, A. W., Erickson, D. G. and Hickman, R. L. (1970). *Am. J. Trop. Med. Hyg.* **19,** 427.

Sayegh, E. S. (1950). *J. Urol.* **63,** 353.

Shamma, A. H. (1955). *Br. J. Surg.* **45,** 240.

Shamma, A. H. and Al-Azzawi, J. H. (1964). *J. Fac. Med. Baghdad* **6,** (N.S.) 57.

Shamma, A. H. and Azzo, B. S. (1966). *J. Fac. Med. Baghdad* **8,** (N.S.) 1.

Shaw, A. F. B. and Ghareeb, A. A. (1938). *J. Path. Bact.* **46,** 401.

Shokeir, A. A., Ibraham, A. M., Hamid, M. Y., Shalaby, M. A., Hussein, H. E. and Badr, M. (1972). *E. Afr. Med. J.* **49,** 312.

Smith, J. H., Elwi, A., Kamel, I. A. and Lichtenberg, F. von (1975). *Am. J. Trop. Med. Hyg.* **24,** 806.

Smith, J. H., Kamel, I. A., Elwi, A. and Lichtenberg, F. von (1974). *Am. J. Trop. Med. Hyg.* **23,** 1054.

Smith, J. H., Kelada, A. S. and Khalil, A. (1977). *Am. J. Trop. Med. Hyg.* **26,** 89.

Smith, J. H., Kelada, A. S., Khalil, A. and Torky, A. H. (1977). *Am. J. Trop. Med. Hyg.* **26,** 96.

Smith, J. H., Torky, H., Kelada, A. S. and Farid, Z. (1977). *Am. J. Trop. Med. Hyg.* **26,** 85.

Straffon, R. A. and Higgins, C. C. (1970). *Urology,* p. 687. W. B. Saunders, Philadelphia.

Sutherland, J. C., Berry, A., Hynd, M. and Proctor, N. S. F. (1965). *S. Afr. J. Obstet. Gynaec.* **3,** 76.

Tannenbaum, M. (1976). *Urology* **7,** 128.

Trout, G. C., Gillman, J. and Prates, M. D. (1962). *Acta. Un. Inst. Cancer* **18,** 575.

Umerah, B. C. (1977). *Br. J. Radiol.* **50,** 105.

Walt, F. (1954). *S. Afr. Med. J.* **28,** 89.

Webbe, G., James, C. and Nelson, G. S. (1974). *Ann. Trop. Med. Parasit.* **68,** 187.

Wilkins, H. A. (1977). *Ann. Trop. Med. Parasit.* **71,** 179.

Wilkins, H. A., Goll, P., Marshall, T. F. de C. and Moore, P. (1979). *Trans. R. Soc. Trop. Med. Hyg.* **73,** 74.

Wright, C. A. and Knowles, R. J. (1972). *Trans. R. Soc. Trop. Med. Hyg.* **66,** 108.

Young, S. W., Farid, Z., Bassily, S. and El-Masry, N. A. (1973a). *Trans. R. Soc. Trop. Med. Hyg.* **67,** 417.

Young, S. W., Farid, Z., Bassily, S. and El-Masry, N. A. (1973b). *Trans. R. Soc. Trop. Med. Hyg.* **67,** 417.

Young, S. W., Farid, Z., Bassily, S. and El-Masry, N. A. (1978). *Trans. R. Soc. Trop. Med. Hyg.* **72,** 627.

Young, S. W., Farid, Z., Bassily, S. and El-Masry, N. A. (1979). *Trans. R. Soc. Trop. Med. Hyg.* **73,** 249.

Zaher, M. H. and El Deeb, A. A. (1969). *J. Urol.* **101,** 870.

Zahran, M. M., Kamel, M., Mooro, H. and Issa, A. (1976). *Urology* **8,** 73.

5 Infection with *S. mansoni*

Aluizio Prata

S. mansoni infection affects people in different ways. Some are asymptomatic carriers of the parasite, while others develop severe disease. Reasons for these variations are unclear, but there is evidence that parasite load may be of prime importance in the development of pathological conditions. The worm burden in the human population increases with age, usually reaching a maximum between 10 and 20 years, after which it declines. In 124 patients with hepatosplenomegaly subjected to extracorporeal filtration of portal blood, a mean of 749 worms was recovered per patient (Prata, 1970). Patients under 20 years old had a mean worm load of 1057, compared with 503 in patients above 30 years. While various reports relate severe forms of the disease to intensity of infection, some people have high levels of egg excretion but appear not to show or develop severe disease. As discussed in Chapter 10, in different localities other factors, besides the parasite load, may influence the development of severe manifestations.

PATHOGENIC EFFECTS OF THE PARASITE

Cercariae

Swimmer's itch is generally associated with penetration of the skin by non-human cercariae, but may rarely occur with *S. mansoni* (Barlow, 1936). The pruritus has been ascribed to local anaphylaxis, and reagin-like skin-sensitising antibodies have been demonstrated in experimental animals (Ogilvie *et al.*, 1966). The inflammatory exudate of round cells in the papules suggests the lesions are a form of cell-mediated hypersensitivity (Warren, 1973).

Adult worms

Live adult worms in the portal system are apparently well tolerated by the host and produce no mechanical, irritative or inflammatory side-effects. The antigenic metabolic products of the worms, both excretory and secretory, are eliminated or deposited in various organs, but the pathogenic role of any of these products is not clear. The schistosomal hepatitis seen in the acute phase of the infection appears to be related to the presence of living worms and not eggs, since it may appear before oviposition (Bogliolo, 1967).

(In chimpanzees, fibrosis in the larger portal spaces precedes egg laying, although the pathogenesis of this fibrosis is unclear. In contrast, fibrosis in the small portal spaces is associated with granulomas which form around eggs (Sadun *et al.*, 1970).)

Dead adult worms promote a focal inflammatory lesion with necrosis causing vessel obstruction and, eventually, scarring. These lesions are principally in the liver and lungs (Menezes, 1967). Some authors believe that such dead worms promote Symmer's fibrosis and they advise against specific treatment. However, treated mice have longer lives than infected controls and lesions produced by dead worms resolve completely (Warren, 1962). Moreover, after treatment of thousands of patients, many with heavy worm loads, hepatosplenomegaly commencing after specific treatment has not been described. In a few patients, worm death has been associated with the development of signs of acute hepatic insufficiency, elevated portal pressure and haematemesis, pneumonitis, asthma, acute cor pulmonale, anaphylactic shock or generalised vasculitis resulting in death (Coutinho, 1975).

Schistosome eggs

Dead immature eggs in tissues are removed by phagocytosis in the same manner as any foreign body and, when viable, do not produce a reaction in the host (Prata, 1957a). When mature (from day 6 after oviposition), they can survive in host tissue for 11–12 days. They contain a complex miracidium and secrete an antigenic histolytic substance. They stimulate an extensive host defence reaction, considered to be a form of delayed hypersensitivity (Warren, 1973) and probably T-lymphocyte dependent (von Lichtenberg, 1978), resulting in the formation of a granuloma or pseudotubercle. In an early infection, granulomas may be 100 times the size of the contained egg and have a central area of necrosis with or without a hyaline eosinophilic band (Hoeppli phenomenon)—possibly the result of an antigen–antibody reaction, as suggested by immunocytochemical studies (Koppish, 1941; Andrade *et al.*, 1961). The area of necrosis is surrounded by an exudative cellular reaction, with many eosinophils and lymphocytic infiltration about the periphery. With the death of the ovum, foreign body giant cells appear and reparative fibrosis occurs.

Granulomas vary depending on the phase of the disease, their location and possibly the nutritional state of the host (Fig. 5.1; Akpon and Warren, 1975). Compared with those produced in the early stage of infection, those forming later are much smaller, with an apparently more rapid rate of destruction of schistosome eggs. These differences are thought to be due to a form of endogenous desensitisation or modulation (Warren, 1977).

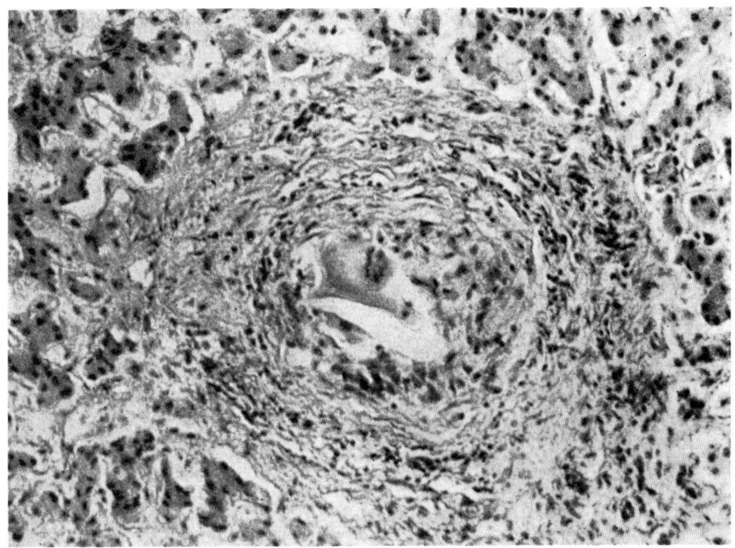

Fig. 5.1 Well-developed granuloma containing an egg of *S. mansoni*. The lateral spine can be clearly seen. A multinucleate cell is prominent, the cellular reaction is being replaced by fibrous tissue.

In man, it has been calculated that each day one egg per worm pair is retained in the tissues (Cheever, 1968). The removal of eggs is a continuous process, but in certain circumstances their accumulation surpasses the capacity of the host to remove them. Most authors agree that formation of egg granulomas is the principal process responsible for severe forms of the disease. Perhaps because of this, studies of egg granulomas and their character and immunological basis have been important facets of recent research (see Chapter 7).

Of interest is the recent report that no reaction to eggs was found in an autopsy study of tissue from an *S. mansoni*-infected person after immunosuppressive therapy for a non-schistosomal disease (Hillyer and Cangiano, 1979), and the demonstration (Michaels, 1970) that guinea-pigs lack one of several substances essential for promoting egg maturation—these animals do not develop hepatitis, fibrosis or vascular lesions of schistosomiasis (Andrade, 1964).

ACUTE SCHISTOSOMIASIS

In the vast majority of infections, reaction to cercarial penetration goes unnoticed, but fever, allergic manifestations with eosinophilia, diarrhoea, hepatosplenomegaly and lymphadenopathy may occur. The incubation period can be as short as two to three weeks or up to eight, and severity is usually related to intensity of infection (Hiatt *et al.*, 1979).

Pathology

Pathological changes have been noted 15–25 days after exposure to infection—prior to the commencement of egg laying. The liver may show evidence of hepatitis on needle biopsy, and the spleen may display characteristics of acute infectious splenitis, with intense eosinophilic infiltrates. The intestinal mucosa, including the jejunum and ileum, may show superficial necrotic and haemorrhagic ulcers (Bogliolo, 1967).

The acute phase is, however, characterised by large granulomas, found principally in the liver and the intestines and less frequently in other organs.

In the enlarged liver, intralobular foci of necrosis and destruction of hepatocytes occur with portal infiltration of histiocytes, eosinophils, lymphocytes, and hyperplasia and hypertrophy of the Kupffer cells (Bogliolo, 1959). The spleen enlarges and there is hyperplasia of the cords of Bilroth, with intense eosinophilia and congestion of the sinuses. In severe cases, a necrotising arteritis may occur in the lungs, with miliary dissemination of eggs and granulomas with exudate and necrosis in the liver, intestines, peritoneum, abdominal and pulmonary lymphatic glands, pleura, lungs and pancreas (Raso and Bogliolo, 1970). In the rectum and sigmoid, severe oedema, erythema, haemorrhages, petechiae, small ulcerations, and punctate elevations occur (Tonelli and Neves, 1969).

Clinical features

Rarely, there may be an irritating macular, papular rash lasting for several days. In a study of 120 acute cases, these skin reactions depended not on the quantity of cercariae gaining access to the skin but on host response (Neves, 1970; see Chapter 7).

Symptoms of the acute phase are due to hypersensitivity (Bogliolo, 1967), and patients with chronic schistosomiasis can have similar symptoms suggesting re-infection or reactivation of the disease (Katz and Bittencourt, 1965).

Constitutional symptoms typical of many infections may occur—asthenia, headache, anorexia, lassitude and nausea. The onset is generally abrupt and complaints may include headache, weakness, anorexia and muscle pain; intermittent increases in body temperature may occur—frequently reaching 39°C. It can continue for one or two months and disappears by lysis. Occasionally there may be delirium. Sweating and chills may be marked and bronchospasm can produce asthmatic crises or be followed by pneumonia. Nausea and vomiting are common. Diarrhoea or dysentery may be prolonged, with a sensation of epigastric discomfort, abdominal pain and distension. Signs of hypersensitivity include urticaria, facial oedema, erythematous or purpuric lesions.

Patients lose weight, and there is a tender hepatomegaly. (Liver enlargement can also occur in the absence of symptoms.) Generally, the spleen is palpable but soft, but does not attain the size seen in chronic cases. The hepatosplenomegaly regresses within a few months. There is discreet generalised enlargement of the lymph nodes. It is unusual for death to occur during the acute phase of schistosomiasis and only rarely do patients develop severe forms of the disease straight away. Exceptionally, serious complications such as coma or an acute abdomen (Neves, 1970) and jaundice may develop, and spinal cord complications have been reported (Neves et al., 1973).

Blood examination reveals a leucocytosis which can reach 50 000/mm^3 and eosinophilia can reach 70%. The erythrocyte sedimentation rate is elevated. The bone marrow shows eosinophilic hyperplasia. The serum globulin may be 6 g% (Diaz-Rivera *et al.*, 1956); IgG and IgE levels are positively correlated with egg output but IgM level is not (Hiatt *et al.*, 1979). The Paul–Bunnel reaction may be positive.

In an outbreak of schistosomiasis in Puerto Rico (Clark *et al.*, 1970), fluorescent, complement-fixing and flocculating antibodies were present 8 weeks after exposure, whereas circumoval percipitin reactions were not positive for 20 weeks. Skin test positivity increased from 56% to 100% between the eighth and twenty-second week after exposure.

Sigmoidoscopy or liver biopsy may demonstrate the changes described above. Rectal biopsy may be negative at the start of oviposition. Stool examination is essential but may be negative in the early stages.

Differential diagnosis

Typhoid fever, brucellosis, mononucleosis, and miliary tuberculosis may resemble acute schistosomiasis but may be excluded by the presence of the high eosinophilia. The acute phase of other helminth infections may cause confusion. In invasive ancylostomiasis, fever and hepatosplenomegaly are uncommon.

CHRONIC SCHISTOSOMIASIS

The majority of patients are asymptomatic but others have been categorised into so-called intestinal (Type I) or hepatointestinal (Type II) cases. The division is, however, artificial as hepatic changes are the same (Polak *et al.*, 1959). With the development of hepatosplenomegaly, the disease is considered potentially more severe, though in the compensated (Type III) patients prognosis is good compared with the uncompensated (Type IV) subjects. Pulmonary hypertension with cyanosis is an evolutionary form of Type III. Pseudoneoplastic and other forms of disease are reported but are uncommon.

Intestinal and hepatointestinal

Pathology
The liver shows variable degrees of fibrosis in the portal tracts

with eggs, granulomas and cellular infiltrations; which are also found in the intestines and, less frequently, in the lungs and other organs of the body.

Clinical features

Intermittent diarrhoea is probably the most common symptom reported. Episodes alternate with periods of normal bowel movement or constipation and faeces often contain blood and mucus; tenesmus is not uncommon. While a variety of abdominal symptoms have been attributed to *S. mansoni*, recent morbidity studies suggest such complaints are not necessarily due to the infection.

On palpation, the abdomen may be tender, particularly along the course of the descending colon and sigmoid; the liver may be enlarged and hardened. Especially in endemic areas, patients commonly present a nodular liver but without portal hypertension or splenomegaly.

Liver biopsy may show granulomas, portal inflammation, septal fibrosis, and at times inflammation invading the borders of the hepatic parenchyma, but hepatic function tests are invariably normal.

Barium studies of the large intestine may show spasm, mucosal oedema and intestinal atony. Sigmoidoscopy is normal in about half the patients. The main abnormal findings are a granular appearance of the mucosa (27%), hyperaemia (15%), exaggerated pattern (12%), punctate haemorrhages (9%) and a tendency to bleed (7%). Other rarer rectal findings are ulceration, polyps and sigmoid stenosis. Although not specific, these findings are suggestive of the disease. Polyps in some series can affect 20% of patients (Dimmete and Sproat, 1955). They are rare in the Western hemisphere (Hernandez-Morales, 1945; Vargas, 1945; Candia and Louis, 1955), but very common in Egypt where they are associated with loss of intestinal protein and chronic blood loss, depleting the body iron stores (Biggam *et al.*, 1934; Ata *et al.*, 1970; Lehman *et al.*, 1970).

Rectal biopsy material taken from the valves of Houston and compressed between two slides for examination show eggs in 80% of cases. The stage of egg development enables an estimate to be made of the duration of egg deposition. In a biopsy fragment of 0·33 cm^2, there may be 200 eggs (Prata, 1957a).

Hepatosplenic schistosomiasis and portal hypertension

Symmer's fibrosis of the liver, which may result in portal hypertension and congestive splenomegaly, occurs in the 6- to 20-year age group or 5 to 15 years after the onset of infection (Prata and Bina, 1968; Fig. 5.2). The liver and spleen are palpable, the liver eventually becoming hard and nodular. The portal pressure rises from 190 to 440 mmH$_2$O. Two to four years after the onset, hepatosplenomegaly is firmly established, but patients are frequently unaware of the condition.

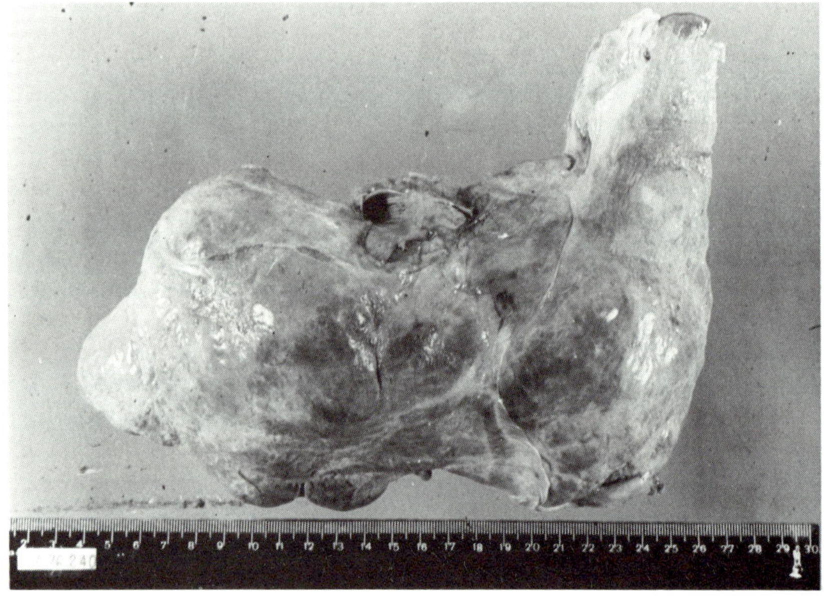

Fig. 5.2   Symmer's fibrosis of the liver: left lobe increased in size; surface with protuberances.

Pathology

The left lobe of the liver is often affected more than the right. The basic lesion is fibrosis in the portal tracts, with phlebitis and periphlebitis caused by schistosome ova. Fibrosis is interstitial and invasive and is accepted as being unique to schistosomiasis. It is unlike that of cirrhosis, when fibrosis follows degeneration of the liver cells (Hashem, 1947). On cross-section of the organ, the large fibrous portal spaces appear as white areas surrounded by normal hepatic parenchyma, although lobules at the edge of the liver may show some distortion (Fig. 5.3). Fibrosis also

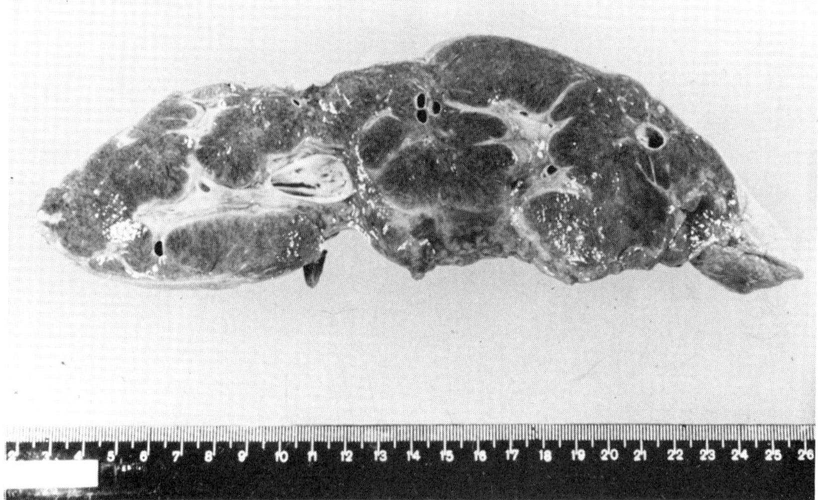

Fig. 5.3 Symmer's fibrosis: cross-section of the liver showing large fibrous portal spaces.

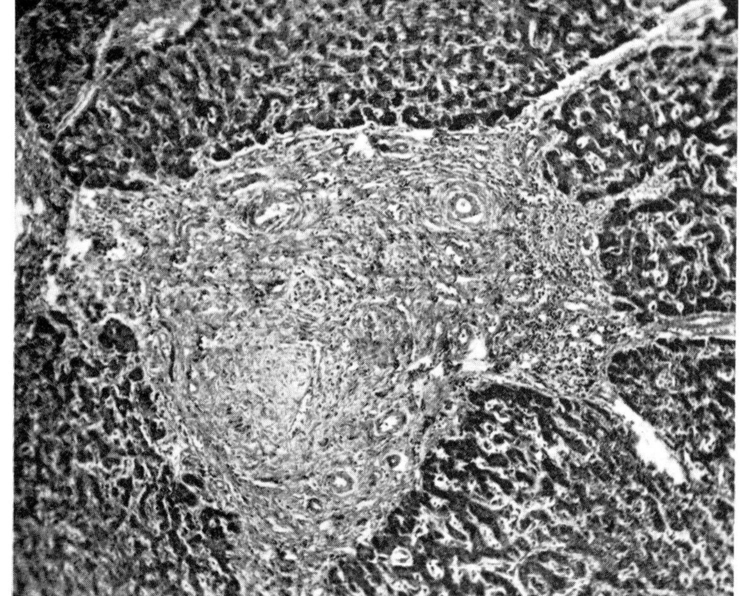

Fig. 5.4 Pipe-stem fibrosis of liver due to *S. mansoni*, showing obliteration of portal radicle. (Photograph by courtesy of Dr F. von Lichtenberg.)

extends along the smaller divisions of Glisson's capsule and, on contraction, gives the liver the typical nodular appearance.

Granulomas around ova can be seen in abundance in the portal spaces and more rarely in the lobules; they are much smaller than in the early stages of the infection. After cessation of parasitic activity, they may disappear completely, although fibrosis remains as an irreversible lesion (Fig. 5.4). At autopsy, it is not rare to find thrombosis of the principal trunk of the portal vein.

There may be sinusoidal dilatation and proliferation of bile ducts in the thickened periportal tracts and lobules. Schistosomal pigment derived from blood ingested by the adult worm is deposited in Kupffer cells, portal tracts and lobules. It cannot be distinguished from malaria pigment by histochemical methods but, under the electron microscope, differences in the ultrastructure have been reported (Stenger *et al.*, 1967).

The liver parenchyma remains intact except in cases with focal areas of necrosis or regenerative nodules, probably produced by intrahepatic thrombi or by ischaemia after massive gastrointestinal haemorrhage (Andrade *et al.*, 1962), and at the edge of the liver where some distortion of lobules may occur (Cheever and Andrade, 1967).

Vinyl acetate injected into the portal system of livers removed at autopsy showed obstruction in the portal tracts (particularly near the periphery of the liver), leading to a reduction in the portal bed and intrahepatic presinusoidal block to blood flow with the development of portal hypertension (Andrade and Cheever, 1971). An increase in the periportal capillary system (Bogliolo, 1957) communicates with the hepatic artery and the portal vein and provides collateral circulation to portions of the liver having a deficient portal supply (Andrade and Cheever, 1971).

The portal hypertension in turn produces oesophageal varices.

The spleen in many cases of Symmer's fibrosis increases in size due to congestion caused by portal hypertension; hyperplasia of the reticulo-endothelial elements results. The microscopic lesions found are indistinguishable from those seen in the sclero-congestive splenomegalies.

In Brazil, 1% of spleens removed for hepatosplenic schistosomiasis showed a giant follicle or nodular lymphoma, apparently primary and limited to the spleen (Fig. 5.5). The relationship of this follicle to *S. mansoni* has yet to be elucidated (Andrade and Abreu, 1971).

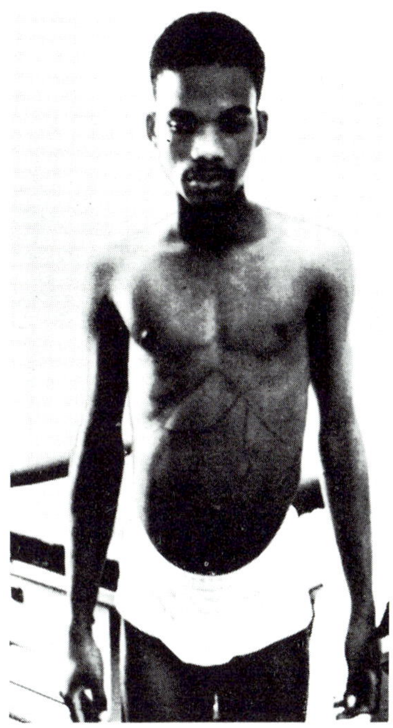

Fig. 5.5 Hepatosplenomegaly in a St Lucian aged 21 years. (Photograph by courtesy of Dr R. E. M. Lees.)

The kidneys have attracted increasing attention in recent years, with disease being found in some patients with hepatosplenic schistosomiasis; glomerulosclerotic changes were found in 36% of 50 patients with hepatosplenic schistosomiasis (and in 27% of cirrhotic patients). A progressive worsening of these changes leads to glomerulonephritis, which was found in 10% of hepatosplenic patients but was absent in mild cases of *S. mansoni* and in cases with cirrhosis (Andrade *et al.*, 1971). Complexes of IgG and IgM were found in deposits in basement membranes and in laminated bodies near mesangial cells during electron-microscopy studies but there was no clinical evidence of renal disease (Da Silva *et al.*, 1970). In a further renal biopsy study (Queiroz *et al.*, 1973), of 15 patients with schistosomal hepatosplenomegaly, 11 showed a membranous-proliferative glomerulonephritis, a glomerular sclerotic focal lesion was present in 3, and a membranous glomerulonephritis in 1. Serum cholesterol was normal in 5 and, in spite of an increase in serum globulin being usual in hepatosplenic cases, no such rise was demonstrated in 11 of the 15. While most reports of renal complications refer to Brazil, workers in the Sudan have also reported focal sclerosing glomerulonephritis and secondary amyloidosis. After treatment, amyloid deposits decreased (Veress *et al.*, 1978).

It is not clear why renal lesions are found only in hepatosplenic schistosomiasis; duration of infection, worm burden and immunological reactivity of the host may all play a part.

Clinical features

Amongst patients in hospital in Brazil, symptoms were melaena, left hypochondrial tumour, haematemesis, small alveolar oedema, epistaxis, abdominal fullness, fever, ascites and pallor.

Haematemesis is the most important clinical manifestation, and is generally directly related to the degree of portal hypertension. It may occur without prodromal symptoms or it may be preceded by asthenia or epigastric discomfort. Occasionally, it commences after ingestion of aspirin tablets (Kelner *et al.*, 1966). The usual signs and symptoms of haemorrhage occur, followed in another day by fever, 'coffee grounds' faeces, and later, in patients with severe blood loss, oedema and ascites. The haematemesis may be fulminating but in the majority of cases it is repeated, at intervals, over a period of years.

Hepatomegaly and splenomegaly may be minimal or severe. A hard liver is characteristic of schistosomiasis with portal hypertension. The organ has a sharp border and frequently has a nodular surface. The left lobe may be prominent—a sign of diagnostic significance. The size of the liver apparently decreases with evolution of the disease.

The occurrence of ascites varies with geographical location. It is common in Egypt, but in Brazil it is usually a consequence of blood loss and responds promptly to treatment. Superficial collateral circulation may be seen particularly when ascites is present. Icterus, spider angiomas, palmar erythema, gynaecomastia and other manifestations of severe hepatic insufficiency are rare but may develop in the terminal stage of the disease or as a consequence of portocaval surgical procedures.

Portal thrombosis may develop as a complication and is particularly common after surgery (Cheever and Andrade,

1967). It may pass undetected or produce intense abdominal pain, distension and ascites regressing after a few days.

Endocrine dysfunction may lead to delayed growth, absence of secondary sexual characteristics and genital hypoplasia; gonadotrophin deficiency is found in these cases of infantilism (Ferreira, 1957; Fayez *et al.*, 1970). Amenorrhea is common.

Peritoneoscopy shows the typical liver morphology and an increased portal circulation.

Barium swallow and oesophagoscopy show oesophageal varices in 80% of patients. The varices are found principally in the lower third and sometimes in the fundus of the stomach. The transparietal splenic pressure is 100–200 mm H_2O in 5%, 200–300 mm H_2O in 26%, 300–400 mm H_2O in 45% and over 400 mm H_2O in 24% of patients. Splenoportography shows evidence of dilatation, tortuosity, and thrombosis of the extrahepatic vessels, while uptake of contrast medium by the liver is patchy, as in cirrhosis. The most characteristic findings are in the intrahepatic circulation—occlusion with or without recanalisation, thin venules or intricate vascular plexuses alongside dichotomous branches with enlargement of the left lobe (Almeida and Luz, 1970). The hepatic vein wedge pressure is normal or slightly raised showing that, in contrast to Laennec's cirrhosis, the obstruction is presinusoidal. The portorectopulmonary and duodenopulmonary circulation times are delayed.

The gall bladder may be thickened, with fat deposition in its walls, and adherent to the liver but the cholecystogram is usually normal (Prata, 1957b; Hassab, 1962).

Scintiography shows an enlarged left liver lobe.

The blood may show a leucopenia (affecting mainly the neutrophils) and a mild eosinophilia. Anaemia occurs and is microcytic and hypo- or normochromic. Less frequently, macrocytic cells are found in poor and undernourished persons (Jamra *et al.*, 1964; Katz and Bittencourt, 1965). Apart from anaemia following haematemesis, it is associated with iron deficiency, increased plasma volume, reduced life span of erythrocytes and a slow plasma albumin turnover (Woodruff *et al.*, 1963).

Severe anaemia, unresponsive to iron, may be due to hypersplenism and associated with leucopenia and thrombocytopenia in different combinations. Such cases usually respond to splenectomy (Farid *et al.*, 1966), which restores the blood picture to normal.

The bone marrow is hyperplastic, with increased production of red cells and eosinophil precursors; megakaryocytes are normal or diminished, mononuclear cells are usually within the normal range.

The erythrocyte sedimentation rate is increased. Coagulation disorders include an abnormal prothrombin time and an increase in fibrinolytic activity (El-Attar *et al.*, 1972).

A lowered serum albumin is attributed to reduced synthesis and an increase in plasma volume (Fayez *et al.*, 1970) or to intestinal loss (El-Saadani *et al.*, 1968). There is an increase in serum globulins (principally the gamma fraction). The alkaline phosphatase level may be raised and there may be retention of bromsulphthalein. The urinary urobilinogen level is altered. After repeated haemorrhages in the final phase of the diseases, there may be frank hepatic insufficiency.

Glucose intolerance (Ghanem *et al.*, 1971) and alterations in exocrine activity of the pancreas (Michaels, 1970; Mott *et al.*, 1972) may occur, although the latter does not affect glucose and xylose absorption (Bettarello and Mott, 1971). The gastric secretion of acid and pepsin may be reduced, as in other types of portal hypertension (Firky, 1964).

When there is renal involvement, the patient may develop a type of nephrotic syndrome, with arterial hypertension or proteinuria (Rocha *et al.*, 1976).

Rectal biopsy in patients with advanced disease is often negative, possibly because the worms are predominant in the upper regions of the intestine (Meira, 1951).

Two forms of hepatosplenic involvement are recognised—compensated and decompensated.

In patients with compensated disease, the collateral circulation and liver function are adequate and liver function tests show only slight changes, but some abnormalities have been reported from a modified radioactive rose bengal test (Razzak, 1966). Normal detoxication of ingested ammonium hydrochloride occurs with no, or only slightly raised levels of blood ammonia and, following the absorption of large amounts of protein after intestinal bleeding from varices, compensated patients show little rise in blood ammonia levels, as compared with decompensated cases. In compensated cases, high blood ammonia levels follow haemorrhages (Warren and Rebonças, 1966). The classing of patients with haematemesis or malaena as decompensated would seem, therefore, to be unjustified, but decompensated disease carries a poor prognosis.

Differential diagnosis

Kala-azar, prolonged salmonellosis, tropical splenomegaly syndrome, leukaemia, lymphoma, Laennec's cirrhosis and post-necrotic cirrhosis must all be considered.

In kala-azar, the liver is without nodules and the fever, anaemia, leucopenia and hypergammaglobulinaemia are all more marked; bone marrow or liver biopsy is typical and shows leishmania.

Prolonged salmonellosis is due to an association of schistosomiasis with *Salmonella*, principally *S. typhi* (Teixeira, 1960). It is characterised by prolonged fever, leucocytosis with neutrophilia and eosinophilia, positive Widal reaction and persistent and positive blood culture for *Salmonella*. This form of salmonellosis is cured by specific treatment for schistosomiasis, either with niridazole (Neves *et al.*, 1969) or with hycanthone (Macêdo *et al.*, 1970), oxamniquine or praziquantel.

Tropical splenomegaly syndrome, the result of chronic malaria infection, is characterised by high titres of malaria fluorescent antibody and IgM and absence of a nodular liver or marked portal hypertension.

In leukaemia and certain lymphomas, the lymphadenopathy, the white cell count and bone marrow pattern allow the diagnosis to be made.

In Laennec's and post-necrotic cirrhosis, signs of hepatic insufficiency may be marked with jaundice, spider angiomas, hepatic fetor, palmar erythema and ascites. The superficial collateral circulation may be marked and the patient wasted. Hepatic insufficiency dominates, with liver function tests being markedly abnormal.

In its early stages, hepatosplenomegaly is curable with effective chemotherapy, but even if it persists, progression of the condition is not inevitable. Many patients with portal hypertension live normal lives unaware of their condition. In others, the condition progresses with haematemesis as a terminal event. An annual mortality from schistosomiasis of 44·8 per 100 000 people infected was reported in an area in north-east Brazil (Barbosa and Voss, 1961).

Surgical treatment

The main indication for surgery is repeated haematemesis.

Splenectomy with splenorenal anastomosis is the preferred operation, as complications of encephalopathy and jaundice are less common than after portacaval shunts. The reduction in portal pressure is similar with the two operations (Shiroma *et al.*, 1963). Some surgeons favour gastro-oesophageal decongestion with splenectomy; postoperative complications are fewer and liver, cardiac, lung and gastric functions are improved (Hassab, 1962).

PULMONARY HYPERTENSION WITH CYANOSIS

Deposition of eggs in the lungs is not customary but, with the development of portal hypertension, increased communications between the portal and systemic circulations lead to the passage of eggs into the pulmonary vessels. The eggs cause an allergic arteritis with a paravascular granulomatous reaction resulting in obstructive pulmonary vascular disease, pulmonary hyperten-

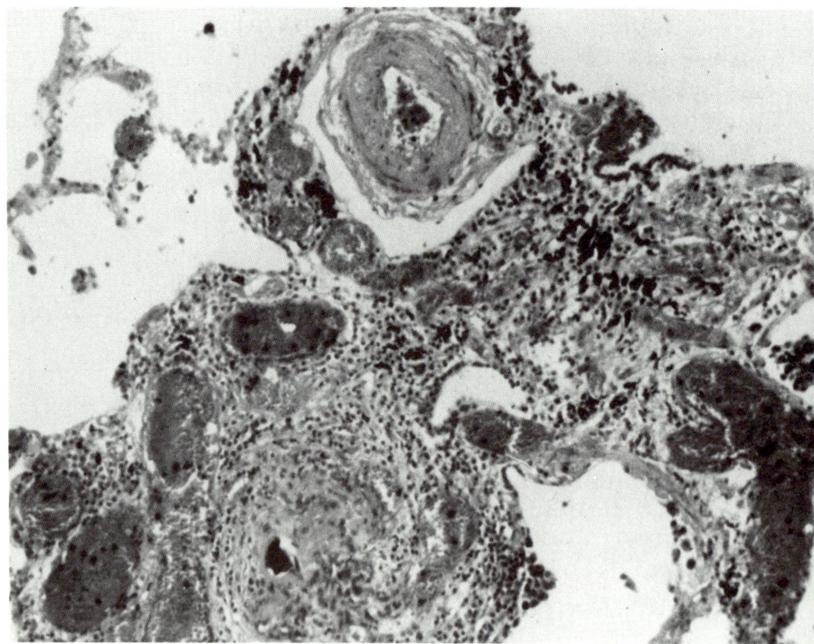

Fig. 5.6 Schistosomal pulmonary arteritis: artery obstructed and angiomatoid lesion.

sion and a rise in right intracardiac pressure with right ventricular hypertrophy (Fig. 5.6). Arterial dilation, aneurysm and
thrombotic occlusion of the great vessels may also occur.

Miracidial secretions from the egg seem to be the causative
agent of the necrotising arteriolitis which destroys the intima and
causes vascular obstruction. The occluding tissue recanalises and
the newly formed vessels dilate, at times exceeding the original
size of the artery to produce an angiomatoid lesion. Vessels
localised near this area of the artery exhibit hypertrophy of the
media, hyaline thrombi, arterial fibrosis and necrosis. These
findings are similar to the anatomical–pathological picture
relating to Ayerza's disease (Shaw and Ghareeb, 1938) but were
demonstrated to be different, suggesting the designation of
schistosomal pulmonary arteritis (Meira, 1942).

In Egypt, 7·5% of patients with hepatosplenomegaly developed cor pulmonale (Kenawy, 1950), and in Brazil, 23% of
hepatosplenic patients had a mean pulmonary arterial pressure
above 20 mmHg (Vinhaes, 1974).

As portal hypertension increases, so does the chance of
developing pulmonary hypertension (Guimarães, 1972). Patients
complain of dyspnoea, at first only on exercise and then continuously. Exercise can produce giddiness and mental clouding
followed by loss of consciousness.

Clinical and radiological findings are similar to those associated with other causes of pulmonary hypertension.

Haemodynamic studies show a raised arteriolar resistance of
92·5 μN/sec per cm^5 (Cavalcanti *et al.*, 1962). A normal arteriolar
wedge pressure rises after exercise, as does the arteriolar pulmonary resistance, and there is a slight rise in pulmonary blood flow.
Initially, the intracardiac pressure is normal, even in patients
with a dilated pulmonary conus (Ramly *et al.*, 1953). Later there
is a rise in systolic and diastolic pressures which may exceed the
levels of the systemic pressure. The degree of pulmonary hypertension is not necessarily proportional to the degree of arterial
dilatation as this depends on other factors as well, such as the
elasticity of the pulmonary conus (Ramly *et al.*, 1953).

The arterial oxygen saturation is normal, but due to left-to-
right shunts (Zaky *et al.*, 1962), may not reach 100% after
inhaling pure oxygen.

The electrocardiogram is normal until right ventricular hypertrophy appears. The pulmonary P wave is usually absent and the
QRS complex of low voltage, in contrast to the findings in cor

pulmonale associated with parenchymal lung disease. Arrhythmia is rarely seen (Marchand *et al.*, 1957).

The differential diagnosis must exclude other diseases causing cor pulmonale—principally primary pulmonary hypertension (difficult to diagnose), parenchymatous lung disease, multiple pulmonary emboli and other organic cardiopathies. The hepatosplenomegaly of schistosomiasis is not present in these other diseases. Blood gas estimations, pressure studies, angiography, radioscopic scanning and pulmonary biopsy can be of use in differential diagnosis. Examinations of populations in endemic areas show that schistosomal pulmonary hypertension is not always a severe disease but can be present in a benign asymptomatic manner. Histopathological studies have confirmed this clinical impression.

A cyanotic syndrome with clubbing of the fingers is rarely reported in patients with portal hypertension and hepatosplenomegaly; cardiac failure is not a feature of the condition and pulmonary hypertension is minimal (Faria *et al.*, 1957 and 1959). Many such patients have dyspnoea on exertion, a low cardiac output, alveolar hypotension and a decrease in arterial saturation even after breathing pure oxygen. There is no rise in systolic pressure in the right ventricle and arteriolar resistance in the lungs is diminished. The cyanosis may be due to pulmonary arteriovenous fistulas (Faria, 1956), or portopulmonary anastomoses, or a diminution in the affinity of haemoglobin for oxygen (Zaky *et al.*, 1964). Half the cases mentioned in the literature developed cyanosis after splenectomy.

PSEUDONEOPLASTIC FORM

Pseudoneoplastic lesions are principally localised in the descending colon and sigmoid. A hard mass grows from the serosa to the abdominal cavity or from the submucosa protruding into the bowel lumen or intramural space (Wydell, 1958; Raso and Bogliolo, 1970). These lesions can obstruct the intestinal lumen. Within the fibrotic tissue are masses of eggs, both calcified and in granulomas.

Analysis of 26 cases (Raso and Bogliolo, 1970) showed the following distribution: descending colon and sigmoid 50%, terminal ileum 10·3%, small intestine 11·4%. The patients present with abdominal pain and delayed intestinal transit or occlusion. The tumour may get very large and involve other organs; a hard mass can be palpated in the line of the intestine. In Egypt, abdominal masses are frequently seen due to tumours located in the omentum, mesentery or pericolically (Ata *et al.*, 1970). Pericolic masses are rare in Brazil (Andrade and Melo, 1974). They can appear at any point in the large intestine. Polyps and bloody stools may often be present, as may finger clubbing. A similar tumour can develop in the female genital tract (Chaves and Palitot, 1964) or medulla (Gama and Sá, 1945).

OTHER CLINICAL FORMS

Of 40 cases of myelitis due to schistosomiasis in America and Africa, 24 were due to *S. mansoni*, 9 to *S. haematobium*, 1 to both forms, and 6 were unidentified (Kugler and Solis, 1969). The paraplegia can begin rapidly, with sphincter disturbances and sensory alterations. Cells and protein may be present in the cerebrospinal fluid. As well as transverse myelitis, other central nervous system syndromes, such as the cauda equina syndrome, may develop and there are well-documented cases of myocarditis (Barros *et al.*, 1956; Carvalhal *et al.*, 1965). There have also been descriptions of cases where eggs were widely disseminated through the body—the pan visceral form. Such patients may have portal and pulmonary hypertension, infantilism and pseudoneoplasms.

There are many references in the literature to ectopic egg deposition in different organs, but these are not always sufficient to suggest a clinical syndrome.

S. *mansoni* and its association with other diseases

Schistosomiasis can modify the development of various infections, but the mechanisms of this are not clear.

The course of *Salmonella* infections in patients with schistosomiasis is unusual; the infection becomes chronic with prolonged fever and blood cultures which remain positive for months; it can only be cured by antischistosomal treatment. The same phenomenon occurs with *Escherichia* infections (Teixeira *et al.*, 1976). Australia antigen can be found in the serum of patients with hepatosplenic schistosomiasis long after the onset of disease

(Lyra *et al.*, 1976), but it is not known whether the virus affects the development of the parasitic disease. In mice lightly infected with *S. mansoni*, the effects of hepatitis virus (MHV_3) were enhanced (Warren *et al.*, 1969), but *Toxoplasma gondii* was found to protect these animals from *S. mansoni* (Mahmoud *et al.*, 1976). A synergistic relationship between *S. mansoni* and *Entamoeba histolytica* in mice has also been demonstrated (Knight and Warren, 1973).

The importance of other infections and malnutrition in influencing the course of schistosomiasis in man requires further investigation.

REFERENCES

Akpon, C. A. and Warren, K. S. (1975). *Am. J. Path.* **79,** 435.

Almeida, F. C. and Luz, F. F. C. (1970). *Graz. Méd. Bahia* **70,** 1.

Andrade, Z. A. (1964). *Revta Inst. Med. Trop. S. Paulo* **6,** 277.

Andrade, Z. A. and Abreu, W. N. (1971). *Am. J. Trop. Med. Hyg.* **20,** 237.

Andrade, Z. A., Andrade, S. G. and Sadigursky, M. (1971). *Am. J. Trop. Med. Hyg.* **20,** 77.

Andrade, Z. A. and Cheever, A. W. (1971). *Am. J. Trop. Med. Hyg.* **20,** 425.

Andrade, Z. A. and Melo, I. S. (1974). *Revta Pat. Trop.* **3,** 143.

Andrade, Z. A., Paronetto, F. and Popper, H. (1961). *Am. J. Path.* **39,** 589.

Andrade, Z. A., Santana, F. S. and Rebouças, G. (1962). *Revta Inst. Med. Trop. S. Paulo* **4,** 170.

Ata, A. A., El-Raziky, S. H., El Hawey, A. M. and Rafla, H. (1970). *J. Egyptian Med. Ass.* **53,** 762.

Barbosa, F. S. and Voss, H. (1961). *Bull. Wld Hlth Org.* **40,** 966.

Barlow, C. M. (1936). *Am. J. Hyg.* **24,** 587.

Barros, O. M., Giannoni, F. G., Marigo, C. and Frizzo, F. J. (1956). *Arq. Hosp. Santa Casa de São Paulo* **2,** 1.

Bettarello, A. and Mott, C. B. (1971). *Arq. Gastroenterd* **8,** 63.

Biggam, A. G., Hashim, M. and Ghalioungui, P. (1934). *Trans. R. Soc. Trop. Med. Hyg.* **27,** 409.

Bogliolo, L. (1957). *Ann. Trop. Med. Parasit.* **51,** 1.

Bogliolo, L. (1959). *Revta Bras. Malar. Doenç. Trop.* **11,** 359.

Bogliolo, L. (1967). In *Bilharziasis*, p. 184. Ed. F. K. Mostofi, Springer-Verlag, Berlin.

Candia, E. C. and Louis, C. E. (1955). *G.E.N. Caracas* **10,** 347.

Carvalhal, S., Lichtig, C., Saad, F. A. and Bocanegra, J. (1965). *Arq. Bras. Card.* **18,** 225.

Cavalcanti, I. L., Tompson, G., Souza, N. and Barbosa, F. S. (1962). *Br. Heart J.* **24,** 363.

Chaves, E. and Palitot, P. (1964). *Am. J. Obst. Gyn.* **89,** 1000.

Cheever, A. W. (1968). *Am. J. Trop. Med. Hyg.* **17,** 38.

Cheever, A. W. and Andrade, A. Z. (1967). *Trans. R. Soc. Trop. Med. Hyg.* **61,** 626.

Clark, W. D., Cox, P. M., Ratner, L. H. and Correa-Coronas, R. (1970). *Ann. Int. Med.* **73,** 379.

Coutinho, A. (1975). *Bras. Med.* **11,** 69.

Da Silva, L. C., De Brito, T., Carmago, M. E., De Boni, D. R., Lopes, J. D. and Gunji, J. (1970). *Bull. Wld Hlth Org.* **42,** 907.

Diaz-Rivera, R. S., Ramos-Morales, F., Koppisch, E., Garcia-Palmieri, M. R., Cintron-Rivera, A. A., Marchani, E. J., Gonzalez, O. and Torregrose, M. V. (1956). *Am. J. Med.* **21,** 918.

Dimmete, R. M. and Sproat, H. (1955). *Am. J. Trop. Med. Hyg.* **4,** 1057.

El-Attar, O., Shaheen, H., El-Saadani, A. M., Madwar, K., Erfan, A., Kinawi, M. and El-Saif (1972). *J. Egyptian Med. Ass.* **55,** 512.

El-Saadani, A. M., Habib, S. M., El-Gengehy, M. T. and Fayez, M. A. (1968). *Am. J. Trop. Med. Hyg.* **17,** 844.

Faria, J. L. (1956). *Am. J. Trop. Med.* **5,** 860.

Faria, J. L., Barbas, J. V., Fujioka, T., Lion, M. F., Silva, U. A. and Decourt, L. V. (1959). *Am. Heart J.* **58,** 556.

Faria, J. L., Czapski, J., Leite, M. O. R., Penna, D. O., Fujioka, T. and Cintra, A. B. U. (1957). *Am. Heart J.* **54,** 196.

Farid, Z., Schubert, A. R., Bassily, S., Nichols, J. H., Guindz, S., Sherif, M. and Raasch, F. (1966). *Brit. Med. J.* **2,** 153.

Fayez, M. A., Habib, E. M., El-Saadany, A. M. and El-Gengehy, M. T. (1970). *J. Egyptian Med. Ass.* **52,** 595.

Ferreira, J. M. (1957). *Aspectos endócrinos da esquistossomose mansonica hepato-esplenica.* Thesis, University of São Paulo.

Firky, M. (1964). *J. Trop. Med. Hyg.* **67,** 204.

Gama, C. and Sá, J. M. (1945). *Arq. Neuro-Psiq* **3,** 334.

Ghanem, M. H., Said, M. and Guirgis, F. K. (1971). *J. Trop. Med. Hyg.* **74,** 189.

Guimarães, A. C. (1972). *Estudo da hemodinamica da circulação pulmonar e dos gases sanguieos na hipertensão portal esquistossomótica.* Thesis, University of Bahia.

Hashem, M. (1947). *J. Egyptian Med. Ass.* **30,** 48.

Hassab, M. A. (1962). *Proceedings of the 1st National Symposium on Bilharziasis. Cairo* **2,** 47.

Hernandez-Morales, F. (1945). *Puerto Rico J. Publ. Hlth Trop. Med.* **20,** 492.

Hiatt, R. A., Sotomayor, Z. R., Sanchez, G., Zambrana, M. and Knight, W. B. (1979). *J. Inf. Dis.* **139,** 659.

Hillyer, G. V. and Cangiano, J. L. (1979). *Trans. R. Soc. Trop. Med. Hyg.* **74,** 331.

Jamra, M., Maspes, V. and Meira, D. A. (1964). *Revta Inst. Med. Trop. S. Paulo* **6,** 126.

Katz, N. and Bittencourt, D. (1965). *Hospital (Rio de Janeiro)* **67,** 847.

Kelner, S., Ferraz, E. and Wanderley, F. (1966). *Revta Ass. Méd. Bras.* **12,** 99.

Kenawy, M. R. (1950). *Am. Heart J.* **39,** 678.

Knight, R. and Warren, K. S. (1973). *Trans. R. Soc. Trop. Med. Hyg.* **67,** 644.

Koppish, E. (1941). *Puerto Rico J. Pub. Hlth Trop. Med.* **16,** 395.

Kugler, H. and Solis, A. P. (1969). Bilharziasis requidea. Experiences con dos casos. Discusion de algunos problemas. II. *Reunion del Caribe Pro-Investigacion de la bilharziasis. Maracay 1969,* p. 91.

Lehman, J. S., Farid, Z., Bassily, S., Haxton, J., Abdel Wahab, M. F. and Kent, D. C. (1970). *Gastroenterology* **59,** 433.

Lichtenberg, F. von (1978). *S.E. Asian J. Trop. Med. Hyg.* **9,** 186.

Lyra, L. G., Rebonças, G. and Andrade, Z. A. (1976). *Gastroenterology* **71,** 641.

Macêdo, V., Bina, J. C. and Prata, A. (1970). *Gaz. Méd. Bahia* **70,** 194.

Mahmoud, A. A. F., Warren, K. S. and Strickland, G. T. (1976). *Nature, London* **263,** 56.

Marchand, E. J., Marcial-Rojas, R. A., Rodriques, R., Polango, G. and Diaz-Rivera, R. S. (1957). *Arch. Intern. Med.* **100,** 965.

Meira, J. A. (1942). *Arq. Circ. Clin. Exp.* **6,** 3.

Meira, J. A. (1951). *Esquistossomiase mansoni hepato-esplenica* Thesis, University of São Paulo.

Menezes, H. (1967). In *Bilharziasis,* p. 175. Ed. F. K. Mostofi. Springer-Verlag, Berlin.

Michaels, R. M. (1970). *Expl Parasit.* **27,** 217.

Mott, C. B., Neves, D. P., Ukumura, M., Britto, T. and Bettarello, A. (1972). *Am. J. Dig. Dis.* **17,** 583.

Neves, J. (1970). *Quadro Clínico de Esquistossomose Mansoni,* p. 131. Ed. Aloisio Sales da Cunha. Editora de Universidade de São Paulo.

Neves, J., Marinho, R. P., de Araujo, P. K. and Raso, P. (1973). *Trans. R. Soc. Trop. Med.* **67,** 782.

Neves, J., Marinho, R. P., Martins, N. R. L. L., de Araujo, P. K. and Lucciola, J. (1969). *Trans. R. Soc. Trop. Med. Hyg.* **63,** 79.

Ogilvie, B. M., Smithers, S. R. and Terry, R. J. (1966). *Nature, London* **209,** 1221.

Polak, M., Montenegro, M. R., Meira, J. A., Conte, V. P., Espejo, H., Franchini, F. and Pontes, J. F. (1959). *Revta Inst. Med. Trop. S. Paulo* **1,** 18.

Prata, A. (1957a). *Biopsia retal na esquistossomose mansoni.* Thesis, University of Bahia.

Prata, A. (1957b). In *I Simpósio Sobre Esquistossomose.* Eds A. Prata and E. Aboim. Brazilian Navy.

Prata, A. (1970). In *II Simpósio Sobre Esquistossomose.* Eds A. Prata and E. Aboim. Brazilian Navy and University of Bahia.

Prata, A. and Bina, J. C. (1968). *Gaz. Méd. Bahia* **68,** 49.

Queiroz, F. P., Brito, E., Martinelli, R. and Rocha, H. (1973). *Am. J. Trop. Med. Hyg.* **22,** 622.

Ramly, Z., Sorour, A., Serif, A., Loutfy, M. and Ibrahim, M. (1953). *J. Egyptian Med. Ass.* **36,** 567.

Raso, P. and Bogliolo, L. (1970). Patologia. In *Esquistossomose mansoni,* p. 77. Ed. Aloisio Sales da Cunha. Editora de Universidade de São Paulo.

Razzak, M. A. (1966). *Am. J. Trop. Med. Hyg.* **15,** 37.

Rocha, H., Cruz, T., Brito, E. and Susin, M. (1976). *Am. J. Trop. Med. Hyg.* **25,** 108.

Sadun, E. H., von Lichtenberg, F., Cheever, A. W. and Erickson, D. G. (1970). *Am. J. Trop. Med. Hyg.* **19,** 258.

Shaw, A. F. B. and Ghareeb, A. A. (1938). *J. Path. Bact.* **46,** 401.

Shiroma, M., Ferneira, J. M. and Meira, J. A. (1963). *Revta Hosp. Clin. Fac. Med. S. Paulo* **18,** 462.

Stenger, R. J., Warren, K. S. and Johnson, E. A. (1967). *Am. J. Trop. Med. Hyg.* **16,** 473.

Teixeira, R. (1960). *Revta Inst. Med. Trop. de S. Paulo* **2,** 65.

Teixeira, R., Bina, J. C. and Barreto, S. H. (1976). *Revta Méd. Bahia* **22,** 70.

Tonelli, E. and Neves, J. (1969). *Revta Ass. Méd. Minas Gerais* **20,** 107.
Vargas, E. E. V. (1945). *Revta Pol. Caracas* **14,** 133.
Veress, B., Musa, A. R., Osman, H., Asha, A., Saddig, E. W. and El Hassan, A. M. (1978). *Ann. Trop. Med. Parasit.* **72,** 357.
Vinhaes, L. S. A. (1974). *Estudo da circulacao pulmonar na síndrome de hipertensão portal esquistossomótica Interrelacona radiológico-hemodinâmica.* Thesis, University of Bahia.
Warren, K. S. (1962). *Trans. R. Soc. Trop. Med. Hyg.* **56,** 510.
Warren, K. S. (1973). *Helm. Abstr.* **42,** 592.
Warren, K. S. (1977). *Am. J. Trop. Med. Hyg.* **26,** 113.
Warren, K. S. and Rebonças, G. (1966). *Am. J. Trop. Med. Hyg.* **15,** 32.
Warren, K. S., Rosenthal, M. S. and Domingo, E. O. (1969). *Bull. N.Y. Acad. Med.* **45,** 2.
Woodruff, A., Shafei, A. Z., Awward, H. K., Pettitt, L. E. and Abaza, H. H. (1963). *Trans. R. Soc. Trop. Med. Hyg.* **60,** 343.
Wydell, S. (1958). *E. Afr. Med. J.* **35,** 413.
Zaky, H. A., El-Heneidy, A. R. and Foda, M. T. (1962). *Brit. Med. J.* **1,** 367.
Zaky, H. A., El-Heneidy, A. R. and Khalil, M. (1964). *Brit. Med. J.* **1,** 1021.

6 *S. japonicum* and *S. japonicum*-like Infections

Kenneth E. Mott

S. japonicum represents the extremes of biological characteristics of the human schistosomes. The developmental stages in the snail require the longest period of time, up to 10 weeks; a longer exposure to light is necessary before cercariae are shed, and yet the daily rate of cercarial shedding is the lowest. The adult worms are the largest, yet the eggs are the smallest. In man, the female worm excretes eggs in clumps, not singly, and in greater numbers than other human schistosomes. The worm is found in a wider range of wild and domestic animals than the other human schistosomes and at least one strain from Taiwan, morphologically indistinguishable from the human strains of *S. japonicum*, is zoophilic and will not infect man. Teleologically, these characteristics of *S. japonicum* might be interpreted to indicate that it is a parasite which is poorly adapted to man and even to its intermediate host.

Although the life-cycles of these parasites are, in general, similar to those of *S. haematobium* and *S. mansoni* and the clinical manifestations comparable in many ways to those of the latter, some details of the life-cycle and some responses of the human body to *S. japonicum* are very different, resulting in differences in the epidemiology, disease processes and control of *S. japonicum*.

GEOGRAPHICAL DISTRIBUTION

At least 5% of the world's population is estimated to reside in *S. japonicum*-endemic areas. The distribution in man in south-east Asia closely follows the distribution of *Oncomelania* snails; the most northerly endemic area is the Tone River basin in Japan, located 36°N and the southern-most focus is in Lake

Lindu in Central Sulawesi which, at 1200 m, is also the highest known transmission site of *S. japonicum*.

China remains the largest endemic area. The marshes and lowlands in the regions of the Taiku, Poyang and Tongtin lakes of the Yangtze River basin and the Yangtze delta, as well as the provinces bordering this immense river, remain infected areas. In 1950, 350 counties in 13 provinces were endemic for schistosomiasis. Presently, about half of these counties are still endemic; however, in the southern provinces of Kwangtung, Kwangsi and Fukien schistosomiasis is no longer considered a public health problem. In the 1950s, 10 million people were estimated to be infected but the number is now possibly much less due to successful control (Cross, 1976).

Schistosomiasis is endemic in five areas in two of Japan's five islands. Four of these areas are on the main island of Honshu, including the Katayama district in Hiroshima and Okayama prefectures in the south and on the coast of the Inland Sea; the Kofu basin in Yamanashi prefecture and the Numazu district in Shizuoka prefecture; the Tone River basin in Chiba, Saitama and Ibaraki prefectures; and in small foci in the Arakawa and Edogawa basins of Tokyo. On the southern island, Kyushu, the Chikugo river basin of the Fukuoka and Saga prefectures is also an endemic area.

In the Philippines, 6 of the 13 main islands, or 129 towns, are endemic for *S. japonicum*; 16·5% of the population is thought to be infected, involving an estimated 655 000 persons (Santos, 1976). In Luzon, the Irosin valley, a rice farming area of about 4500 hectares in area, is the only endemic focus. In Mindoro, the endemic area is limited to around Lake Naujan. On Samar, only the southern portion of the island is not endemic. On Leyte, the infection is endemic on the east coast. Bohol has the most recently discovered endemic area on the northern side of the island. Mindanao has endemic foci in all provinces.

In Lake Lindu and the Napu valley in Central Sulawesi, western Indonesia (geologically related to the Philippine island chain), *S. japonicum* has been known to be endemic since 1937 (Brug and Tesch, 1937). Prevalence rates above 50% have been recorded but the populations affected are comparatively small.

S. japonicum-like infections

The status of schistosomiasis in Laos has recently been reviewed

(Sornmani, 1976). The first case of *S. japonicum*-like infection was reported in a Laotian student in Paris. He was from Khong Island, in the Mekong River, the home of five other infected Laotian students (Barbier, 1966). The island was confirmed as an important endemic area and in the limited surveys completed, the prevalence has been shown to be about 15% (Iijima *et al.*, 1973). Aside from man, only dogs have been found to be infected. The Hmong people in northern Laos are also known to be infected (Westermeyer, 1978).

In Cambodia, the same parasite has been identified near Kratie, a floating village on the lower Mekong River. The overall prevalence of infection in this village was about 10% (Audebaud *et al.*, 1968; Schneider, 1976).

In Peninsular Malaysia, schistosomiasis has been found at autopsy or on rectal biopsy. Rarely, and never consistently, have *S. japonicum*-like eggs been found in the stool of Orang Asali aborigines (Murugasu and Dissanaike, 1973; Leong *et al.*, 1975; Murugasu *et al.*, 1978). Experimental infection in mice has been achieved successfully and a naturally infected *Rattus mulleri*, excreting viable *S. japonicum*-like eggs, has been captured (Greer 1980).

In Thailand, a *S. japonicum*-like infection was found at autopsy in the presence of hepatosplenomegaly (Nidtayasudthi *et al.*, 1975), and in North Borneo, crab-eating macaques but not humans were found to be infected (Kuntz, 1978).

THE LIFE-CYCLE

Snail intermediate hosts

Details of the snail intermediate hosts of *S. japonicum* have been described in Chapter 2. They may be contrasted with the snail hosts of *S. mansoni* and *S. haematobium* as shown in Table 6.1.

The snail intermediate host of the *S. japonicum*-like infection (*S. mekongi*) in Laos is *Tricula aperta*, which is probably the host in nearby Cambodia. In Malaysia, a new snail species initially classified as *Robertsiella kaporensis* has been found infected with a *S. japonicum*-like parasite (Greer *et al.*, 1980).

Intra-molluscan development

The details of the intra-molluscan development of *S. japonicum*

Table 6.1 A comparison of the genera *Oncomelania* and *Bulinus/Biomphalaria*.

Oncomelania	*Bulinus/Biomphalaria*
Gills	Pulmonate
Operculum	No operculum
Maximum size 10 mm	Maximum size 20–25 mm
Amphibious	Aquatic
Separate sexes	Hermaphrodite
Eggs laid single or in short chains	10–30 eggs in masses
Hatch in 10–25 days	Hatch in 9–11 days
Mature in 4–6 months	Mature in 2–3 months

have not been studied in as much detail by modern techniques as those of *S. mansoni* in *B. glabrata*.

In general, there is no difference between the sexes of *Oncomelania* in susceptibility to *S. japonicum* infection, although the maturation and survival of female infected snails have been reported to be lower (Moose, 1963) and are reduced following infection in both sexes (Okamoto, 1963; Hairston, 1973). Heavy infections reduce survival, and cercarial output will thus be decreased (Yasuraoka, 1970). Infected snails may live for up to $1\frac{1}{2}$ years; 50% die within 8 months.

The miracidium penetrates the snail within a few minutes at the point of contact. By the seventh day, the miracidium can no longer be recognised as such and migrates as an elongated form to the distal lymph spaces or perinephric region where it develops primary and secondary sporocysts. The cercariae leave the secondary sporocysts, move into the surrounding lymph spaces between the liver lobules and the hermaphroditic organs and hence penetrate to the outside.

Experiments in the Philippines indicate that from single and multiple infections relatively few cercariae are shed daily (Pesigan, Hairston *et al.*, 1958)—very much fewer than in *S. haematobium* or *S. mansoni*, where the daily total may be counted in hundreds or even thousands.

Cercariae

The few cercariae that emerge swim towards the surface of the water where they may survive for up to 48 hours. Although emergence is facilitated by sunlight or artificial light, peak density of cercariae occurs in the late evening in the Philippines, and in mid-afternoon in China and Japan. The most suitable water temperature is between 20°C and 28°C (range 15°C and 35°C), at pH of 6·6 to 7·8. In areas with temperate climates, such as China and Japan, the density of *S. japonicum* cercariae is greatest in July. In contrast, in tropical climates, as in the Philippines, cercarial density is dependent on micro-environmental fluctuations of rainfall. In the laboratory, the cercariae are noted to have an adhesive quality with a strong affinity to glass.

Cercariae of *S. japonicum* penetrate more rapidly than those of other *Schistosoma* and the rate varies in different experimental animals (Pan *et al.*, 1954). The processes of penetration and the migration patterns in the host are similar to those of other human schistosomes. The fork-tailed cercariae of *S. japonicum* may be confused with other furocercariae which do not infect man (Ito *et al.*, 1972 and 1977).

The adult worm

Morphological details of different stages of the parasite have been described in Chapter 1.

In the initial stages of experimental infection, as early as three weeks after the cercariae penetrate, adult worms migrate to the distal venules of the portal, superior and inferior mesenteric veins (Stirewalt, 1973). Eggs are released in large numbers in clumps in the submucosa and mucosa of the small intestines; eggs that get trapped in the tissue tend to calcify if not excreted. In contrast, *S. mansoni* adult females lay daily about a tenth of the number of eggs produced by *S. japonicum* and these are laid in different parts of the small and large intestines near the ileocaecal junction.

The lack of a prominent spine on the *S. japonicum* egg does not hinder its rapid penetration of the mucosa.

At least five reports of congenital infection of *S. japonicum* in experimental animals are described in the literature (Morishita *et al.*, 1964); this occurrence has never been documented in *S. mansoni* or *S. haematobium* infections. It is assumed that congenital infection occurs when the infection is acquired during the course of pregnancy.

Different strains of *S. japonicum* have been defined according to the geographical origin of the isolate and their different inter-mediate snail hosts. There are basically five major strains referred to in the literature, from Japan, the Philippines, China, Indonesia and Formosa. Some morphological and biological differences between strains have been reported (Hsu and Hsu, 1958a and 1958b); however, the isoenzyme patterns and electron-micrographs of the integument are similar. The strain found in Formosa does not infect man. These different strains interbreed without change in fertility or infectivity. Heterologous mating between *S. japonicum* and *S. incognitum* has also been observed (Stafford *et al.*, 1979).

Selected aspects of energy metabolism of the adult *S. japonicum* have been studied (Huang, 1980). The major energy source is anaerobic glycolysis. The tricarboxylic cycle activity is reduced and citrate synthetase, isocitrate dehydrogenase and malate dehydrogenase activities are generally similar to those of *S. mansoni* (Oya *et al.*, 1970; Smith and Brown, 1977). Succinic dehydrogenase activity is twice as high in *S. japonicum* paired adults as in *S. mansoni*. The same enzyme is found in *S. japonicum* eggs and is the basis of a technique to measure viability of the egg in tissue by specific staining with triphenyl tetrazolium chloride (TTC) (Yoshizumi and Ota, 1957).

Although similar in weight, the female *S. japonicum* appears to contain less protein than the male. Marked differences in amino acid metabolism between *S. mansoni* and *S. japonicum*, as well as between male and female *S. japonicum*, have been reported (Bruce *et al.*, 1972). Glutamic and aspartic acid are metabolised at a lower rate in *S. japonicum*. Whereas neither proline nor histidine has been shown to be utilised by *S. mansoni*, proline and tyrosine are utilised by the *S. japonicum* female worm and histidine is utilised by the *S. japonicum* male worm.

Cyclic adenosine monophosphate (cAMP) phosphodiesterase activities are similar in *S. mansoni* and *S. japonicum*; however, their importance in the metabolism or effect on hormonal reactivity, as is known in mammalian cells, remains unexplored (Brown and Smith, 1977).

The *S. japonicum* adult worms have been maintained *in vitro* for short periods of time for biochemical studies (Bruce *et al.*, 1972). No compatible medium has been developed which permits development of adults from the cercariae, but male schistosomula at 17 days of age have developed in culture to the adult stage. Female schistosomula, however, remained in the larval form (Fu *et al.*, 1976).

The adult *S. japonicum* may survive in the human host residing outside the endemic area and produce viable eggs for up to 47 years (Hall and Kehoe, 1970). In endemic areas, the age–prevalence distribution of *S. japonicum* infection also supports the hypothesis that the parasite survives for longer periods than *S. mansoni* or *S. haematobium*.

Animal reservoirs

Many animal reservoirs of *S. japonicum* have been found; however, the significance of their role in the maintenance of transmission in endemic areas has not been evaluated. In China, at least 31 wild mammals and 13 domestic animals have been found to be infected (Cheng, 1971).

In the Philippines, based on the total animal population, prevalence, mean daily egg output and hatchability, the dog, cow, pig, rat, carabao (water buffalo) and goat (in decreasing order of importance) were considered responsible for about 25% of the total potential environmental contamination, while man contributed the rest (Pesigan, Farooq *et al.*, 1958). The hatchability and viability of *S. japonicum* vary widely among naturally infected animals.

Before effective control measures had been instituted in Japan, many species of rodent were found to be naturally infected, including *Microtus montebelli*, *Apodemus specious specious*, *Rattus norvegicus* and *Eothenomys smithii*. In general, the wild rat and laboratory albino rats are not good hosts and in the latter most of the female worms are infertile.

In Sulawesi, nine species of wild mammal are known to serve as reservoir hosts, including *Rattus exulans*, *R. hoffmanni*, *R. marmosurus*, *R. chyrscomus rallus*, wild deer, wild pig, civet cat, cattle and the domestic dog.

INFECTION IN MAN

In defined populations, peak egg excretion and prevalence are observed in the 15–20 year age groups. Women between 45 and 55 years old have also been noted to have a high prevalence and intensity of infection (Lewert *et al.*, 1979; Domingo *et al.*, 1980; WHO Workshop, 1980). Egg output gradually falls after the age of 20, but prevalence remains high. The pattern of prevalence and/or intensity in these studies was bimodal, unlike that of *S. mansoni*; however, the frequency distribution of *S. japonicum* eggs is similar, with the majority of infected persons excreting low numbers of eggs.

Morbidity

S. japonicum is generally considered to cause more severe disease than *S. mansoni*, but few studies of community morbidity have been reported and these do not support this conclusion. In the pioneer work of Pesigan and his colleagues in the Philippines, about a third of those infected had some complaints but more than half of these were mild. In recent studies in the Philippines, dysentery was the only symptom found to be significantly more common among infected persons and severity was related to intensity of infection; clinically, hepatomegaly and splenomegaly were associated with *S. japonicum* though liver enlargement was found in a large number (67%) of uninfected persons (WHO Workshop, 1980). In infected persons the extent of liver enlargement was directly related to the intensity of infection.

Pathology

As in other schistosome infections, the primary lesion in *S. japonicum* is a granulomatous reaction to the egg, generally considered to be more severe than the reaction to *S. mansoni* and *S. haematobium*. Whether the aetiology of the granuloma in the three infections is the same is uncertain; it has been suggested that while those associated with *S. mansoni* and *S. haematobium* are largely cell-mediated immunological reactions, those associated with *S. japonicum* may be related to immune complex deposition (Warren *et al.*, 1975).

Relative to *S. mansoni* and *S. haematobium*, less information exists on the pathology of *S. japonicum* infection in man, in spite of the fact that the first pathological descriptions were produced some 20 years prior to the discovery of the parasite.

The liver is the organ most affected by *S. japonicum* infection and changes are similar to those in *S. mansoni* infections. In general, the liver surface becomes irregular and may have nodular swellings up to 3 cm or more in diameter. Fissures as deep as 1 cm and fibrosis occur in the parenchyma. The left lobe is often proportionally larger than the right lobe. In the latter stages of the disease, the liver consistency becomes hard and the entire organ may be shrunken.

The appearance of the cut surface of the liver varies with the duration and intensity of infection. In mild cases, sparse scarring is present, whereas in the most severe cases, the parenchymal cells may be displaced by fibrous tissue. Beside the 'pipe-stem' portal fibrosis which is also characteristic of *S. mansoni* infection, extensive intralobular fibrosis may be present.

Histologically,the inflammatory reaction is extensive and the granuloma contain abundant plasma cells, lymphocytes and

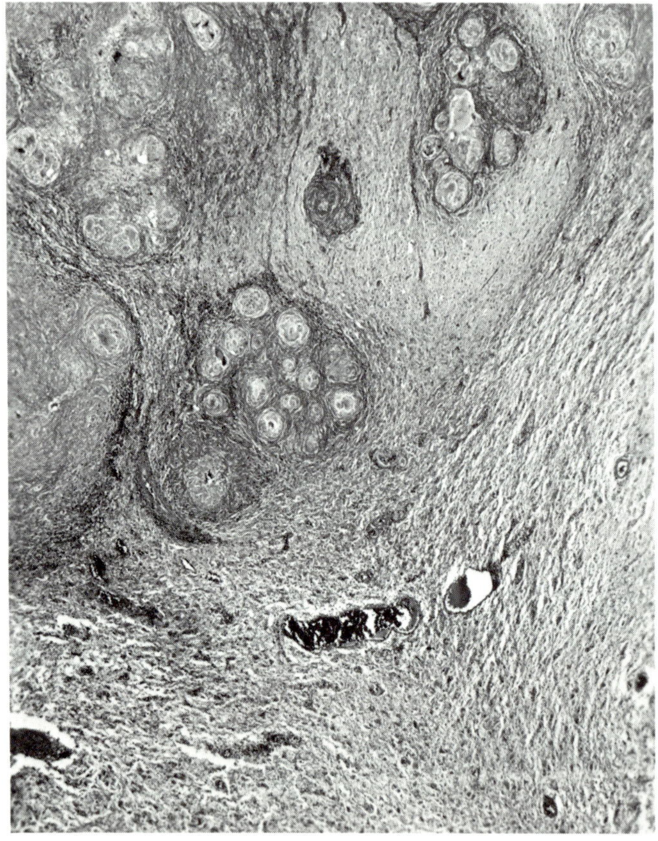

Fig. 6.1(a) *S. japonicum* ova in the brain. Many granulomas forming conglomerate masses enmeshed in scar tissue. (H & E; × 25; AFIP photograph 80-12054.) (By courtesy of Armed Forces Institute of Pathology, Washington DC.)

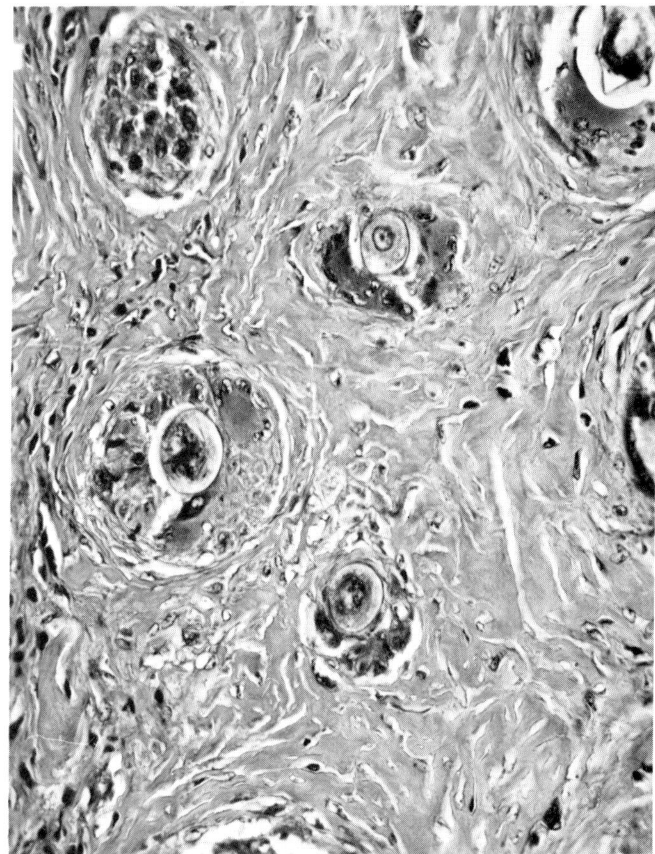

Fig. 6.1(b) *S. japonicum* ova in the brain. Ova surrounded by giant cells of foreign body type and enclosed by hyalinised fibrous tissue. (Movat stain; × 250; AFIP photograph 80-12050.) (By courtesy of Armed Forces Institute of Pathology, Washington DC.)

eosinophils. Compared with other schistosome infections, many eosinophils and neutrophils are present in early granulomas. In the portal tracts, extensive fibrosis, inflammation and neovascularisation are found. The portal veins may be seriously affected, with focal endothelial or internal proliferation and endophlebitis.

A general correlation was found between the presence and severity of fibrosis and the number of eggs recovered from digested tissue (Tsutsumi *et al.*, 1963); egg recovery increased from the small bowel to the rectosigmoid region. Most of the eggs were found in the submucosa (Tsutsumi and Hasuda, 1964). Compared with *S. mansoni* infection, the gastrointestinal tract lesions tend to be focal, isolated and more proliferate.

Central nervous system involvement of *S. japonicum* infection is a pathological and clinical entity which has been recognised for nearly a century, but its public health significance is unknown. A number of well-documented cases have been reported in the literature (Kane and Most, 1948; Ando *et al.*, 1966; Haedicke, 1972), with complete pathological studies at autopsy or from surgical specimens. The pathogenesis of these lesions is not understood. The source of the eggs found in the brain, whether from worms in the brain itself or embolised from remote worms, is not known (Fig. 6.1).

Ova initiate an intense granulomatous reaction in the cerebral vessels and in the surrounding brain. The pia-arachnoid, cortex, subcortex, basal ganglia, internal capsule and choroid plexuses are most frequently affected, but ova have been found in all areas of the brain. Healing leads to calcification of the ova and scar tissue (Kane and Most, 1948).

CLINICAL MANIFESTATIONS

Acute infection

During the acquisition of infection, the cercariae penetrate the skin and this event may be associated with local pruritis, erythema and swelling. In Japan, the term 'kabure' has been used to describe this phase of infection. The immune status of the host undoubtedly influences the response of the cercariae to penetration; however, most of the current information remains anecdotal. Some Japanese investigators experienced intense itching after self-exposure to cercariae (Faust and Meleney, 1924).

Acute clinical schistosomiasis has been observed only in individuals who have not previously been exposed nor resided in an endemic area. The mean incubation period between exposure and the onset of clinical symptoms is estimated to be 40 days—range 14 to 84 days (Ts'ai and Yu, 1966). 'Katayama fever' is the term used to describe the initial prolonged fever at the onset of infection. Few systemic signs are present; slight tender liver and spleen enlargement have been reported. Eosinophilia ranging from 30–80% of the total white blood cell count was present in 75% of infected US Army personnel in Leyte (Bang *et al.*, 1945). Liver function tests are generally normal.

Chronic infection

Gastrointestinal and hepatic involvement

As in *S. mansoni* infection, the early chronic stages of disease are generally asymptomatic, although diarrhoea and abdominal pain are common and have been associated with intensity of infection (Domingo *et al.*, 1980; WHO Workshop, 1980). The clinical measurement of liver size, as an index of the prevalence of schistosomiasis, has been recognised and used by the Japanese since the 1930s in their field surveys. More recently, epidemiological studies have shown a correlation between the intensity of infection and liver enlargement in all age groups. Most severe liver disease due to *S. japonicum* infection occurs in the second and third decades. The liver scintillation scan pattern is an 'inverted triangle' type, quite distinct from that seen in cirrhosis or other forms of liver disease. Liver function tests are normal.

Hepatic coma, as a terminal event in *S. japonicum* disease, is frequently observed in hospitalised persons, particularly in China (Fu *et al.*, 1965) but in the Philippines the main terminal event is massive bleeding in the upper gastrointestinal tract, rather than hepatic coma (Sulit *et al.*, 1964).

At the onset of ascites, most hospitalised patients have abnormal bromsulphthalein retention and lowered serum albumin. If the urinary sodium is less than 2 meq in 24 hours or if serum albumin falls, the prognosis is poor. Biochemical liver function is usually preserved until this terminal phase. The careful studies on ammonia metabolism which have been completed in *S. mansoni* infection have not been reported for *S. japonicum*.

S. japonicum infection was implicated as a co-carcinogen in carcinoma of the rectum and carcinoma of the liver before the life-cycle of the parasite had been fully described. Granulomatous disease of the rectum and sigmoid colon with mucosal hyperplasis, pseudopolyposis, ulceration, thickening of the bowel wall and stenosis (as reported in mice by Warren, 1969) may occur (Ch'en *et al.*, 1965; Chen *et al.*, 1978). While the prevalence in endemic areas is unknown, these pathological changes may be the substrate for malignant transformation. The mean age of *S. japonicum* infected individuals with carcinoma of the colon or rectum was 10 years lower than those who were not infected (Ch'en *et al.*, 1965). In a large autopsy series from Kurume Medical School in Japan, the rate of carcinoma of the colon in infected persons was 25 times greater than that of non-infected persons. Histologically, the associated carcinoma of the colon has been described as a well-differentiated adenocarcinoma with pseudopolyps, and calcified eggs were identified in the tissues.

An association between *S. japonicum* infection and hepatitis B surface (Hbs) antigen has not been reported. In cases of hepatoma associated with *S. japonicum* infection, the prevalence of antigen has not been reported. In cases of hepatoma associated with *S. japonicum* infection, the prevalence of antigen has been high compared to the general population (Nakashima *et al.*, 1965). The rate of hepatoma in this same autopsy series in Japan in infected individuals was about four times that documented in non-infected individuals. Although the epidemiological information is scarce, *S. japonicum* probably acts as a co-carcinogen.

Anaemia is often found in patients with high egg output (Medado, 1967). Dysentery increased in frequency proportionally with egg output (Lewert *et al.*, 1979; Domingo *et al.*, 1980; WHO Workshop, 1980), and may contribute to clinical anaemia. No data from general populations in endemic areas on the relationships between hematocrit and *S. japonicum* infection are available.

Severe portal hypertension may be associated with shunting of eggs to the pulmonary circulation and cor pulmonale (Jongco and Lee, 1963; Ostrea and Marcelo, 1964). The frequency of this clinical condition will depend on the intensity of infection in any given endemic area, but data from population-based studies are unfortunately not available.

Central nervous system

The brain is principally involved in *S. japonicum*, in contrast to the spinal cord in *S. mansoni* and *S. haematobium* infections.

Clinically, Jacksonian-type paroxysmal seizures in persons over 20 years of age are the first manifestations of cerebral schistosomiasis, followed in many fatal instances by grand mal seizures, which are unresponsive even to intravenous diazepam. Permanent cerebral cortical damage occurs and in the large number of American military personnel infected in Leyte in

1944–5, 2% suffered permanent disability from cerebral schistosomiasis.

Diagnosing cerebral schistosomiasis is complicated by the fact that many patients do not have eggs in the stool. Conversely, as neurological signs or symptoms in a patient with systemic schistosomiasis are treated as schistosomal cerebral involvement, such cases may be over-diagnosed.

Although the cerebrospinal fluid may be abnormal, there do not appear to be any characteristic changes. There may be increased pressure, a mild pleocytosia, increased globulin, total protein content and alteration in the colloidal gold curve. The presence of ova of *S. japonicum* has not been reported but the circumoval precipitin test has been reported to be positive.

Computerised axial tomography has been utilised to demonstrate cerebral masses in individuals with recurrent convulsions from endemic areas, and the significant reduction in size of the mass after specific chemotherapy (Maramba, personal communication).

No specific EEG pattern is present in cerebral schistosomiasis; however, diffuse alpha and asymmetric theta waves have been frequently observed (Hayashi, 1979). Although the high incidence of convulsions in endemic areas of the Philippines has been attributed to *S. japonicum* infection, two recent population-based studies did not correlate the presence of convulsions with schistosomiasis (Domingo *et al.*, 1980; WHO Workshop, 1980).

DIAGNOSIS

Parasitological

Definitive diagnosis of an active infection can be made only by detecting ova of *S. japonicum* in faeces or tissues.

As the female worm lays eggs in clusters in the faeces, they tend to be aggregated in light infections, but in heavier ones they are more randomly distributed; this means repeated stool examinations may be necessary to detect light infections.

The MIFC (see Chapter 8) has gained wide acceptance but as at least three sediments from each 1 g sample must be examined in order to approximate 95% of eggs present (Santos *et al.*, 1968), the method is not practical for large-scale surveys and precise quantitation is difficult.

The Kato thick smear technique (see Chapter 8) has been modified for quantitative estimation of *S. japonicum* eggs (WHO Workshop, 1980). Cellophane coverslips are soaked in a 50% malachite-green glycerine preparation, or in a solution consisting of 0·3 ml of a saturated solution of methylene blue in sodium acetate buffer (pH 3·8), diluted to 100 ml with 25% glycerine.

After turning the slide upside down and pressing it against a flat surface, the preparation is allowed to clear for 15–30 minutes: 3–5 drops of 1% aqueous eosin solution are added gently over the cellophane square, left for 2–4 minutes and then wiped off with absorbent paper.

Rectal biopsy specimens may contain eggs when they are not found in the stools. When 2,3,5-triphenyl tetrazolium chloride in the presence of sodium succinate is added to the biopsy material, a colour reaction occurs with viable eggs (Yoshizumi and Ota, 1957).

Serodiagnosis

The repeated clinical observation that infection may occur yet eggs remain undetected in faeces has encouraged research in this area. However, as for *S. mansoni* and *S. haematobium*, immunodiagnostic tests are neither sensitive nor specific enough to warrant general acceptance outside research laboratories.

The circumoval precipitin (COP) test (see Chapter 8) is probably the most sensitive and specific of the immunodiagnostic tests for schistosomiasis, but is the least standardised and there is no concensus on the preparation of eggs, the procedure, nor the criteria for reactivity.

In spite of these deficiencies, the test is more sensitive and specific than the intradermal test but is frequently negative in infected persons over 40 years of age. It was negative amongst persons in Taiwan who showed positive intradermal tests presumably due to infection with the local zoophilic strain of *S. japonicum*. Sera from *S. japonicum* infections react with *S. mansoni* eggs but individuals infected with *S. mansoni* or *S. haematobium* do not react with *S. japonicum* eggs. Sera from patients with *Clonorchis* or *Paragonimus* infections give negative reactions to *S. japonicum* eggs.

Using cerebrospinal fluid, the COP test is reported to be positive in cases of cerebral *S. japonicum* infection (Reyes and Yogore, 1963).

The complement fixation test and other serological tests have been used but, as with other schistosome infections, their lack of specificity and sensitivity limits their usefulness.

Skin tests using various antigens derived from adult *S. japonicum* worms have been advocated (Garcia *et al.*, 1969; Sawada *et al.*, 1969, 1970). Sensitivity is higher in infected adults than in children, but cross-reactions occur with other parasitic infections including *Capillaria* (Yogore and Lewert, 1974).

Precipitins to *S. japonicum* antigens have been demonstrated in dialyzed urine of infected individuals (Okabe and Ono, 1962; Ts'ai and Yu, 1966) but this has not been used clinically to assess infection.

IMMUNOPATHOLOGY

Cellular immune response

As early as 1916, Fujinami noted that immunopathology related to the egg was associated with full maturation of the contained miracidium, and that the granuloma surrounding it diminished in size as the duration of the infection increased.

Based on comparative studies, the lesions associated with *S. japonicum* eggs have been described as more exudative and destructive than those of other schistosomes (Hsu *et al.*, 1972, 1973; Lichtenberg *et al.*, 1973; Erickson *et al.*, 1974). The granuloma contains more neutrophils and plasma cells, necrosis and exudation occur and the Hoeppli phenomenon is frequently present.

The Hoeppli phenomenon (Lichtenberg *et al.*, 1966) is an eosinophilic corona radiating around usually viable *S. japonicum* eggs within a small proportion (10%) of the granuloma observed in heavily infected man or experimental animals. The precipitate is an antigen–antibody complex with a gradient to antibody excess at the periphery, similar to the *in vitro* circumoval precipitin phenomenon. Hoeppli observed this phenomenon only in rabbits but it is seen in other infected animals and man and surrounds *S. mansoni* and *S. haematobium* eggs as well, though less frequently.

Central necrosis in granuloma of *S. japonicum* has been frequently reported in mice (Warren and Moore, 1966). These severe lesions have been attributed to the clustering of eggs and a direct toxic effect on the liver parenchyma. This lesion may be associated with the Hoeppli phenomenon.

Single egg granulomas of *S. mansoni* were observed to be larger than those of *S. japonicum* in naturally infected *Aotus* monkeys (Erickson *et al.*, 1971). Experimentally, after injection of viable eggs through the tail vein (Warren and Domingo, 1970; Warren *et al.*, 1975), single egg granulomas of *S. mansoni* in pulmonary vasculature were larger than those of *S. japonicum* in unsensitised mice and in mice sensitised by prior intraperitoneal *S. japonicum* eggs; if the animal is sensitised by a subcutaneous injection of eggs, granulomas of *S. japonicum* and *S. mansoni* are similar in size (Warren *et al.*, 1975). These findings are in contrast to those in naturally infected mice (Meleney *et al.*, 1953).

A slight tissue cellular response has been observed (Meleney *et al.*, 1952) in unisexual infections, probably due to embolisation of adult worms.

Soluble circulating immune complexes have been detected in *S. japonicum*-infected rabbits with decreased C_3 (third component of complement) concentration, and renal lesions were detected in animals with persistently high levels of circulating immune complexes (Jones *et al.*, 1977). In infected chimpanzees with surgical portocaval shunts, renal lesions occurred which were similar to those observed in the unshunted control animals (Sadun *et al.*, 1975). The epidemiological significance of these lesions in man is not known. In man, lymphocyte responsiveness to phytohaemagglutinin (PHA) is depressed but not related to egg output or to duration of infection (Lewert *et al.*, 1979). In the same study, no differences in response to adult or egg antigens between infected individuals and controls were detected.

Humoral immune response

Specific antibodies to *S. japonicum* are found in the experimental host approximately at the onset of egg laying by female worms (Kawasaki *et al.*, 1968). Antibody to gut-associated proteoglycan (GASP) has been detected in unisexual infections with *S. japonicum* (Nash 1978). During the course of experimental infection, the albumin:globulin ratio decreased due primarily to an initial rise in IgG and IgE. The IgE response in inbred mice is controlled by H-2 genes (Kojima and Yokogawa, 1979).

In young infected persons excreting viable eggs, IgE levels exceeding 1000 mg/ml are not uncommon (Ishizaki *et al.*, 1974); however, in older persons these high levels were not observed. Serum levels of specific *S. japonicum* IgE have been suggested to correlate with skin reactivity to the *S. japonicum* adult worm (Miyamoto *et al.*, 1975) and to egg antigens (Ishii *et al.*, 1978). After specific treatment, the IgE levels and the total globulin may return to normal (Ito *et al.*, 1972). Recently, it has been suggested that IgM antibodies to GASP may indicate active infection (Nash, 1978).

Uncharacterised precipitating antibodies have been found in the urine of infected experimental animals and rarely in patients; these precipitins disappear after specific treatment (Okabe and Tanaka, 1958).

A variety of autoantibodies has been documented in experimental *S. japonicum* infections, including anti-DNA (Hillyer, 1976), anti-immunoglobulin (Ig) (Wistar *et al.*, 1975), anti-liver, anti-colon and anti-sheep red blood cell antibodies (Kurata, 1966; Jones *et al.*, 1976). Anti-DNA antibodies have been observed in sera from infected man (Hillyer, 1971).

Antigens

Compared with *S. mansoni*, relatively little has been published on the antigenic composition of *S. japonicum*. The availability of newer labelling techniques, particularly involving monoclonal antibodies, and affinity binding will rapidly add to our present knowledge on this subject.

As with other schistosome eggs, the shell of the egg is probably immunologically inert and it is the metabolic products or secretions of the viable eggs which are immunogenic. Soluble egg antigens of *S. japonicum* have been recently used to assess immediate hypersensitivity in man and experimental animals (Ishii *et al.*, 1978). The surface of cercariae has been observed (Sato *et al.*, 1964), using the fluorescent antibody technique; however, specific antigens have not been isolated. The characteristics of antigens of the other developmental stages of *S. japonicum* have not been reported.

The antigenic mosaic of the adult *S. japonicum* has been shown to include at least 10 antigens which cross-react with *S. haematobium* and *S. mansoni* in experimental infections (Capron *et al.*, 1966). A number of soluble antigens have been purified for skin tests, complement fixation (CF) and indirect haemagglutination (IHA) immunodiagnostic tests (Matsuyama, 1968; Sato *et al.*, 1969; Sawada *et al.*, 1969 and 1970). Both live and lyophilised worms have been used and antigens have been isolated by isoelectric focusing, zone or disc electrophoresis, or various column separations.

Circulating *S. japonicum* antigen similar to the *S. mansoni* antigen (Berggren and Weller, 1967) has been described (Hirata and Akusawa, 1975; Hillyer, 1976; Hirata *et al.*, 1977), but further characterisation has not been completed. Antigenic substances have been reported in the faeces (Okabe *et al.*, 1971) and the urine (Okabe and Akusawa, 1971) but neither the epidemiological nor the clinical importance of these observations has been pursued.

REFERENCES

Ando, S., Okaniwa, T. and Takeuchi, K. (1966). *Brain and nerve (Tokyo)* **18,** 553.

Audebaud, G., Tournier-Lasserve, C., Brumpt, V., Jolly, M., Mazaud, R., Imbert, X. and Brazilo, R. (1968). *Bull. Soc. Path. Exot.* **61,** 778.

Bang, F. B., Ferguson, M. S., Hairston, N. G. and Graham, O. H. (1945). *Am. J. Trop. Med.* **25,** 407.

Barbier, M. (1966). *Bull. Soc. Path. Exot.* **59,** 974.

Berggren, W. L. and Weller, T. (1967). *Am. J. Trop. Med. Hyg.* **16,** 606.

Brown, J. N. and Smith, T. M. (1977). *Trans. R. Soc. Trop. Med. Hyg.* **71,** 356.

Bruce, J. I., Ruff, M. D., Belusko, R. J. and Werner, J. K. (1972). *Int. J. Parasit.* **2,** 425.

Brug, S. L. and Tesch, J. W. (1937). *Geneesk T. Med. Ind.* **77,** 2151.

Capron, A., Vernes, A., Biguet, J., Rose, F., Clay, A. and Adenis, L. (1966). *Ann. Parasit. Hum. Comp.* **41,** 123.

Ch'en, Ming-Chai *et al.* (1965). *Chinese Med. J.* **84,** 513.

Chen, M., Wang, S., Chang, P., Chuang, G., Chen, Y., Tang, Y. and Chou, S. (1978). *Chinese Med. J.* **4,** 371.

Cheng, T. H. (1971). *Am. J. Trop. Med. Hyg.* **20,** 26.

Cross, J. H. (1976). *S.E. Asian J. Trop. Med. Publ. Hlth* **7,** 167.

Domingo, E. O., Tu, E., Peters, P. A., Warren, K. S., Mahmoud, A. A. F. and Houser, H. B. (1980). *Am. J. Trop. Med. Hyg.* **29,** 858.

Erickson, D. G., Jones, C. E. and Tang, D. B. (1974). *Am. J. Trop. Med. Hyg.* **23,** 449.

Erickson, D. G., von Lichtenberg, F., Sadun, E. H., Lucia, H. L. and Hickman, R. L. (1971). *J. Parasit.* **57,** 543.

Faust, E. C. and Meleney, H. E. (1924). *Am. J. Hyg.* Monograph Series 3.

Fu, H. M. *et al.* (1965). *Chinese Med. J.* **84,** 166.

Fu, H. M., Chow, K., Chiu, J. K. (1976). *Int. J. Zoon.* **3,** 105.

Garcia, E. G., Cabrera, B. D., Cristi, Z. A. and Silan, R. B. (1969). *J. Philipp. Med. Ass.* **45,** 86.

Greer, G. J., Ow-Yang, C. K., Sing, K. I. and Lim, H. K. (1980). *Trans. R. Soc. Trop. Med. Hyg.* **74,** 425.

Haedicke, T. A. (1972). *Minnesota Med.* **55,** 1105.

Hairston, N. (1973). In *Epidemiology and Control of Schistosomiasis (Bilharzia),*

p. 250. Ed. N. Ansari. World Health Organization/University Park Press, Baltimore, London, Tokyo.

Hall, S. C. and Kehoe, E. L. (1970). *California Med. J.* **113,** 75.

Hayashi, M. (1979). *Bull. Tokyo Med. Dentl University* **26,** 287.

Hillyer, G. V. (1971). *Proc. Soc. Exp. Biol. Med.* **136,** 880.

Hillyer, G. V. (1976). *Am. J. Trop. Med. Hyg.* **25,** 432.

Hirata, M. and Akusawa, M. (1975). *Jap. J. Microbiol.* **24,** 250.

Hirata, M., Takamori, K. and Tsutsumi, H. (1977). *Kurme Med. J.* **24,** 139.

Hsu, H. F. and Hsu, S. Y. L. (1958a). *Trans. R. Soc. Trop. Med. Hyg.* **52,** 363.

Hsu, H. F. and Hsu, S. Y. L. (1958b). *Am. J. Trop. Med. Hyg.* **7,** 125.

Hsu, S. Y. L., Hsu, H. F., Davis, J. A. and Lust, G. (1972). *Ann. Trop. Med. Parasit.* **66,** 89.

Hsu, S. Y. L., Hsu, H. F., Lust, G. L., Davis, J. R. and Eveland, L. K. (1973). *Ann. Trop. Med. Parasit.* **67,** 349.

Huang, Tso-Yueh (1980). *Int. J. Biochem.* **12,** 457.

Iijima, T., Garcia, R. G. and Lo, C. T. (1973). *Jap. J. Parasit.* **22,** 338.

Ishii, A., Owhashi, M. and Hashiguchi, J. (1978). *Jap. J. Parasit.* **28** (Suppl.), 56.

Ishizaki, T., Kobayakawa, T., Ito, Y., Hosaka, Y., Katsumi, H., Minai, M., Kajihara, N. and Mitsugi, A. (1974). *Jap. J. Parasit.* **23,** 201.

Ito, J., Yasuraoba, K., Santos, A. T. and Blas, B. L. (1977). *Jap. J. Exp. Med.* **47,** 141 and 151.

Ito, K., Sawada, T. and Sato, S. (1972). *Jap. J. Exp. Med.* **42,** 115.

Jones, C. E., Lewert, R. M. and Ozcel, A. A. (1976). *Am. J. Trop. Med. Hyg.* **25,** 613.

Jones, C. E., Rachford, F. W., Ozcel, M. A. and Lewert, R. M. (1977). *Expl. Parasit.* **42,** 221.

Jongco, A. and Lee, W. (1963). *J. Philipp. Med. Assoc.* **39,** 54.

Kane, C. A. and Most, H. (1948). *Arch. Neurol. Psychiat.* **59,** 141.

Kawasaki, H., Nakamo, H., Kojira, M. and Shuido, M. (1968). *Kurume Med. J.* **15,** 243.

Kojima, S. and Yokogawa, M. (1979). *Jap. J. Parasit.* **28,** 105.

Kuntz, R. E. (1978). *Am. J. Trop. Med. Hyg.* **27,** 208.

Kurata, M. (1966). *Kurume Med. J.* **13,** 177.

Leong, S. H., Murugasu, R. and Chong, K. C. (1975). *Proc. 10th Malaysian/Singapore Congress of Medicine* **10,** 21.

Lewert, R. M., Yogore, M. G. Jr. and Blas, B. L. (1979). *Am. J. Trop. Med. Hyg.* **28,** 1010.

Lichtenberg, F. von, Erickson, D. G. and Sadun, E. H. (1973). *Am. J. Path.* **72,** 149.

Lichtenberg, F. von, Smith, J. H. and Cheever, A. W. (1966). *Am. J. Trop. Med. Hyg.* **15,** 886.

Matsuyama, S. (1968). *Jap. J. Parasit.* **17,** 90.

Medado, P. M. (1967). *J. Philipp. Med. Ass.* **43,** 374.

Meleney, H. E., Moore, D. V., Most, H. and Carney, B. M. (1952). *Am. J. Trop. Med. Hyg.* **1,** 263.

Meleney, H. E., Sandground, J. H., Moore, D. V., Most, H. and Carney, B. M. (1953). *Am. J. Trop. Med. Hyg.* **2,** 883.

Miyamoto, T., Ito, K., Ishizaki, T., Hosaka, Y., Kutsumi, H., Ohtomo, H. and Minai, M. (1975). *Jap. J. Parasit.* **24,** 220.

Moose, J. W. (1963). *J. Parasit.* **49,** 151.

Morishita, K., Komiya, Y. and Matsubayashi, H. (1964). *Progress of Medical Parasitology in Japan*, Vol. 1. Meguro Parasitological Museum, Tokyo.

Murugasu, R. and Dissanaike, A. S. (1973). *Trans. R. Soc. Trop. Med. Hyg.* **67,** 880.

Murugasu, R., Wang, F. and Dissanaike, A. S. (1978). *Trans. R. Soc. Trop. Med. Hyg.* **72,** 389.

Nakashima, T., Okuda, K., Kajiro, M., Sakamoto, K., Kubo, Y. and Shimokawa, Y. (1975). *Cancer* **36,** 1483.

Nash, T. E. (1978). *Am. J. Trop. Med. Hyg.* **27,** 939.

Nidtayasudthi, T., Jaroonvesama, N. and Dharamadhach, A. (1975). *J. Med. Ass. Thailand* **58,** 542.

Okabe, K. and Akusawa, M. (1971). *Kurume M. J.* **18,** 51.

Okabe, K., Akusawa, M. and Hanamura, T. (1971). *Kurume Med. J.* **18,** 201.

Okabe, K. and Ono, N. (1962). *Kurume Med. J.* **8,** 95.

Okabe, K. and Tanaka, T. (1958). *Kurume Med. J.* **5,** 45.

Okamoto, K. (1963). *Jap. J. Parasit.* **12,** 497.

Ostrea, E. M. and Marcelo, F. B. (1964). *Acta Med. Philipp.* **1,** 5.

Oya, H., Hayashi, H. and Aoki, T. (1970). In *Recent Advances in Researches on Filariasis and Schistosomiasis in Japan*, p. 393. Ed. M. Sasa. University Park Press, Baltimore, and Manchester.

Pan, C. T., Williams, R. R. and Ritchie, L. S. (1954). *Am. J. Trop. Med. Hyg.* **3,** 136.

Pesigan, R. P., Farooq, M., Hairston, N. G., Jauregui, J. J., Garcia, E. G., Santos, A. T., Santos, B. C. and Besa, A. A. (1958). *Bull. Wld Hlth Org.* **18,** 345.

Pesigan, T. P., Hairston, M. G., Jauregui, J. J., Garcia, E. G., Santos, B. C. and Besa, A. A. (1958). *Bull. Wld Hlth Org.* **18,** 481.

Reyes, V. A. and Yogore, M. G. (1963). *Philipp. J. Surg.* **18,** 172.

Sadun, E. H., Reid, W. A., Cheever, A. W., Duvall, R. H., Swam, K. G., Kent, K. N., Bruce, J. I. and von Lichtenberg, F. (1975). *Am. J. Trop. Med. Hyg.* **24,** 619.

Santos, A. T. (1976). *S.E. Asian J. Trop. Med. Publ. Hlth* **7,** 133.

Santos, A. T., Blas, B. L. and Portillo, G. (1968). *Bull. Wld Hlth Org.* **38,** 825.

Sato, S., Imamura, S. and Yoneyamak, K. (1964). *Gunma J. Med. Sci. (Maebashi)* **13,** 199.

Sato, S., Sawada, T. and Takei, K. (1969). *Jap. J. Exp. Med.* **39,** 355.

Sawada, T., Sato, K. and Sato, S. (1969). *Jap. J. Exp. Med.* **39,** 339.

Sawada, T., Sato, K. and Sato, S. (1970). In *Recent Advances in Researches on Filariasis and Schistosomiasis in Japan*, p. 365. Ed. M. Sasa. University Park Press, Baltimore, and Manchester.

Schneider, C. R. (1976). *S.E. Asian J. Trop. Med. Publ. Hlth* **7,** 155.

Smith, T. M. and Brown, J. N. (1977). *Trans. R. Soc. Trop. Med. Hyg.* **71,** 329.

Sornmani, S. (1976). *S.E. Asian J. Trop. Med. Publ. Hlth* **7,** 149.

Stafford, E. E., Carney, W. P., Tanudjaja and Purnomo (1979). *S.E. Asian J. Trop. Med. Publ. Hlth* **10,** 149.

Stirewalt, M. A. (1973). In *Epidemiology and Control of Schistosomiasis*, p. 17. Ed. N. Ansari. World Health Organization/University Park Press, Baltimore, London, Tokyo.

Sulit, Y. S. M., Domingo, E. O., Dalmacio-Guz, A. E., de Peralta, D. S. and Imperial, E. S. (1964). *J. Philipp. Med. Ass.* **40,** 1021.

Ts'ai, Ch'un and Yu, Wei (1966). *Chinese Med. J.* **85,** 183.

Tsutsumi, H. and Hasuda, A. (1964). *Kurume Med. J.* **11,** 80.

Tsutsumi, H., Wantanbe, A. and Nakashima, T. (1963). *Kurume Med. J.* **10,** 269.

Warren, K. S. (1969). *Gastroenterology* **57,** 697.

Warren, K. S., Boros, D. L., Hang, L. M. and Mahmoud, A. A. F. (1975). *Am. J. Path.* **80,** 279.

Warren, K. S. and Domingo, E. O. (1970). *Am. J. Trop. Med. Hyg.* **19,** 292.

Warren, K. S. and Moore, D. E. (1966). *Am. J. Trop. Med. Hyg.* **15,** 22.

Westermeyer, J. (1978). *J. Am. Med. Ass.* **240,** 2152.

Wistar, R., Murrel, K. D., Lewert, R. M., Yogore, M. C., Cole, C. and Clutter, W. G. (1975). *Am. J. Trop. Med. Hyg.* **24,** 632.

WHO Workshop (1980). *Bull. Wld Hlth Org.* **58,** 513.

Yasuraoka, K. (1970). In *Recent Advances in Researches on Filariasis and Schistosomiasis in Japan*, p. 291. Ed. M. Sasa. University Park Press, Baltimore, and Manchester.

Yogore, M. G. and Lewert, R. M. (1974). *Am. J. Trop. Med. Hyg.* **23,** 393.

Yoshizumi, Y. and Ota, T. (1957). *Jap. J. Parasit.* **6,** 261.

7 Immunology

Kenneth S. Warren

The immunology of schistosomiasis can be divided into three major areas: immunity, immunopathology and immunodiagnosis. With respect to immunity in man, although it is probable that under certain circumstances some degree of resistance to re-infection occurs, there is no definitive evidence for its existence. If the presence of immunity is demonstrated, however, it is likely to be only partial and it probably does not play a significant role in controlling the prevalence and intensity of infection. Nevertheless, recent remarkable work has contributed greatly to the elucidation of possible mechanisms of immunity and suggests that effective vaccines might be available in the future (Smithers, 1976). Several years ago, schistosomiasis was claimed to be an immunological disease due to granulomatous hypersensitivity to the parasite eggs (Warren, 1975). More and more evidence has been gathered over the intervening years verifying this hypothesis (Colley, 1977). Furthermore, immunoregulatory mechanisms modulating the disease have been described in experimental animals and man, and several possible mechanisms have been established (Warren, 1974; Pelley and Warren, 1978). Finally, an antigen has been isolated in pure form from the schistosome egg, which may play a major role in the host's immunopathological responses (Pelley *et al.*, 1976). For the last decade, the immunodiagnosis of schistosomiasis has been in a state of decline because of inadequate sensitivity (particularly in children) and lack of specificity (Warren *et al.*, 1973), and because of the development of rapid, simple quantitative parasitological means of diagnosis via egg counts. Recently, however, the utilisation of new technology, such as the ELISA test (McLaren *et al.*, 1978) and automated radio-immunoassay (Pelley *et al.*, 1977), and of purified antigens has greatly improved the immunodiagnosis of schistosomiasis.

IMMUNITY

To begin to understand the unique aspects of immunity in schistosomiasis, it must clearly be realised that schistosomes, as with the vast majority of other helminths, do not replicate within the definitive human host. The worms have a finite life span which, as in the case of *S. haematobium* (Wilkins and Capron, 1977), may be less than one year, and in *S. mansoni* averages well less than 10 years (Warren *et al.*, 1974). Worm burdens are dependent upon the degree of exposure to contaminated waters, and they follow an over-dispersed distribution in populations in which only a small proportion of individuals are heavily infected (Warren, 1973). The latter appear to be those in which morbidity and mortality tend to occur.

The recent burgeoning in knowledge of the ecology of schistosomiasis suggests that the degree of exposure to contaminated water is probably the major factor controlling the prevalence and intensity of this infection (Dalton and Pole, 1978). The statement, made only about 17 years ago, that man survives 'under conditions of constant re-exposure such as those experienced by the Egyptian felaheen and rice farmers of the Orient who have been in almost daily contact with cercaria-containing waters since childhood'—as quoted in Warren (1973)—is no longer tenable. We now know that the percentage of infected snails in most environments is exceedingly low (although the total snail populations have not been established), that cercarial output is intermittent on a daily basis and is usually seasonal, that the cercariae are usually widely dispersed in large volumes or in rapidly moving water, that contact with contaminated water in time and space is often circumscribed and is dependent on age, sex and occupation, and that the life span of the worms is much shorter than was originally believed (Warren, 1973).

Other factors that must be taken into consideration in the survival of populations in endemic areas include the presence of innate immunity (i.e. that only a relatively small proportion of an infecting inoculum of cercariae will develop into adult worms), the possible occurrence of non-specific immunity (e.g. in patients with tuberculosis), the development of only partial degrees of specific immunity (as demonstrated in many experimental animals), and the occurrence of immunoregulatory phenomena that suppress immunopathology and hence disease.

Several direct attempts have been made to prove the presence of immunity in man, and these have been discussed in detail elsewhere (Warren, 1973). In summary, a study done in 1934 on six fishermen in the Belgian Congo involved *Schistosoma intercalatum* (Fisher, 1934). Another report from Ghana in 1963 involved a single individual exposed repeatedly to unidentified cercariae shed by naturally infected snails (Gothe, 1963). The third, from Zimbabwe, involved two volunteers exposed to cercariae which were probably *S. mattheei*, a schistosome of cattle and sheep (Clarke, 1966). More recently, a series of passive transfer studies was performed in children with *S. mansoni* infections in St Lucia. These studies included the therapeutic effect of large doses of hyperimmune anti-schistosome serum given to children with moderate infections (Warren *et al.*, 1972), the preventive effect of repeated doses of such antiserum administered to uninfected young children in an area of high incidence (Cook *et al.*, 1972), and the injection of 'transfer factor' (to induce cell-mediated immunity) from infected, constantly exposed field workers into moderately infected children (Warren, Cook *et al.*, 1975). None of these measures had any effect on infection in the treated children. Epidemiological experiments have claimed to demonstrate immunity (Bradley and McCullough, 1973), but they are difficult to perform rigorously, and their results are open to alternative explanations (Jordan *et al.*, 1974).

Many studies of immunity to schistosomes have been performed in experimental and domestic animals.* Most laboratory animals, whether rodents or primates, are highly resistant to *S. haematobium*; in contrast, many experimental, domestic and wild animals are susceptible to *S. japonicum. S. mansoni* falls somewhere in between, and this is the organism that has been studied most extensively. Basically, four different states of immunity occur to *S. mansoni*. It is virtually impossible to infect some animals, including primitive primates, with this organism (Sadun *et al.*, 1966; Warren and Jane, 1967). Some rodents and primates develop partial immunity after relatively prolonged

---

* Partial resistance has been stimulated against *S. bovis* in cattle in field conditions in the Sudan. Single intramuscular injections of 10 000 3 Krad irradiated schistosomula led to worm burdens and tissue egg loads being more than 60% lower than in unprotected animals; protection lasted 40 weeks and improved body weights were recorded (Majid *et al.*, 1980). Some control of this economically important parasite might become possible and, although a live vaccine is at present required, irradiated schistosomules can be cryopreserved in an effective form in liquid nitrogen (Bickle and James, 1978)—Jordan and Webbe.

periods of infection (mice, baboons). Some few species undergo a self-cure phenomenon, followed by virtually complete immunity (rats, rhesus monkeys), and no resistance to re-infection has been demonstrated in either vervet monkeys or chimpanzees. It is worthy of note that even in the best hosts a significant proportion of infected organisms do not develop into adult worms. Thus, varying degrees of innate immunity have been described, as well as acquired immunity of two different types—one involving self-cure and virtually complete resistance to re-infection and the other partial resistance to re-infection. No evidence has ever been gathered that a self-cure phenomenon occurs in man, and there certainly does not appear to be complete immunity to re-infection.

The phenomenon of 'concomitant immunity' explains why partial immunity exists to new parasites while the adult worms within the body are unaffected. This has been elegantly studied both *in vivo*, by transferring adult worms to different hosts (Smithers and Terry, 1967), and *in vitro* (Smithers, 1976). Within a few days after penetration, the young schistosomes acquire host antigens on their surface—these include red cell and histocompatibility antigens. These host antigens effectively disguise the parasite as a foreign organism and prevent any immune attack on it.

A key technique in the establishment of the state of immunity in living animals is the use of passive transfer with either cells or serum from infected animals. Extensive studies in rats have revealed a complex series of responses, beginning with transfer of immunity with cells, succeeded by transfer of immunity with serum, and then followed by disappearance of both cellular and humoral immunity (Phillips *et al.*, 1977). The extensively studied partial immunity which occurs in mice has been transferred only with serum (Sher *et al.*, 1975). *In-vivo* studies of this phenomenon in mice have demonstrated two different and separable components: (i) a form of antibody-dependent cellular cytotoxicity, in which the killer cell is the eosinophil (anti-eosinophil serum abrogates immunity, but anti-neutrophil, lymphocyte and macrophage sera do not (Mahmoud *et al.*, 1975); (ii) a much less potent but significant form of antibody-dependent complement-mediated killing has been demonstrated via the use of diffusion chambers and cobra venom factor—a potent inhibitor of complement (Kassis *et al.*, 1979).

In recent years, a series of *in-vitro* systems of immunity has been established. These elegant systems involve the mixing of schistosomula with cells and sera obtained from rodents (mice and rats), primates (baboons), and man. Using this technique, a plethora of immunological mechanisms has been established, including lethal antibody (Smithers, 1976); antibody-dependent cellular cytotoxicity involving neutrophils (Dean *et al.*, 1974) or eosinophils (Butterworth *et al.*, 1975), complement-dependent cellular cytotoxicity (Ramalho-Pinto *et al.*, 1978), and IgE cytophilic antibody on macrophages (Capron *et al.*, 1975). The only systems confirmed *in vivo* are those mentioned above involving antibody-dependent eosinophil and complement-mediated killing. It is worthy of note that innate immunity has recently been demonstrated in that peripheral monocytes obtained from uninfected humans will kill a small proportion of schistosomula *in vitro* (Ellner and Mahmoud, 1979).

Non-specific acquired resistance to schistosomiasis has been studied both *in vitro* and *in vivo* in both rodents (Civil *et al.*, 1978; Maddison *et al.*, 1978) and primates (Maddison *et al.*, 1978). These systems involve activators of the mononuclear phagocyte system, such as BCG (Civil *et al.*, 1978; Maddison *et al.*, 1978), *Corynebacterium parvum* (Mahmoud *et al.*, 1979), and chemical adjuvants, such as trehalose dimycolate and dipalmitate (Olds *et al.*, 1980). Peritoneal macrophages obtained from animals treated with *C. parvum* kill schistosomula *in vitro* by the release of toxic substances into the supernatant (Mahmoud *et al.*, 1979).

IMMUNOPATHOLOGY

The pathogenesis of many of the relatively minor disease syndromes associated with schistosomiasis has both proven and putative immunological associations. The earliest of these is schistosome dermatitis (or swimmer's itch) which is a transient pruritic, papular rash occurring most frequently in insusceptible definitive hosts after penetration of cercariae and their death in the skin. This leads to relatively specific sensitisation (Olivier, 1949), and biopsy evidence in man and studies in experimental animals suggest hypersensitivity reactions of both the immediate and delayed types (Colley *et al.*, 1972). In a small proportion of infected individuals, a syndrome known as acute schistosomiasis may be seen; it consists of fever, eosinophilia, splenomegaly, lymphadenopathy and urticaria and is usually found in primary infections (Warren, 1971). Heavy infection may not be a necessary concomitant, and it is possible that the syndrome may begin prior to the onset of egg laying (Hiatt *et al.*, 1979). This reaction has been postulated to be a form of serum sickness due to immune complexes (Warren, 1971). Another form of immune complex disease—glomerulonephritis—has been reported to occur in patients with schistosomiasis mansoni (Andrade *et al.*, 1971), and IgG and IgM complexes have been observed in kidney biopsies (Silva *et al.*, 1970). Studies in experimental animals have shown the presence of glomerulopathy, and its mechanisms are now being explored. The clinical significance of these findings is not known.

Over the past 15 years, however, it has been clearly shown that the major disease syndromes of schistosomiasis—hepato-splenic and obstructive urinary tract disease—are due to hyper-sensitivity reactions of the host to the schistosome eggs trapped in the tissues. Although both Bilharz (1856) and Symmers (1904) explicitly stated that the schistosome eggs were the cause of the inflammation and fibrosis of hepatic and urinary schis-tosomiasis, it was not until animal models of the respective disease syndromes were developed in rodents (Warren and De Witt, 1958) and primates (Sadun *et al.*, 1970) in the last two decades that the eggs were definitively shown to be the cause of the disease syndromes. This was most clearly demonstrated in a mouse model of hepatosplenic disease in which the host–parasite relationship was manipulated to eliminate the theories of disease caused by toxin secretion by the worms and dead adult worms. Only when egg production was present did hepatomegaly, splenomegaly, portal hypertension and oesophageal varices occur in the mouse (Warren, 1961).

The essential role of the host granulomatous inflammatory response to the eggs in obstruction to portal blood flow within the liver was then demonstrated by microcirculation studies in living mice (Bloch *et al.*, 1972). In the early stages of infection, eggs impacted in the portal venules often did not completely occlude the circulation and had no effect on the surrounding blood vessels. When the large avascular granulomas formed around the eggs, however, not only was local blood flow completely blocked, but a large surrounding area was destroyed. Later, a fibrous scar formed and new blood vessels developed, all of which were arterial. Thus, obstruction to portal blood flow by granulomatous inflammation and fibrosis eventually leads to the syndrome of portal hypertension, congestive splenomegaly, and portal–systemic collateral circulation. Arterialisation of the liver through neovascular formation in the fibrous tissue maintains total liver blood flow within normal limits, leading to adequate perfusion of the liver parenchymal cells and the good liver function associated with the classical hepatosplenic syndrome. Plastic cast studies in cadavers have demonstrated arterialisation of the liver in man (Andrade and Cheever, 1971).

Investigations of the immunological aetiology of the schistosome egg granuloma were greatly facilitated by the development of a technique in which eggs isolated from the livers of infected animals were injected intravenously into tail veins of mice, dispersing the eggs throughout the pulmonary microvasculature (von Lichtenberg, 1962). The key experiments revealed that secondary exposure to schistosome eggs (following primary exposure by intraperitoneal injection of eggs) resulted in marked anamestic reactivity—greatly accelerated and augmented granuloma formation (Warren *et al.*, 1967). This reactivity was shown to be specific (there was no cross-reactivity with *Ascaris* eggs) and transferable with lymph node and spleen cells, but not with serum (Warren *et al.*, 1967). Complete specificity was subsequently demonstrated with *S. japonicum* eggs, but there was partial cross-reactivity with *S. haematobium* eggs (Warren and Domingo, 1970). Studies using the same methodology have demonstrated that the granulomatous inflammation around *S. haematobium* eggs shows similar specificity and is again transferable with cells, but not with serum (Kassis *et al.*, 1978). Interestingly enough, the response to *S. japonicum* eggs appears to be different: histologically, *S. japonicum* eggs are found in aggregates in the tissues, large eosinophilic abscesses form in the early lesions, and many plasma cells are seen. Granulomatous activity is exceedingly meagre around single eggs injected into the pulmonary microvasculature, even in naturally infected animals (Warren, Boros *et al.*, 1975). Furthermore, in early natural infections and following sensitisation with soluble egg antigens, only immediate footpad swelling occurs in *S. japonicum*-infected mice, while only delayed footpad swelling occurs in *S. mansoni-* and *S. haematobium*-sensitised mice (Warren *et al.*, 1978). Thus, the *S. mansoni* and *S. haematobium* egg granulomas seem to be largely immunological reactions of the cell-mediated type, but the aetiology of the *S. japonicum* reaction remains unclear, although there are some indications that antibody-mediated inflammatory responses may be occurring in this lesion.

Extensive studies of the effects of immunosuppressive measures on the *S. mansoni* granuloma strongly support the belief that this lesion is essentially a cell-mediated immunological reaction. Conditions which suppress cell-mediated hypersensitivity—niridazole, cholera toxin, anti-lymphocyte serum, neonatal thymectomy (in mice and chickens), diabetes, Hodgkin's disease (SJL/J mice) and nude mice—strongly inhibited granuloma formation (Warren, 1978). Further evidence supporting the cell-mediated aetiology of the *S. mansoni* egg granuloma and illuminating its mechanism is provided by a series of experiments in which intact granulomas were isolated from the livers of infected animals and maintained *in vitro* (Boros *et al.*, 1973). Both in the presence and absence of added soluble egg antigens the granulomas have been shown to emit the lymphokines, macrophage migration inhibitory factor (Boros *et al.*, 1973) and eosinophil stimulation promotor (James and Colley, 1975). The lesions contain lymphocytes at their earliest stages, and it is probable that secretion of the above lymphokines and others attract or maintain *in situ* the principle cells of the lesions—macrophages and eosinophils. Recent studies using the incorporation of radiolabelled leucine have shown production of proteins by the granulomas *in vitro*, but column purification has revealed that these are not immunoglobulins (Pelley, R. P., personal communication). Finally, an intriguing series of experiments is being performed on the complete formation of granulomas *in vitro* following the addition of leucocytes and eggs (Doughty and Phillips, 1982).

The above findings reveal, therefore, that the schistosome egg is the parasite factor responsible for schistosomal disease, but that the host granulomatous reaction to the eggs is a major factor in the pathogenesis of schistosomiasis. As the granulomas have been shown to be immunological reactions, the chronic syndromes of schistosomiasis are perforce immunological diseases. Another interesting aspect of the host response is the demonstration *in vitro* that the egg is destroyed by eosinophils (James and Colley, 1976). Recent studies *in vivo* have revealed that elimination of eosinophils via anti-eosinophil serum results in the accumulation of large numbers of eggs which, with the addition of the reactions around them, results in increased morbidity and mortality (Olds and Mahmoud, 1980).

In order to carry our knowledge of these diseases to the molecular level, it is necessary to isolate and characterise the antigen or antigens from the eggs which are responsible for the granulomatous hypersensitivity. There is now strong evidence that this has been achieved for the *S. mansoni* egg granuloma. Soluble egg antigens (SEA) produced by homogenisation and ultracentrifugation of the eggs have been shown both to induce (by intraperitoneal injection followed by intravenous injection of eggs) and to elicit (by binding to bentonite particles and intravenous injection) granulomatous hypersensitivity (Boros and Warren, 1970). Using serum from chronically infected animals, SEA has been shown to contain three major serological antigens (Pelley *et al.*, 1976). These antigens have each been isolated in pure form from SEA by desalting on Sephadex G25, affinity chromatography on concanavalin A-Sepharose and ion-exchange chromatography on DEAE cellulose. Major serological antigen$_1$ (MSA$_1$), a glycoprotein of molecular weight 50 000, is the most abundant of the three antigens. This antigen seems to be involved in granuloma formation on the basis of the following evidence: (i) radioimmunoassay using ^{131}I-labelled, purified antigen and inhibition with crude SEA has shown that MSA$_1$ has the same stage and species specific characteristics as intact *S. mansoni* eggs in the induction of granulomatous hypersensitivity (Hamburger *et al.*, 1976); (ii) intraperitoneal injection of antigen–antibody complexes prepared from chronic infection serum and purified MSA$_1$ has resulted in marked sensitisation to subsequent egg injection (Pelley and Pelley, 1976); (iii) the Con A-Sepharose eluate induced by alpha-methyl mannoside, which was rich in MSA$_1$, was markedly more sensitising than crude SEA, while the column drop-through was non-sensitising (Pelley and Pelley, 1976).

The availability of a major granuloma-inducing antigen raises the question of its possible use for the good of the host. This becomes feasible in view of the occurrence of modulation of granulomatous hypersensitivity in chronic schistosomiasis (Warren, 1974; Pelley and Warren, 1978). Thus, granuloma formation reaches its maximal size several weeks after the onset of egg laying, thereafter getting smaller and smaller around eggs newly deposited in the tissues. This phenomenon, originally called endogenous desensitisation (Domingo and Warren, 1968), has been demonstrated in experimental animals to be due largely to suppressor cells (Colley, 1976) but also to antibody (Pelley and Warren, 1978). Such a state has also been found in man and the mechanisms appear to be similar (Colley *et al.*,

1977; Rocklin *et al.*, 1977). Thus, administration of the granuloma-inducing antigen by different routes, in different quantities, and/or with different types of adjuvants may induce the suppressor responses and thereby prevent disease.

IMMUNODIAGNOSIS

Schistosomiasis is usually diagnosed by parasitological means, i.e. the detection of schistosome eggs in the excreta of the host. Because of the highly distinctive appearance of the eggs, these tests are totally specific; counting of eggs in known volumes of excreta also provides quantitative data relating quite well to worm burdens. Recently, parasitological means of diagnosis have been greatly improved in terms of simplicity and rapidity (Peters *et al.*, 1976 and 1980). Thus, aside from fastidiousness, immunological means of diagnosis must either equal or better parasitological means to be worthy of widespread utilisation.

Since 1919, when Fairley described a complement fixation test, and 1927 when he reported an intradermal test (Fairley and Williams, 1927), a wide variety of antigens, including infected snail tissues and *Fasciola hepatica*, as well as crude extracts of worms, cercariae and eggs have been used. The skin tests are really not acceptable in terms of sensitivity and specificity, as clearly shown in studies in St Lucia (Warren *et al.*, 1973), Uganda (Morierty and Lewert, 1974), and Puerto Rico (Hiatt *et al.*, 1978). A vast number of methods of detecting antibodies, from complement fixation to a variety of flocculation tests to chemical methods (enzyme-linked immunosorbent assay, ELISA) and physical methods (fluorescent dye, radio-isotope), have been used. Generally, these techniques have shown inadequate sensitivity, particularly in children, and a lack of specificity, cross-reacting with a wide variety of helminths as well as some other organisms (Warren *et al.*, 1973). In virtually all cases, attempts to increase sensitivity result in decreased specificity. It clearly stands to reason that a crude mixture of many different antigens might suffer from these problems, inhibiting the sensitivity of some antigens and containing cross-reacting antigens which decrease the specificity. Thus, increasing the sophistication and sensitivity of the detection procedures will not necessarily make them more specific.

Recently, several antigens have been isolated from schistosomes in a highly purified state. One of these is a negatively charged polysaccharide excreted from the gut of the adult schistosomes (Nash, 1977), which has been detected as a circulating antigen in heavily infected animals and people. Detection of a circulating antigen, while it may provide a high degree of specificity, has not as yet proven to be a sensitive enough method for general use. This antigen has recently been described in an ELISA test for detecting antibodies (Kelsoe and Weller, 1978). Other purified antigens are a globinase (Senft *et al.*, 1979) from worms, and two glycoproteins and one protein from eggs (Pelley and Pelley, 1976). While it may seem that the availability of purified antigens should result in highly specific and sensitive tests, this is not necessarily so. For instance, an antigen has been isolated from *Fasciola hepatica* which completely cross-reacts with an antigen in schistosome eggs (Pelley and Hillyer, 1978).

Nevertheless, one of the glycoprotein antigens isolated from schistosome eggs mentioned above (MSA_1) has been developed into an unusually sensitive and specific radio-immunoassay (Pelley *et al.*, 1977). With respect to specificity, the antigen does not cross-react with sera from patients with any other known infections, including the helminths. In the case of the different species of schistosomes, a quantitative variant of the test can distinguish among *S. mansoni*, *S. haematobium* and *S. japonicum*, the former producing a greater binding of antigen at comparable levels of infection. Initial reports showed 100% positivity in infected patients of all age groups in a heavily parasitised area of Kenya. In St Lucia, where infections were milder, 64% of infected children, 83% of adolescents and 98% of adults were positive. Specificity using a matching population on the adjacent uninfected island of St Vincent was 100% (Pelley *et al.*, 1977). Follow-up studies on St Lucia, using a finger-prick filter-paper blood sample, showed improved sensitivity, with 92% of children, 100% of adolescents and 91% of adults positive. All those with egg counts greater than 20/g were positive (Pelley, R. P., personal communication). Comparison on St Lucia of the radio-immunoassay with two parasitological methods (Kato and Bell) and the ELISA test revealed the greatest reliability in the radio-immunoassay and the Kato (Long *et al.*, 1981). Comparison tests in Puerto Rico revealed that the MSA_1 radio-immunoassay had a sensitivity of 95%, with 100% of those with egg counts greater than 10/g being positive. Specificity in this endemic area was listed as 79%, but this could be due to the presence of exceedingly light infections or persistent low levels of antibodies following cure (Hillyer *et al.*, 1979). Although the initial cost of equipment is high, the radio-immunoassay has been working satisfactorily in St Lucia, and a single technician can process 200 samples per day. Its exceedingly high sensitivity makes it particularly useful for post-control monitoring of infection.

Thus, it cannot be over-emphasised that while modern technology may enable the development of simpler, cheaper and more rapid serological tests, the development of a truly useful test will be dependent upon the isolation and production of certain purified antigens via the most modern techniques of biology: immunochemistry, hybridomas and perhaps even recombinant DNA. If the antigens can be obtained in sufficient quantity, the use of high technology systems such as radio-immunoassay can be superseded by simpler techniques, which can be utilised in the field (see also Chapter 10).

REFERENCES

Andrade, Z. A. and Cheever, A. W. (1971). *Am. J. Trop. Med. Hyg.* **20,** 425.

Andrade, Z. A., Andrade, S. G. and Sadigursky, M. (1971). *Am. J. Trop. Med. Hyg.* **20, 77.**

Bickle, Q. D. and James, E. R. (1978). *Trans. R. Soc. Trop. Med. Hyg.* **72,** 677.

Bilharz, T. (1856). *Win. Med. Wochenschr.* **6,** 49.

Bloch, E. H., Abdel-Wahab, M. F. and Warren, K. S. (1972). *Am. J. Trop. Med. Hyg.* **21,** 546.

Boros, D. L. and Warren, K. S. (1970). *J. Expl. Med.* **132,** 488.

Boros, D. L., Warren, K. S. and Pelley, R. P. (1973). *Nature* **245,** 224.

Bradley, D. J. and McCullough, F. S. (1973). *Trans. R. Soc. Trop. Med. Hyg.* **67,** 491.

Butterworth, A. E., Sturrock, R. F., Houba, V., Mahmoud, A. A. F., Sher, A. and Rees, P. H. (1975). *Nature* **256,** 727.

Capron, A., Dessaint, J. P. and Capron, M. (1975). *Nature* **253,** 474.

Civil, R. H., Warren, K. S. and Mahmoud, A. A. F. (1978). *J. Infect. Dis.* **137,** 550.

Clarke, V. de V. (1966). *Cent. Afr. J. Med.* **12,** 1.

Colley, D. G. (1976). *J. Expl. Med.* **143,** 696.

Colley, D. G. (1977). In *Recent Advances in Clinical Immunology*, p. 101. Ed. R. A. Thompson. Churchill Livingstone, Edinburgh, London and New York.

Colley, D. G., Heiny, S. E., Bartholmew, R. K. and Cook, J. A. (1977). *Am. J. Trop. Med. Hyg.* **26,** 917.

Colley, D. G., Magalhaes-Filho, A. and Coelho, R. B. (1972). *Am. J. Trop. Med. Hyg.* **21,** 558.

Cook, J. A., Warren, K. S. and Jordan, P. (1972). *Trans. R. Soc. Trop. Med. Hyg.* **66,** 777.

Dalton, P. R. and Pole, D. (1978). *Bull. Wld Hlth Org.* **563,** 417.

Dean, D. A., Wistar, R. and Murrell, K. D. (1974). *Am. J. Trop. Med. Hyg.* **23,** 420.

Domingo, E. O. and Warren, K. S. (1968). *Am. J. Path.* **52,** 369.

Doughty, B. L. and Phillips, M. S. (1982). *J. Immunol.* **128,** 30.

Ellner, J. L. and Mahmoud, A. A. F. (1979). *J. Immunol.* **123,** 949.

Fairley, N. J. (1919). *J. Roy. Army Med. Corps* **32,** 449.

Fairley, N. J. and Williams, F. F. (1927). *Med. J. Aust.* **2,** 818.

Fisher, A. C. (1934). *Trans. R. Soc. Trop. Med. Hyg.* **28,** 277.

Gothe, K. M. (1963). *Tropenmed. Parasit.* **14,** 512.

Hamburger, J., Pelley, R. P. and Warren, K. S. (1976). *J. Immunol.* **117,** 1561.

Hiatt, R. A., Barnett, L. C. and Knight, W. B. (1978). *Am. J. Trop. Med. Hyg.* **27,** 535.

Hiatt, R. A., Sotomayor, Z. R., Sanchez, G., Zambrano, M. and Knight, W. B. (1979). *J. Inf. Dis.* **139,** 659.

Hillyer, G. V., Ruiz Tiben, E., Knight, W. B., Gomez de Rios, I. and Pelley, R. P. (1979). *Am. J. Trop. Med. Hyg.* **28,** 661.

James, S. L. and Colley, D. G. (1975). *J. Reticuloendothel. Soc.* **18,** 283.

James, S. L. and Colley, D. G. (1976). *J. Reticuloendothel. Soc.* **20,** 359.

Jordan, P., Cook, J. A. and Davis, A. (1974). *Trans. R. Soc. Trop. Med. Hyg.* **68,** 340.

Kassis, A. I., Warren, K. S. and Mahmoud, A. A. F. (1978). *Cell Immunol.* **38,** 310.

Kassis, A. I., Warren, K. S. and Mahmoud, A. A. F. (1979). *J. Immunol.* **123,** 1659.

Kelsoe, G. H. and Weller, T. H. (1978). *Proc. Natl. Acad. Sci. U.S.A.* **75,** 5715.

Lichtenberg, F. von (1962). *Am. J. Path.* **41,** 711.

Long, E. G., McLaren, M. L., Goddard, M. J., Bartholomew, R. K., Peters, P. and Goodgame, R. (1981). *Trans. R. Soc. Trop. Med. Hyg.* **75,** 365.

McLaren, M., Draper, C. C., Roberts, J. M., Minter-Goedbloed, E., Ligthart, G. S., Teesdale, C. H., Amin, M. A., Omer, A. H. S., Bartlett, A. and Voller, A. (1978). *Ann. Trop. Med. Parasit.* **72,** 243.

Maddison, E. S., Chandler, R. W. and Kagan, I. G. (1978). *J. Reticuloendothel. Soc.* **24,** 615.

Mahmoud, A. A. F., Peters, P. A., Civil, R. H. and Remington, J. S. (1979). *J. Immunol.* **122,** 1655.

Mahmoud, A. A. F., Warren, K. S. and Peters, P. A. (1975). *J. Expl. Med.* **142,** 805.

Majid, A. A., Bushara, H. O., Saad, A. M., Hussein, M. F., Taylor, M. G., Dargie, J. D., Marshall, T. F. de C. and Nelson, G. S. (1980). *Am. J. Trop. Med. Hyg.* **29,** 452.

Morierty, P. I. and Lewert, R. M. (1974). *Am. J. Trop. Med. Hyg.* **23,** 169.

Nash, T. R. (1977). *J. Immunol.* **119,** 1627.

Olds, G. R., Chedid, C., Lederer, R. and Mahmoud, A. A. F. (1980). *J. Infect. Dis.* **141,** 473.

Olds, G. R. and Mahmoud, A. A. F. (1980). *J. Clin. Invest.,* **66,** 1191.

Olivier, L. (1949). *Am. J. Hyg.* **49,** 490.

Pelley, R. P. and Pelley, R. J. (1976). In *Biochemistry of Parasites and Host-parasite Relationships*, p. 283. Ed. H. van den Bossche. Elsevier/North Holland Biomedical Press, Amsterdam.

Pelley, R. P., Pelley, R. J., Hamburger, J., Peters, P. A. and Warren, K. S. (1976). *J. Immunol.* **117,** 1553.

Pelley, R. P. and Warren, K. S. (1978). *J. Invest. Dermatol.* **71,** 49.

Pelley, R. P., Warren, K. S. and Jordan, P. (1977). *Lancet* **ii,** 781.

Peters, P. A., El Alamy, M., Warren, K. S. and Mahmoud, A. D. F. (1980). *Am, J. Trop. Med. Hyg.* **29,** 217.

Peters, P. A., Mahmoud, A. A. F., Warren, K. S., Ouma, J. H. and Siongok, T. K. A. (1976). *Bull. Wld Hlth Org.* **54,** 159.

Phillips, S. M., Reid, W. A., Khoury, P. B. and Doughty, B. L. (1977). *Am. J. Trop. Med. Hyg.* **26,** 48.

Ramalho-Pinto, F. J., McLaren, D. O. and Smithers, S. R. (1978). *J. Expl. Med.* **147,** 147.

Rocklin, R. E., Brown, A. P., Warren, K. S., Pelley, R. P., Houba, V. Siongok, T. K. A., Ouma, J., Sturrock, R. F. and Butterworth, A. E. (1980). *J. Immunol.* **125,** 1916.

Sadun, E. H., von Lichtenberg, F. and Bruce, J. I. (1966). *Am. J. Trop. Med. Hyg.* **15,** 705.

Sadun, D. H., von Lichtenberg, F., Cheever, A. W. and Erickson, D. G. (1970). *Am. J. Trop. Med. Hyg.* **19,** 258.

Senft, A. W., Weltman, J. K., Godgraber, M. B., Egyud, L. G. and Kuntz, R. E. (1979). *Parasite Immunol.* **1,** 79.

Sher, A., Smithers, S. R. and MacKenzie, P. (1975). *Parasitology* **70,** 347.

Silva, L. C., Brito, T. de, Camargo, M. E., DeBoni, D. R., Lopes, L. D. and Gunji, J. (1970). *Bull. Wld Hlth Org.* **42,** 907.

Smithers, S. R. (1976). *Adv. Parasit.* **14,** 399.

Smithers, S. R. and Terry, R. J. (1967). *Trans. R. Soc. Trop. Med. Hyg.* **61,** 517.

Symmers, W. St. C. (1904). *J. Path. Bact.* **9,** 237.

Warren, K. S. (1961). *Am. J. Trop. Med. Hyg.* **10,** 870.

Warren, K. S. (1971). In *Immunological Disease*, 2nd edn., p. 668. Ed. M. Samter. Little, Brown & Company, Boston.

Warren, K. S. (1973). *J. Infect. Dis.* **127,** 595.

Warren, K. S. (1974). In *Parasites in the Immunized Host: Mechanisms of Survival*, p. 234. Ciba Foundation Symposium, 25. Ed. by Ruth Porter and Julie Knight. Elsevier Excerpta Medica, North Holland.

Warren, K. S. (1975). *Bull. N.Y. Acad. Med.* **51,** 545.

Warren, K. S. (1978). *Nature* **273,** 609.

Warren, K. S., Boros, D. L., Hang, L. M. and Mahmoud, A. A. F. (1975). *Am. J. Path.* **80,** 279.

Warren, K. S., Cook, J. A., David, J. R. and Jordan, P. (1975). *Trans. R. Soc. Trop. Med. Hyg.* **69,** 488.

Warren, K. S., Cook, J. A. and Jordan, P. (1972). *Trans. R. Soc. Trop. Med. Hyg.* **66,** 65.

Warren, K. S. and De Witt, W. B. (1958). *Proc. Soc. Exp. Biol. Med.* **98,** 99.

Warren, K. S. and Domingo, E. O. (1970). *Am. J. Trop. Med. Hyg.* **19,** 292.

Warren, K. S., Domingo, E. O. and Cowan, R. B. T. (1967). *Am. J. Path.* **51,** 735.

Warren, K. S., Grove, D. I. and Pelley, R. P. (1978). *Am. J. Trop. Med. Hyg.* **27,** 271.

Warren, K. S. and Jane, J. A. (1967). *Trans. R. Soc. Trop. Med. Hyg.* **61,** 534.

Warren, K. S., Kellermeyer, R. W., Jordan, P., Littell, A. S., Cook, J. A. and Kagan, I. G. (1973). *Am. J. Trop. Med. Hyg.* **22,** 189.

Warren, K. S., Mahmoud, A. A. F., Cummings, P., Murphy, D. J. and
    Houser, H. B. (1974). *Am. J. Trop. Med. Hyg.* **23,** 902.
Wilkins, H. A. and Capron, A. (1977). *Ann. Trop. Med. Parasit.* **71,** 187.

8 Diagnostic and Laboratory Techniques

Peter Jordan (with assistance from Michael Goddard)

Methods of diagnosis can be parasitological or immunological. Parasitological techniques are necessary for providing a definitive diagnosis of an active infection: schistosome ova are demonstrated in urine or stools, less frequently in tissues; rarely, diagnosis may be made by finding adult worms in histological sections.

Qualitative techniques for detection of ova are used in clinical practice. Quantitative techniques are used mainly for research in the fields of epidemiology, control, clinicopathology and drug trials. In general, they require more equipment than do qualitative procedures, and those suitable for large-scale epidemiologic investigations are of comparatively recent design. Sensitivity of the methods vary and while there are pleas for standardisation of techniques in investigations in different (research) institutions, the one most suited to the requirements of a particular area will inevitably continue to be used.

In epidemiological studies (including evaluation of control), where many thousands of specimens are to be examined by semi-skilled workers, high standards of microscopy must be maintained. Quality control is important in any technique used, and becomes of particular importance with effective transmission control or in drug trials when infections may be only infrequently found. Microscopists lose interest if specimens are monotonously negative.

PARASITOLOGICAL TECHNIQUES

The type of container provided for samples of urine or stool, particularly if these are for epidemiological studies, is important. Containers must be large enough to hold adequate-sized samples and for identification marks (names or numbers or both) to be clearly written on them. For collecting urine specimens (particularly from women), it is essential that containers have a wide opening—plastic bags were used successfully in the control scheme on Lake Volta.

In quantitative studies, a scribed glass disc (graticule) inserted into the microscope eyepiece facilitates precise vertical positioning of the slide when scanning, and ensures accurate coverage of the preparation. A hand tally counter is essential for egg counting.

S. haematobium

As ova for *S. haematobium* are 'suspended in a liquid in pure culture' (Bradley, 1963), their detection is comparatively simple. The greatest number of eggs is in urines collected around midday (Stimmel and Scott, 1956), when daily variation in egg output is least (Bradley, 1964), or early afternoon (Pugh, 1979). The highest concentration is claimed to be in the terminal part of the stream (Weber *et al.*, 1967). This has been contested and routine examination of terminal specimens may not be justified (Grove, 1970). There is no evidence that exercise will increase egg output (Jordan, 1962).

For qualitative data, the deposit of a centrifuged or sedimented urine can be examined under a low-power microscope objective. Live eggs can be identified in a fresh urine by flame-cell movement in the miracidia. Patients with active infections frequently also excrete calcified or black eggs from the bladder wall, their number depending more on the activity of the infection than the extent of bladder calcification (Cheever *et al.*, 1975). Infrequently, only calcified eggs are found. They are usually smaller than live eggs and have a less distinct spine. Malformed eggs are seen. They may contain some granular material and, while their origin is in doubt, they may be from unfertilised female worms.

For accurate quantitative studies, 24-hour urine samples over a number of days should be collected for examination. If this is not practicable, the bladder should be emptied at 11 a.m. or midday, the urine discarded and at 2 p.m. a specimen collected for examination.

If a known volume of sediment from a measured volume of urine (10 ml) is examined, the number of eggs counted can be related to the total urine volume. Egg output is usually expressed in terms of ova/10 ml urine. This simple method can be adopted to provide information on hatching of ova (Davis, 1968). Urine specimens of 10 ml in graduated centrifuge tubes were centrifuged at 2000 rpm for 3 min; 9 ml of supernatant were pipetted off or removed by Venturi pump, discarded, and 5 ml freshly boiled cooled water added to the sediment. *S. haematobium* ova hatched when the tube was exposed to artificial light (72°F) for 30 min, when 2 ml absolute or methyl alcohol and 7 drops of aqueous eosin were added, and thoroughly mixed; hatched miracidia were simultaneously killed, fixed and stained. After recentrifuging for 3 min the supernatant was removed to the 0·1 ml level; the miracidia and unhatched ova in this remaining volume represent the content of the original 10 ml urine sample. Hatched and unhatched eggs were counted under the 16 mm objective.

Although requiring more equipment, filtration techniques have now largely replaced the above quantitative sedimentation method. In a WHO research project in Ghana, a modification of an earlier technique (Dazo and Biles, 1974) is used (England, personal communication). One part of Ziehl–Nielsen carbol fuchsin solution is added to 100 parts of distilled water. The stain is added to urine (equal volumes of each) and left for three to four days to allow for satisfactory contrast between ova and background. The sample is filtered through filter paper (Whatman No. 1, cut to 47 mm diameter) on a millipore plastic apparatus connected to a hand or electric vacuum pump. After filtration the paper is dried. For examination it is moistened with distilled water. In the Gambia, equal quantities of urine and a solution of eosin 97·5 mg, thiomersal 1·0 g, spirit 500 ml, and 1000 ml distilled water is used (Wilkins, 1977). Staining with ninhydrin is unsatisfactory unless the eggs are dead. Storage of urine with 2% formalin in saline for a day or two before staining has been recommended (Bradley, 1967).

Nucleopore polycarbonate filters are gaining popularity as the technique is rapid, accurate, sensitive and reproducible (Peters *et al.*, 1976 and 1981). Although the original technique used an 8 μm pore size (and 13 mm diameter filter), other workers find the technique improved with the use of 25 mm diameter filters and a 12 or 14 μm pore size (Klumpp, personal communication; Feldmeir *et al.*, 1979). A further modification is the staining of eggs with trypan blue, which differentiates viable and non-viable eggs—staining the latter blue but not staining those that are viable (Feldmeir *et al.*, 1979).

In the Caribbean, 15% of *S. mansoni* patients investigated were found to have low numbers of eggs in their urine (Cook and Jordan, 1970).

S. mansoni

As the concentration of eggs on the surface of a formed stool has been found to be higher than within, examination of scrapings of the outside of the body of a formed stool has been advocated (Blair *et al.*, 1969); other workers found eggs randomly distributed throughout the stool (Martin and Beaver, 1968; Woodstock *et al.*, 1972).

Egg output varies considerably from day to day, but no pattern has been recognised. The use of single stools may result in the failure to detect many light infections and for detailed quantitative studies of individuals a mean of egg output of at least three different stool specimens is calculated. Amongst groups of persons, the mean egg output (from a single stool) gives useful epidemiological data (see Chapter 10).

A simple direct faecal smear will enable moderately and heavily infected persons to be detected but concentration techniques are necessary for detection of light infections—techniques are based on sedimentation or centrifugation; flotation methods are not suitable for schistosome ova.

The sedimentation method is dependable and simple, it requires a minimum of equipment and reagents and is suitable for the field (Hoffman *et al.*, 1934; Barbosa, 1969). Other concentration methods such as the formol-ether (Ritchie, 1948), acid ether (Hunter *et al.*, 1948) and merthiolate–iodine-formaldehyde concentration (MIFC) (Blagg *et al.*, 1955) techniques involve removal of fat, faecal debris and mucus by centrifugation and require more equipment and chemicals. All the original methods have been modified to improve sensitivity but they are generally not suitable for large-scale epidemiological studies, although in Egypt a modification of the formol-ether method is being used in a research scheme. This method is considered to be the most sensitive for the detection of light infections in Puerto Rico, but in spite of this, it was established that about 50% of eggs are lost with egg levels above 100/g (Knight *et al.*, 1976).

The sedimentation technique is frequently recommended for trematode ova; it requires a minimum of reagents but is time consuming. Approximately 10 g of faeces are well mixed with at least 10 times their volume of tap water and the sediment allowed to settle in urinalysis glasses. After an hour, the top part of the supernatant fluid is poured off and the material is resuspended. This is repeated until the supernatant fluid is clear, when the final sediment is examined. The addition of 0·5% glycerol to the tap water improves the yield of eggs.

In the formalin-ether technique, a portion of the stool is homogenised in about 10 ml of saline and the suspension is strained through two layers of wet surgical gauze into a centrifuge tube. After centrifuging, the supernatant fluid is pipetted off and the residue repeatedly resuspended until the supernatant is clear. Finally, the residue is mixed with 10 ml of 4% formaldehyde and allowed to stand for 5 min, 3 ml of ether is added and the mixture capped and shaken vigorously, then centrifuged at 1500 r/min for 2 min. Four layers should be seen—the topmost clear layer of ether with dissolved fats, a plug of faecal debris and fat layer is freed from the side of the tube and carefully decanted. The sediment is placed on a glass slide and examined under the microscope.

In the AMS III method, hydrochloric acid of specific gravity 1·089 is mixed with an equal volume of sodium sulphate of the same specific gravity (916 g of the anhydrous salt in 100 ml water). This mixture is used for emulsifying the faeces. After centrifuging, the supernatant is clear; it is removed and 5 ml of the acid-sulphate mixture, 3 drops of Triton NE (detergent) and 5 ml refrigerated ether are added. The mixture is shaken and centrifuged. The ring on the top of the column is broken and all but the sediment is removed. This is then put onto a slide and examined in the usual way.

In the MIFC method, 2·35 ml of MF solution (200 ml tincture of merthiolate No. 99 Lilly 1:1000, 25 ml formaldehyde, 5 ml glycerol and 250 ml distilled water) are added to 0·15 ml Lugol's iodine and approximately 1 g of faeces is immediately mixed in. The specimen is strained through two layers of surgical gauze into a 15 ml centrifuge tube. Cold ether (4 ml) is added and well shaken for 15 s. After standing for 2 min, centrifuge for 1 min at 1600 r/min. Four layers appear, the sediment contains the eggs and is examined in the usual way. The MIFC method is used extensively in the Philippines for *S. japonicum* investigations.

Two quantitative methods have been introduced in recent years and now have mainly superseded the original Stoll technique, used extensively in Scott's epidemiological studies in Egypt and Venezuela.

The filtration staining method—Bell's technique (Bell, 1963)—was designed for quantitative examination of 24-hour faecal specimens in drug trials, but has been adapted for smaller quantities. A proportion of the eggs is lost in processing; thus, when *S. mansoni* eggs were seeded into negative stools to densities of 560 e/g and 100 e/g respectively, 18·6% and 67·5% were recovered (Katz and Chaia, 1968). This method has been used in epidemiological studies but it is time consuming and needs specially made equipment. The method gave counts of 69%–83% of those obtained with a dilution method (Cheever and Powers, 1968).

The Kato thick smear (Kruatrachue *et al.*, 1964; Komiya and Kobayashi, 1966) was not originally designed for schistosome investigations but has become popular with many workers. As originally described, a 50-mg stool sample was weighed and, if it contained coarse fibres or seeds, it was passed through a 105-mesh sieve before weighing.

The 50-mg sample is placed on a glass slide and covered by a wettable cellophane coverslip soaked for 24 h in a glycerine–malachite green solution (100 ml pure glycerine, 100 ml water, 1 ml% aqueous malachite green). The preparation is inverted and pressed against an absorbent surface until the faecal mass covers an area of 20–25 mm in diameter.

The need to weight accurately the 50-mg stool sample minimised its use in the field. The technique was modified (Katz and Chaia, 1968; Katz *et al.*, 1972); all stools were sieved and, to obviate weighing, sieved stool was level filled into a 6-mm diameter hole in cardboard, the stool 'plug' was then treated as described above. The cardboard was later replaced by a steel template 1 mm thick, with a hole which, when filled, was found to hold approximately 50 mg of sieved stool (Siongok *et al.*, 1976). In addition, the clearing time was extended from 1–2 h to at least 48 h (Warren *et al.*, 1974). Although a 50-mg sample is the standard, some workers consider the resulting preparation to be too thick for accurate reading and use 25 mg (Hiatt, 1976; Hiatt *et al.*, 1976). A 20-mg sample is easier to examine and gives results proportional to the 50-mg smear (Peters *et al.*, 1981).

Using a 50-mg sample, the recovery rate from stools seeded with *S. mansoni* eggs was between 103% and 128%—the increase being due to sieved stool (as opposed to 'whole' stool) being measured for purposes of calculating eggs/g (Katz and

Chaia, 1968). Other workers (Knight *et al.*, 1976) found sieving increased the egg content of unsieved stool by 38%.

Although similar results have been obtained by the Bell and Kato techniques (Martin and Beaver, 1968; Teesdale and Amin, 1976), in a small study in Brazil (Chaia *et al.*, 1968) the Kato (Katz) was found to give 7·1 times the number of eggs detected by the Bell method. In a community study in St Lucia where over 300 infected persons were examined by the two methods (Kato—2 slide preparations, Bell—3 filter papers), the former method gave an overall mean count 8·2 times the Bell count but the ratio varied inversely with the intensity of infection, being 17 with egg counts less than 25 eggs/g (by Bell) and 6·4 with counts greater than 200 eggs/g (Bartholomew *et al.*, 1981). It was suggested that diet could affect results of the Kato technique, owing to variable quantities of fibrous material, seeds etc. being sieved from the stool.

Particularly in drug trials, the hatchability of ova is important. For *S. mansoni* and *S. japonicum* this is not as easily investigated as in *S. haematobium* infections, but in extensive investigations the following technique was used. Approximately 10 g of stool was emulsified in 250 ml water (freshly collected, filtered spring water). The emulsion was passed through a bank of sieves with meshes of 1 mm, 0·250 mm and 0·125 mm respectively. The filtrate was diluted to 1 litre in a measuring cylinder and placed in the dark for 20 min. The sediment 50–100 ml was rewashed or poured into a 1-litre conical side-arm flask. The flask was filled to the top with water and placed immediately below a 20-W bulb to provide illumination and heat; at suitable intervals (up to 26 h), 50 ml surface water were removed through the side-arm; contained miracidia were killed and stained with aqueous iodine and their numbers counted (Upatham *et al.*, 1976).

Whereas all, or a very high proportion of *S. haematobium* eggs hatch rapidly, those of *S. mansoni* hatch more slowly—in the laboratory not all eggs had hatched by the sixth day (Blair *et al.*, 1969) and in semi-field conditions infections in snails were obtained for up to 3 days (Upatham, 1972).

BIOPSY TECHNIQUE

In spite of efforts to devise an efficient concentration technique for *S. mansoni* ova, it is generally found that rectal biopsy is more effective in recovering eggs in light infections (Kruatrachue *et al.*, 1964). Scraping the rectal mucosa with a curette has been considered more effective by some workers (Turner, 1962).

Biopsy specimens of the rectal mucosa are examined under a microscope as a crush preparation between two slides. The addition of a drop of water or saline prior to crushing improves the preparation. Histological sectioning of the tissue is not required.

S. haematobium ova may also be found in rectal biopsies but even in the presence of an active urinary infection such eggs are invariably black and non-viable, unlike those of *S. mansoni* and *S. japonicum*. In South Africa, *S. mattheei* ova are frequently seen and in parts of West Africa ova of *S. intercalatum*.

It is rarely necessary to resort to liver biopsy for diagnosing *S. mansoni* or *S. japonicum* infections but, where this has been done, it has been found that the examination of fresh hepatic tissue in a crush preparation is better than sectioning of the material. Using a Menghini needle, cores of tissue 25×19 mm may be obtained, which allow for half to be sectioned and the rest crushed (Rosenberg and Black, 1959).

Differentiation of ova in histological sections is frequently difficult or impossible unless a well-marked terminal or lateral spine is seen. Where there is doubt as to the species involved, staining by the Ziehl–Nielsen method may distinguish between *S. mansoni* and *S. haematobium* ova (Lichtenberg and Linderberg, 1954; Brygoo and Randriamala, 1959).

In rare cases, the urine may be consistently negative for *S. haematobium* ova, but cytoscopic examination of the bladder may show evidence of schistosomal infection. Biopsy of the mucosa may reveal eggs, and those of *S. mansoni* may also be recovered in this way.

AUTOPSY INVESTIGATIONS

Adult worms may occasionally be observed in the course of routine post-mortem examinations, but intensive search and specialised techniques are generally required before they can be found in any number.

The pioneering study of Cheever (1968) in Brazil and later studies in Egypt (Cheever *et al.*, 1977) have added greatly to our knowledge of the quantitative aspects of *S. mansoni* infections.

The most satisfactory method of obtaining adult *S. mansoni* worms appears to be the perfusion of mesenteric veins after the intestines have been removed from the cadaver and after removal of the intestines from the mesentery. Perfusion with water is carried out, with the delivery cannula inserted into the proximal end of the superior and inferior mesenteric veins; any adult worms present are then collected from the severed venules at the distal end. The intestinal wall was examined by hand massage to displace adults near the severed ends of the veins and subsequently by separating the mucosa and submucosa from the rest of the wall and examining each between pressed plate glass. The liver was also perfused through the hepatic and portal veins.

Such investigations do not form part of a routine autopsy, but it is desirable that more information relating to adult worm loads should be obtained from different endemic areas, and now that a suitable technique has been devised, it is hoped that such studies will be carried out. The use of the method in areas where *S. japonicum* is endemic should also provide interesting results.

For the recovery of *S. haematobium* adult worms, water was injected into the walls of the bladder and ureters until they were two or three times normal thickness. The tissue was compressed gently with a glass plate and slices 0·1–0·2 cm in thickness were cut. These were compressed between a glass plate and the stage of a dissecting microscope and searched for adult worms (Kamel *et al.*, 1977).

Information on the number of eggs in tissues can be obtained by digestion—particularly of portions of the intestines, liver, bladder and lung. Different areas of these organs should be examined; weighed portions (larger than 10 g) are minced and digested in 5% potassium hydroxide for 24–28 h at 56°C. Digestates are centrifuged and resuspended in a known volume of neutral buffered 10% formalin. After mixing in a vortex mixer, 0·05-ml aliquots are placed on a slide under a coverslip and examined for ova. Very large numbers of ova may be found, particularly in the bladder, and serial dilution of the digestates may be necessary for counting (Smith *et al.*, 1974).

An alternative technique may be used for tissue egg counts (Nelson and Saoud, 1966); 5-g samples of tissue are chopped into small pieces with scissors, or macerated in a domestic mixer; 50 ml of digestive fluid (1% HCl, 1% pepsin) are added, incubated for 16 h at 37°C, centrifuged at 3000 r/min for 5 min and the supernatant discarded. The volume is made up to 50 ml with 0·5% NaOH, then left to clear for 3 h, with occasional shaking; three samples of 0·1 ml should be examined. A 'macdonald' pipette ensures that the suspension is completely agitated before each examination; the mean egg count of 3 samples × 100 equals eggs/g of tissue.

Less exact quantitative information can be obtained from routine histological sections—part of most autopsy examinations. The number of eggs (and/or granulomas) in sections can be counted and related to the number of fields examined and the histological findings.

Quantitative studies are in their infancy, but such information is required from different endemic areas.

IMMUNOLOGICAL TECHNIQUES

Many serological tests of varying complexity have been investigated, but in general they are less satisfactory for field workers than parasitological methods and lack sensitivity and specificity (WHO memoranda, 1974; see Chapter 11), and may be of little value where mixed human or animal schistosomes occur—as in Africa.

As positive results may be obtained for some years after the schistosome infection has died out, they should probably not be the basis of treatment in the absence of parasitological evidence of infection: an exception to this is when central nervous system involvement is suspected. The tests are likewise unreliable for assessing results of chemotherapy.

The skin test has been used in the past in epidemiological studies because of its simplicity (see Chapter 10).

The *WHO reference skin test* (Melcher's antigen) prepared from adult *S. mansoni* worms and standardised to contain 20–40 g/N per ml has been shown to give reproducible results when used in conjunction with the WHO control of merthiolated-buffered-saline (Kagan, 1968).

The area of the wheel which develops after the injection of 0·5 ml of antigen is best measured by outlining it with a ball-point pen 15 min after the injection, transferring the outline to paper moistened with spirit and measuring it with a cellophane template. This immediate reaction is antibody-mediated compared with the delayed intradermal test—read after 24 h— which is a cell-mediated immunologic reaction.

Criteria for interpreting positivity have varied with different workers, but positive immediate reactions can generally be considered when the wheel area is $1{\cdot}1$ cm^2.

The sensitivity and size of the wheel in both immediate and delayed reactions have been shown to correlate with intensity of infection—as assessed by quantitative egg counts (McKay *et al.*, 1973). However, although the immediate test was used in many studies in the past, recent experiences in Puerto Rico, Uganda and St Lucia have shown it to lack sensitivity (particularly amongst children) and specificity. The delayed intradermal test, on the other hand, is specific but lacks sensitivity (Warren *et al.*, 1973).

Complement fixation is one of the best serological tests when conducted under optimum conditions. It is a complicated and highly delicate technique and unsuitable for field operations. There are no reports of it being successfully performed on dried blood samples from a finger prick, although the test has been adopted for microtechniques (Casey, 1965).

An antigen prepared from *Schistosoma spindale* was used to evaluate the complement fixation test on a group of patients from Africa who were shown to be passing ova of *S. mansoni* or *S. haematobium*. It was found that all of those with less than three years residence in the Tropics were positive, but the test was positive in only 44·7% of patients who had been resident for more than ten years in Africa (Schofield, 1959). The sensitivity of this test would seem to differ from that of the intradermal test, where adults with prolonged exposure to infection show a greater response than do young children.

Similar results were found using the *Cercarien Hullen Reaction* (CHR; Papirmeister and Bang, 1948); highest reactivity rates (86%) were found in the younger age groups (Jordan and Goatley, 1963).

This test, while being relatively simple, requires live infectious cercariae—a requirement which severely limits its usefulness as these are generally only available in laboratories maintaining infected snails. The test involves the suspension of cercariae in the serum to be tested. A pericercarial 'envelope' develops in 3 h if the serum is positive. *S. mansoni* cercariae gave better results than *S. haematobium*, whether the patient suffered from *S. mansoni* or *S. haematobium* (Jordan und Goatley, 1963).

The *circumoval precipitin* (COP) test (Oliver-Gonzalez, 1954) is sensitive and specific in *S. mansoni* infections (Hillyer *et al.*, 1979). It is being extensively investigated in the Philippines, where it is considered to be the most sensitive and specific test of a number evaluated (Garcia *et al.*, 1969), but whole serum was 92% positive as opposed to 49% when eluted from dried blood on filter paper (Yogore *et al.*, 1980). This result needs confirmation as other workers obtained good results with the two samples (Cabrera *et al.*, 1968). The test was positive in animals with one pair of worms—it is not positive in unisexual infections (Bruijning, 1964). *S. mansoni* and *S. haematobium* eggs react with sera of patients with *S. japonicum* but not vice versa. In the Far East, there is no cross-reaction of *S. japonicum* with *Clonorchis* or *Paragonimus*.

The method of preparing the ova for the test is important, but like the criteria for positivity, is not standardised. The preparation of lyophilised eggs (Sala *et al.*, 1962) may lead to more reliable results.

The test is performed by mixing 0·05 ml of serum with an equal volume of egg suspension on a slide. A coverslip ringed with vaseline is used to prevent drying, and the slide incubated at 37°C for 24 h. In positive sera, a globular or long-chain type of precipitate is seen around the egg.

Of particular importance is the finding that this test is positive when ova are incubated in cerebrospinal fluid (Reyes and Yogore, 1963) in some suspected cases of cerebral schistosomiasis due to *S. japonicum*.

The *fluorescent antibody test* (FAT) has been developed so that it may be performed on plasma extracted from dried blood-soaked filter paper (Anderson *et al.*, 1961). This enables capillary blood samples to be collected and mailed to a central laboratory for testing. However, the technique is complex and liable to error unless carefully standardised. Positive reactions may also occur in persons who have been exposed to avian and other non-human schistosomes (Sadun and Biocco, 1962; Moore *et al.*, 1968).

Two recently introduced tests show promise of being more satisfactory than earlier serological tests, but both are in the investigational phase of development. The ELISA (enzyme-linked immunosorbent assay) is more likely to be of use in well-equipped laboratories in developing countries, but the RIA (radio-immunoassay), which requires a radioactive antigen and sophisticated equipment, will probably only be of use in the developed countries.

As both tests can be performed on blood collected on filter paper (Whatman No. 3 Chromatography) from a finger prick, they can be considered potentially suitable for large-scale epidemiological investigations, particularly as 200–300 specimens can be processed in a day.

With the ELISA, patients with new infections reacted more positively to cercarial antigen than adult worm antigen: the reverse was found in sera from chronic infections (Lunde *et al.*, 1979). No difference was found in the reactivity of serum from patients with intestinal *S. mansoni* infections and those with hepatosplenic involvement (Goodgame *et al.*, 1978).

A recent development in the field of indirect labelled antibody assays has been the enzyme-linked immunosorbent assay (Engvall and Perlman, 1971). This system involves the passive absorption of soluble antigen on to the surface of a polystyrene tube or plate forming an immunosorbent assay for the subsequent attachment of antibody. The amount of specific antibody bound is measured by drenching it with an enzyme-labelled anti-globulin conjugate. After removal of unbound conjugate, a specific enzyme substrate is added. The enzyme and substrate are chosen so that the product of enzyme substrate breakdown is coloured, the intensity of colour assayed photometrically being proportional to the amount of antibody in the test sample.

Initial results using a highly purified *S. mansoni* egg antigen (Dunne *et al.*, 1981) certainly suggest that this antigen, as well as possessing a higher degree of species specificity and sensitivity than the crude antigens previously used, may be of use as a monitor of chemotherapeutic cure (McLaren *et al.*, 1981).

In the RAI test, radiolabelled antigen (usually major soluble antigen—MSA_1) and normal rabbit serum are added to the serum to be examined. After agitation, incubation and cooling, globulins are precipated by the addition of ammonium sulphate. After centrifugation, the supernatant is decanted and the radioactivity in the precipitate (formed by interaction of antigen and antibody) and that in the supernatant fluid are separately determined in a gamma counter.

Limits of the tests were established: approximately 30% of the radioactivity was precipitated by the ammonium sulphate in the absence of antisera, and excess antibody to MSA_1 could bind only about 85% of total radioactivity. From these data, the normalised antibody bonding (NAB) to the labelled MSA_1 could be calculated (Pelley *et al.*, 1977).

QUALITY CONTROL OF PARASITOLOGICAL INVESTIGATIONS

The validity of the parasitological results of any epidemiological study depends on many factors, one of which is the ability of a diagnostic laboratory to perform accurately the daily tasks of collecting samples, preparing and reading slides, and recording the results. As these are fairly mundane duties, care must be taken to ensure that as few errors as possible are introduced; that is, supervision of all steps is necessary. Attention is focused herein to the checking of slides and recording of data, and although no mention is made of other sources of error such as the mislabelling of specimens or the contamination of apparatus, these factors too should be carefully and routinely checked. The aim of quality control in the current context is to systematise the supervision of microscopy in order to detect inadequate performance rapidly, and to describe simple means of reporting the results to indicate a microscopist's or a laboratory's performance. The fact that checks are made and records are kept and displayed should itself lead to improved microscopy.

The design of the system of checking borrows several ideas from the design of clinical trials. There is no useful general scheme, as problems of design vary between the laboratories and the diagnostic tests employed, and specific statistical advice should be sought for each situation. The aim is to concentrate equally on all microscopists and arrange that each slide read has a constant chance of being checked. It is important that, where possible, the choice of who and what to check is not determined by an individual, but rather by objective means. For example, a chief technician may choose to check the least competent microscopists between 11 and 12 o'clock in the morning. The results of a microscopist who is distracted shortly after arriving or before leaving each day would thus be missed and, if the microscope of a good microscopist began to malfunction slightly, many errors would be committed before trouble was suspected. A properly randomised design would avoid such difficulties.

After a suitable design has been developed, a record-keeping scheme is required which permits large numbers of observations to be kept, yet facilitates rapid assessment. When microscopists are noting more than just the egg count for schistosomiasis (for example, presence or absence of hookworm), then it is important that the same system of writing the results is used by the microscopists, chief technician and main records. Thus, once it is decided that hookworm results appear to the left of schistosomiasis egg counts, then the occurrence of '0–1' is not ambiguous. When a microscopist has studied a slide, the sample number and results should be entered in a separate book, such as a stenographer's shorthand pad. The chief technician takes a slide to be checked, deliberately ignoring the original count, and writes the sample number and his count in his own book. At the end of the day, the microscopists' books are collected and results entered in a master register for checking.

The master register should have separate sections for each microscopist, for which a binder is well suited. For each checked slide, the date, microscopist's count and checked count (and possibly the sample number) are entered in the appropriate sections. The accuracy of each microscopist's count is 'marked' as right or wrong. (Throughout this section, the word 'count' is implicitly taken in a quantitative sense. The methodology applies as well, however, to qualitative results as the variable ultimately considered is itself qualitative: was the slide correctly or incorrectly read?) The set of rules as to which errors are acceptable and which are not is crucial to the operation of the scheme: it should be determined at the outset by the chief technician, epidemiologists, clinicians and other staff if warranted. An explicit set of rules facilitates the chief technician's task and will enable assessment of the performance of the laboratory when compared to others. With the two counts, one also enters whether or not the microscopist's result is in error, as well as the running sum of errors and slides checked.

The entries for each microscopist in the master file provide sufficient information to assess the quality of microscopy, but by preparing graphs, one can more readily appreciate the results. The simplest approach is to plot the running sum of errors against the running number of slides checked. This will provide a step-like diagram that will rise rapidly for poor microscopists and stay level for good performances. An 'acceptable performance' line can be superimposed to provide a quick visual estimate of a microscopist's ability.

An alternative is to assign different scores to correct counts and errors, and then tabulate the cumulative score (or 'cuscore') with the number of slides checked. By a suitable choice of scores, a good performance produces a descending curve, and a poor performance an ascending curve. For example, say it is decided that one error in six or more slides checked is deemed acceptable; then, by taking a score of -1 for a correct check, and $+5$ for an error, a good technician will have more than five -1s for each $+5$ and his graph will descend. The proportion of errors is less readily obtained than in the former case, but it can be calculated. There is a possible dividend to be realised when the graphs are displayed in the laboratory, as microscopists may experience some social pressure to avoid producing the most rapidly rising curve. An example is displayed of the two methods in Fig. 81.

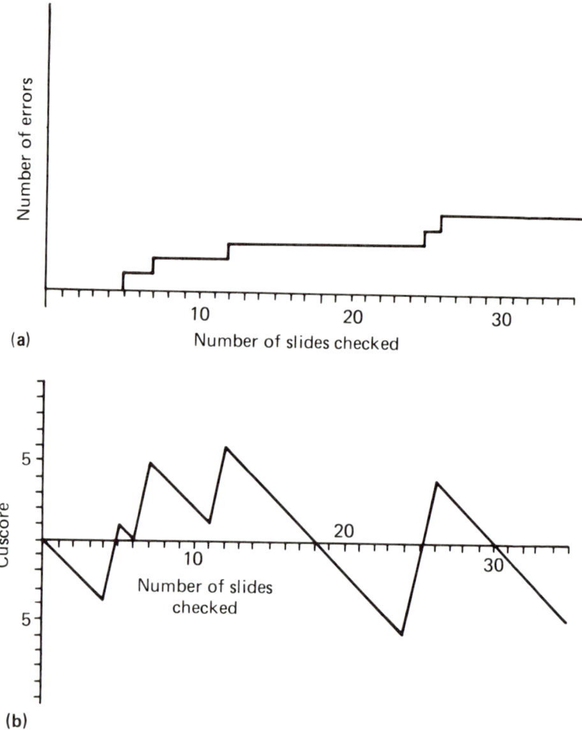

Fig. 8.1 Diagrammatic representation of results of checking the work of microscopists. (a) Cumulative number of errors made; (b) cumulative score (cuscore).

The introduction of cuscore to quality control charts facilitates the performance of simple statistical tests of whether or not a microscopist's results are acceptable. A fuller description of the two graphical techniques and some statistical tools is to be found elsewhere (Bartholomew and Goddard, 1978; Goddard, 1979).

REFERENCES

Anderson, R. I., Sadun, E. H. and Williams, J. E. (1961). *Expl Parasit.* **11,** 111.

Barbosa, F. S. (1969). *Revta Inst. Med. Trop. S. Paulo* **11,** 442.

Bartholomew, R. K. and Goddard, M. (1978). *Bull. Wld Hlth Org.* **56,** 655.

Bartholomew, R. K., Peters, D. A. S. and Jordan, P. (1981). *Ann. Trop. Med. Parasit.* **75,** 401.

Bell, D. R. (1963). *Bull. Wld Hlth Org.* **29,** 525.

Blagg, W., Schaegel, E. L., Mansour, N. S. and Khalaf, G. I. (1955). *Am. J. Trop. Med. Hyg.* **4,** 23.

Blair, D. M., Weber, M. C. and Clarke, V. de V. (1969). *Cent. Afr. J. Med.* **15** (Oct. Suppl.), 2.

Bradley, D. J. (1963). *E. Afr. Med. J.* **40,** 240.

Bradley, D. J. (1964). *Trans. R. Soc. Trop. Med. Hyg.* **58,** 291.

Bradley, D. J. (1965). *Bull. Wld Hlth Org.* **33,** 503.

Bradley, D. J. (1967). In *Bilharziasis*, p. 301. Ed. F. K. Mostofi. Springer-Verlag, Berlin, Heidelberg, New York.

Bruijning, C. F. A. (1964). *Trop. Geogr. Med.* **16,** 256.

Brygoo, K. R. and Randriamala, J. C. (1959). *Bull. Soc. Path. Exot.* **52,** 26.

Cabrera, B. D., Garcia, E. G. and Silan, R. B. (1968). *Acta Med. Philipp.* **4,** 168.

Casey, H. (1965). *Public Health Monograph* No. 74.

Chaia, G., Chaia, A. B. Q., McAullife, J., Katz, N. and Gasper, D. (1968). *Revta Inst. Med. Trop. S. Paulo* **10,** 349.

Cheever, A. W. (1968). *Am. J. Trop. Med. Hyg.* **17,** 38.

Cheever, A. W., Kamel, I. A., Elwi, A. M., Mosimann, J. E. and Danner, R. (1977). *Am. J. Trop. Med. Hyg.* **26,** 702.

Cheever, A. W. and Powers, K. G. (1968). *J. Parasit.* **54,** 632.

Cheever, A. W., Young, S. W. and Shehata, A. (1975). *Trans. R. Soc. Trop. Med. Hyg.* **69,** 410.

Cook, J. A. and Jordan, P. (1970). *Trans. R. Soc. Trop. Med. Hyg.* **64,** 793.

Davis, A. (1968). *Bull. Wld Hlth Org.* **38,** 197.

Dazo, B. C. and Biles, J. E. (1974). *Bull. Wld Hlth Org.* **51,** 399.

Dunne, D. W., Lucas, S., Bickle, Q., Pearson, S., Madgwick, L., Bain, J. and Doenhoff, M. J. (1981). *Trans. R. Soc. Trop. Med. Hyg.* **75,** 54.

Engvall, E. and Perlman, P. (1971). *Immunochemistry* **8,** 871.

Feldmeir, H., Bienzle, U. and Dietrich, M. (1979). *Tropenmed. Parasit.* **30,** 417.

Garcia, E. C., Cabrera, B. D., Criste, Z. A. and Silan, R. B. (1969). *J. Philipp. Med. Assoc.* **45,** 86.

Goddard, M. (1979). *Bull. Wld Hlth Org.* **58,** 313.

Goodgame, R. W., Colley, D. G., Draper, C. C., Lewis, F. A., McLaren, M. L. and Pelley, R. P. (1978). *Am. J. Trop. Med. Hyg.* **27,** 1174.

Grove, R. B. (1970). *Trans. R. Soc. Trop. Med. Hyg.* **64,** 431.

Hiatt, R. A. (1976). *Am. J. Trop. Med. Hyg.* **25,** 808.

Hiatt, R. A., Barnett, L. C. and Knight, W. B. (1976). *Am. J. Trop. Med. Hyg.* **27,** 235.

Hillyer, G. V., Ruiz Tiben, E., Knight, W. B., de Rios, I. G. and Pelley, R. (1979). *Am. J. Trop. Med. Hyg.* **28,** 661.

Hoffman, W. A., Pons, J. A. and Janer, J. H. (1934). *Puerto Rico J. Publ. Hlth Trop. Med.* **9,** 283.

Hunter, G. W. III, Hodges, E. P., Jahnes, W. G., Diamond, L. S. and Ingalls, J. W. (1948). *Bull. U.S. Army Med. Dept.* **8,** 128.

Jordan, P. (1962). *Ann. Rep. E. Afr. Inst. Med. Research*, 1961/62.

Jordan, P. and Goatley, K. D. (1963). *Trans. R. Soc. Trop. Med. Hyg.* **57,** 184.

Kagan, I. G. (1968). *Bull. N.Y. Acad. Med.* **44,** 262.

Kamel, I. A., Cheever, A. W., Elwi, A. M., Mosimann, J. E. and Danner, R. (1977). *Am. J. Trop. Med. Hyg.* **26,** 696.

Katz, N. and Chaia, G. (1968). *Revta Inst. Med. Trop. S. Paulo* **10,** 295.

Katz, N., Cheves, A. and Pellegrino, J. (1972). *Revta Inst. Med. Trop. S. Paulo* **14,** 497.

Klumpp, R. K. (1980). Personal communication.

Knight, W. B., Hiatt, R. A., Cline, B. L. and Ritchie, L. S. (1976). *Am. J. Trop. Med. Hyg.* **25,** 818.

Komiya, Y. and Kobayashi, A. (1966). *Jap. J. Med. Hyg.* **19,** 59.

Kruatrachue, M., Bhaibulaya, M. and Harinasuta, C. (1964). *Am. J. Trop. Med. Parasit.* **58,** 276.

Lichtenberg, F. von and Linderberg, M. (1954). *Am. J. Trop. Med. Hyg.* **3,** 1066.

Lunde, M. N., Ottensen, E. A. and Cheever, A. W. (1979). *Am. J. Trop. Med. Hyg.* **28,** 87.

McKay, D., Warren, K. S., Cook, J. A. and Jordan, P. (1973). *Am. J. Trop. Med. Hyg.* **22,** 205.

McLaren, M. L., Lillywhite, J., Dunne, D. and Doenhoff, M. J. (1981). *Trans. R. Soc. Trop. Med. Hyg.* **75,** 72.

Martin, L. K. and Beaver, P. C. (1968). *Am. J. Trop. Med. Hyg.* **17,** 382.

Moore, G. T., Kaiser, R. L., Lawrence, R. S., Putman, S. M. and Kagan, I. G. (1968). *Am. J. Trop. Med. Hyg.* **17,** 79.

Nelson, G. S. and Saoud, M. F. A. (1966). *Trans. R. Soc. Trop. Med. Hyg.* **60,** 429.

Oliver-Gonzalez, J. (1954). *J. Infect. Dis.* **95,** 86.

Papirmeister, B. and Bank, F. B. (1948). *Am. J. Hyg.* **48,** 74.

Pelley, R. P., Warren, K. S. and Jordan, P. (1977). *Lancet* **ii,** 781.

Peters, P. A., El'Alemy, M., Warren, K. S. and Mahmoud, A. A. F. (1980). *Am. J. Trop. Med. Hyg.* **29,** 217.

Peters, P. A., Warren, K. S. and Mahmoud, A. A. F. (1976). *J. Parasit.* **62,** 154.

Pugh, R. N. H. (1979). *Ann. Trop. Med. Parasit.* **73,** 89.

Reyes, V. A. and Yogore, M. G. (1963). *Philipp. J. Surg.* **18,** 172.

Ritchie, L. S. (1948). *Bull. U.S. Army Med. Dept.* **8,** 326.

Rosenberg, E. and Black, H. (1959). *Am. J. Clin. Path.* **32,** 472.

Sadun, E. H. and Biocco, E. (1962). *Bull. Wld Hlth Org.* **27,** 810.

Sala, A. R., Cancio, M. and Rodriquez-Molina, R. (1962). *Am. J. Trop. Med. Hyg.* **11,** 199.

Schofield, F. D. (1959). *Trans. R. Soc. Trop. Med. Hyg.* **53,** 64.

Smith, J. H., Kamel, I. A., Elwi, A. and von Lichtenberg, F. (1974). *Am. J. Trop. Med. Hyg.* **23,** 1054.

Siongok, T. K. A., Mahmoud, A. A. F., Ouma, J. H., Warren, K. S., Muller, A. S., Handa, A. K. and Houser, H. B. (1976). *Am. J. Trop. Med. Hyg.* **25,** 273.

Stimmel, C. M. and Scott, J. A. (1956). *Texas Rep. Biol. Med.* **14,** 440.

Teesdale, C. H. and Amin, M. A. (1976). *J. Helminth.* **50,** 17.

Turner, J. A. (1962). *Am. J. Trop. Med. Hyg.* **11,** 620.

Upatham, E. S. (1972). *S.E. Asian J. Trop. Med. Publ. Hlth* **3,** 600.

Upatham, E. S., Sturrock, R. F. and Cook, J. A. (1976). *Parasitology* **73,** 253.

Warren, K. S., Cook, J. A., Littell, A. S., Kegan, I. G. and Jordan, P. (1973). *Am. J. Trop. Med. Hyg.* **22,** 199.

Warren, K. S., Mahmoud, A. A. F., Cummings, P., Murphy, D. J. and Houser, H. B. (1974). *Am. J. Trop. Med. Hyg.* **23,** 902.

Weber, M. C., Blair, D. M. and Clarke, V. de V. (1967). *Cent. Afr. J. Med.* **13,** 75.

WHO memoranda (1974). *Bull. Wld Hlth Org.* **51,** 553.

Wilkins, H. A. (1977). *Am. Trop. Med. Hyg.* **71,** 53.

Woodstock, L., Cook, J. A., Peters, P. A. and Warren, K. S. (1972). *J. Inf. Dis.* **124,** 613.

Yogore, M. G., Lewert, R. M. and Blas, B. L. (1980). In *Proceedings of the Philippine—Japan Joint Conference on Schistosomiasis Research and Control*, p. 49. Japan International Cooperation Agency, Tokyo.

9 Management of the Patient with Schistosomiasis

Andrew Davis

GENERAL CONSIDERATIONS

Despite a multiplicity of confounding factors, it is usually possible to treat the individual patient with high expectations of cure of the infection and improvement in functional or structural damage if this is not too far advanced.

In few other parasitic diseases have there been advances in therapy comparable to those which have occurred in the treatment of schistosomal infections during the last 15 years. A variety of alternative drugs has become available—curative efficacy has improved markedly and side-effects of treatment have diminished in frequency and severity. That this should have occurred in a period of steadily rising research and development costs and increasingly stringent national and international standards of drug safety, combined with uncertain prospects of market returns, is surprising, yet, one hopes, indicates that the chemotherapy of schistosomiasis and, indeed, parasitic infections generally, still commands the interest of certain specialised sectors of the pharmaceutical industry.

Compared with the therapeutic scene a decade ago, treatment nowadays is a relatively simple procedure and increasing attention is being paid to the more complex clinical situations encountered.

The primary four stages in case management are:

(i) the clinical history followed by physical examination, establishment of the diagnosis and ancillary radiographic, biochemical, endoscopic, haematologic or other appropriate investigations to assess the physiopathological state of the patient;

(ii) specific chemotherapy of the proven (or, in a small minority, suspected) infection;

(iii) any appropriate and essential surgical measures;

(iv) the education of the patient in the prevention of further exposure to infection.

A decisive diagnosis can be made only by the direct demonstration of the eggs of the parasite in stool or urine or in biopsy or surgical tissue specimens (see Chapter 8).

Hatching tests are particularly useful since the demonstration of swimming miracidia originating from excreted eggs indicates beyond any doubt that the eggs are viable and therefore originate from living fertilised female schistosomes. An active infection is therefore proven.

Having established a qualitative parasitological species diagnosis by direct demonstration of eggs (for species characteristics see Chapter 1), the quantitative excretal egg output (see Chapter 8) of all patients should ideally be estimated to assess, however roughly, the category of infection intensity into which the patient can be classified.

In any individual patient, the extent of structural and/or functional damage (as described elsewhere) caused by schistosome infection should be assessed. Where facilities are available, a variety of ancillary investigations may be employed. It is not possible to list general rules of management; indications for further investigation lie at the individual patient level and the attending physician is responsible for decisions on which ancillary procedures should be used, and when.

Aims of chemotherapy

Chemotherapy has two broad objectives: in the individual patient, to eradicate the infection—successful treatment will stop further deposition of eggs preventing further tissue damage and existing lesions will often regress; for the community, the cessation of egg excretion will block the egg/miracidium/snail stage of the biological cycle, thereby reducing transmission.

Justification for and priorities in chemotherapy

There are two basic categories of patients with schistosomiasis: those not subject to re-exposure to infection and those living in endemic areas where re-exposure is probable, or even inevitable.

While there is no doubt that patients not subject to re-exposure should be given curative treatment, for even 'light' infections can lead to serious complications (e.g. hydro-ureter, neurological sequelae), there has, in the past, been a body of opinion which held that treatment in endemic areas was largely unjustified. This view was based on the propositions that the drugs available were cumbersome to use, that they produced numerous severe side-effects and occasionally fatalities, that they were by no means certain to cure and that re-infection was inevitable. This attitude has been changed by the advent of new chemotherapeutic compounds but was always suspect for the following reasons: schistosomiasis causes insidious complications with cumulative pathological structural and functional damage and, although its deleterious effects are difficult to evalute, there is a mass of circumstantial evidence to show that, in population terms, the infection may cause serious functional changes and impose a socio-economic burden on the bread-winners of the family; and the individual patient is the unit which, in mass, constitutes 'the population' (see Chapter 10).

Schistosomiasis is an infection of childhood, adolescence and young adulthood—those periods of maximum physiological growth, activity and effort, both mental and physical. Treatment benefits these young age groups in terms of the individual's improvement in health and by the diminution of transmission potential.

Finally, it should be recalled that schistosomes do not multiply within the human host. Treatment will eradicate completely or considerably reduce the body's population of resident flukes, with obvious benefit to the patient.

While on medical grounds there are abundant justifications for treatment, there frequently exist, in endemic areas, many non-medical factors which may force physicians to establish priorities. Among these factors are the high prevalence of the infection, which indeed may be practically universal, the high cost of drugs, lack of purchasing funds at governmental level, bed shortages and paucity of personnel.

Priorities for treatment might then fall into a ranking order which may, of course, vary in different local situations. For example:

(i) children, adolescents and young adults with acute symptoms;

(ii) adults with acute symptoms;

(iii) patients of any age with a heavy excretal egg output, regardless of their symptomatic history;

(iv) patients of educational standard sufficient to benefit from health education designed to prevent re-exposure to infection.

AVAILABLE CHEMOTHERAPEUTIC COMPOUNDS

A variety of highly effective drugs now exists for the treatment of schistosomiasis. Traditionally, drugs were either antimonials or non-antimonials, but since the use of the former has declined markedly in parallel with the advent of new compounds, the classification has outlived its utility. This review will concentrate on those drugs of relatively recent origin for which experience of their use has accumulated in the last 10 years; less emphasis will be given to the older compounds for which there has existed for many years a large body of knowledge.

Drugs effective against one species of schistosome

Oxamniquine (Mansil®, Vansil®, Pfizer Inc.)

Oxamniquine is 6-hydroxymethyl-2-isopropylaxinomethyl-7-nitro-1, 2, 3, 4-tetrahydroquinoline, a light orange-coloured crystalline solid, slightly soluble in water, with a molecular weight of 279·3 and the structural formula shown in Fig. 9.1.

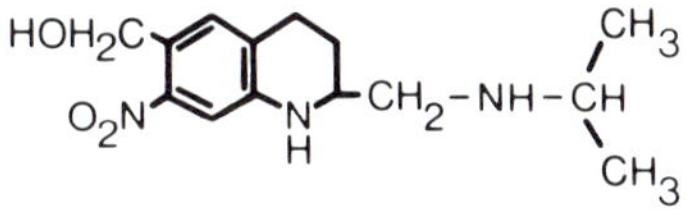

Fig. 9.1 Oxamniquine.

It is formulated as capsules of 250 mg or as a syrup containing 50 mg/ml and marketed under the trade names Mansil, in South America, and Vansil in the African continent (Pfizer Inc. manufacturers' data, 1978). Given by mouth, oxamniquine is one of the drugs of first choice in all forms of *S. mansoni* infection.

Experimentally, it is inactive against *S. japonicum* in mice, hamsters and monkeys. In animals the drug is highly active against *S. mansoni*, male worms being more susceptible than females. Activity against immature parasites has been observed in both mice and primates (Foster, 1973; Foster and Cheetham, 1973; Foster *et al.*, 1973).

The drug has virtually no effect against *S. haematobium* in man

(Clarke *et al.*, 1969; McMahon, 1976; Kale and Lucas, 1978) and no effect was noted when patients with *S. mattheei* were given a total dose of 60 mg/kg (Pitchford and Lewis, 1978).

Metabolic studies in many animals and in man (Kaye and Woolhouse, 1976) show that oxamniquine is well absorbed in all species and is extensively metabolised to inactive acidic metabolites which are mainly excreted in the urine. Two metabolites occur, the major one arising from oxidation of the 6-hydroxymethyl group to a carboxyl group (Metabolite I) and the other by oxidation of the side chain to produce the 2-carboxylic acid (Metabolite II). In volunteer studies in man, only 0·4–1·9% of the dose was excreted as unchanged drug in the urine and 41–73% was excreted as the 6-carboxy metabolite with only traces of the 2-carboxylic acid fraction. Most of the metabolites were excreted in the first 12 hours, indicating that drug-related material is rapidly eliminated.

Clinical use

Clinically, oxamniquine has been used to treat acute, subacute, chronic and complicated cases of *S. mansoni* infection with uniformly good effects. In the toxaemic form of *S. mansoni* infection, treatment of a small number of patients in Brazil with a single oral dose of 20 mg/kg of body weight produced 'cure' in about half, with no significant side-effects (Lambertucci *et al.*, 1980). Numerous trials in Brazil and the African continent have confirmed the drug's efficacy (Silva *et al.*, 1974; Clarke *et al.*, 1976; Katz *et al.*, 1976 and 1977; Omer, 1978) and have shown that the therapeutic response varies with age, and hence surface area of the patient, and with the geographic origin of the infection.

The treatment of advanced or complicated cases with hepatosplenomegaly and/or ascites is rewarding for both patient and physician since improvement is marked and parasitological cure rates very high (Bassily *et al.*, 1978; Farid *et al.*, 1980). Similarly, the treatment of schistosomal polyposis of the colon with anaemia and protein-losing enteropathy has been highly effective and safe (Abaza *et al.*, 1978).

Side-effects

In general, oxamniquine is well tolerated. In a cross-over study in volunteers which compared serum oxamniquine levels following ingestion of the drug either in the fasting stage or shortly after food, the mean maximum serum concentration and the mean time taken to achieve peak levels were reduced significantly when the drug was given after food (Pfizer Inc. manufacturers' data, 1978) and, from clinical experience, tolerance is improved if doses are given at this time.

The most frequent side-effects have been dizziness, drowsiness and headache occurring, predictably, in different proportions of samples treated in South America and Africa. Dizziness is usually mild, frequently occurs about 1–2 hours after dosage, rarely lasts for more than 6 hours, and does not prevent the patient from working, although those whose work involves driving automobiles, ships or aircraft should obviously be kept away from their occupation during treatment and for 24–48 hours after. Dizziness does not deter patients from accepting further doses. Its incidence in some studies increased as unit dosage increased, but was not aggravated by multiple doses. When possible, it would be advantageous to give the drug in the evening.

Vomiting and diarrhoea have also been reported, but their relationship to dosage is more tenuous.

Hallucinations and psychic excitement following oxamniquine are known (Katz *et al.*, 1976), and five cases of epileptiform convulsions in some quarter of a million treatments have been documented (Pfizer Inc. manufacturers' data, 1978). In three of these latter patients, prior histories of convulsions were obtained and a further patient had an EEG consistent with an epileptiform focus.

The orange-red discolouration of the urine occasionally observed after treatment (Omer, 1978) is due to the excretion of a mixture of drug and metabolites and is harmless.

A characteristic fever, occurring 24–72 hours after completion of a three-day course of oxamniquine, associated with both a typical Loeffler-like syndrome of peripheral blood eosinophilia and scattered pulmonary infiltrates and with an increase in serum immune complexes and excretion of schistosomal antigens in the urine, has been observed in Egypt (Higashi and Farid, 1979) but not in other centres where large numbers of patients are treated.

Serial clinicopathological measurements performed in the early clinical trials were reassuring and the safety of the drug has been amply confirmed in the many large-scale field projects in which it has been used, particularly in Brazil where oxamniquine has been the chemotherapeutic base of the national schistosomiasis control plan.

An eosinophilia occurs frequently, is maximal 7–10 days after treatment, and represents a normal reaction to dead or dying worms. No consistent changes are seen in other measurements on the peripheral blood.

Although minor increases in serum glutamic oxalo-acetic transaminase (SGOT) and serum glutamic pyruvic transaminase (SGPT) have been seen in individual studies, these findings are inconsistent and there is no constant pattern of liver enzyme alterations following oxamniquine.

Serial electrocardiograms have not revealed any findings of clinical significance.

Dose

There is a distinct difference in the therapeutic responses of schistosome strains of South American and African origin.

In the New World, a single oral dose of 15 mg/kg of body weight in adults gives high cure rates varying between 60% and 90+% in different samples.

In children under 30 kg in weight, the preferred regime is a total dose of 20 mg/kg given in two divided doses each of 10 mg/kg at a 4–6 hour interval. Tolerance is improved if the drug is given shortly after food.

In African *S. mansoni* infections, the therapeutic responses to 15–20 mg/kg is poor. Various regimes have been used, the most popular being total doses of 40 mg/kg and 60 mg/kg given over two or three days. A total dose of 60 mg/kg given as 15 mg/kg twice daily for two days gave a 95% cure rate in Sudan (Omer, 1978), and this experience is representative of many trials. In all parasitological failures, the excretal egg count is markedly reduced—of the order of 80–90%.

The difference in strain response is not due to differing bio-availability of oxamniquine, since drug serum concentrations in patients from Brazil, South Africa and East Africa were very similar following equivalent doses, thus indicating the variation is truly a property of the schistosome strains.

In experimental studies there were no drug interactions with metrifonate, niridazole, pyrantel or oxantel pamoate or tinidazole. In a small trial in Egypt when patients with double infections with *S. mansoni* and *S. haematobium* were treated concomitantly with oxamniquine and metrifonate, the cure rate was 79%; egg reduction in those not cured was 95%, side-effects were not increased and there were no abnormalities of note in monitoring laboratory tests (Saif *et al.*, 1978).

It is possible to produce resistance of *S. mansoni* to hycanthone and oxamniquine in experimental animal studies and there have been reports of several patients who failed to respond to multiple oral doses of oxamniquine (Pfizer Inc. manufacturers' data, 1978). Furthermore, cases are known who failed to respond to hycanthone or oxamniquine and in which the 'resistance' was maintained in subsequently infected mice (Guimaraes *et al.*, 1979). It is as yet uncertain to what extent this will pose a problem in the treatment of large numbers of patients but, from experience gained to date, it appears unlikely.

Although there are no contraindications to oxamniquine, it should be given under medical supervision in patients with a history of any form of epilepsy and should not be used in early pregnancy.

Metrifonate (Bilarcil®, Bayer A.G.)

Metrifonate is the generic name for the dimethylester of (2,2,2-trichloro-1-hydroxy-ethyl)-phosphoric acid, a white crystalline substance of characteristic odour, soluble in water, diethyl ether, chloroform, and ethanol, of molecular weight 257.5. The structural formula is shown in Fig. 9.2.

$$CH_3O\diagdown \quad \diagup O$$
$$P$$
$$CH_3O\diagup \quad \diagdown CHOHCCl_3$$

Fig. 9.2 Metrifonate.

Metrifonate is formulated as tablets, each containing 100 mg of active substance and marketed under the trade name Bilarcil® (Bayer AG). Given by mouth, metrifonate is a drug of first choice in all forms of *S. haematobium* infections. It possesses some activity against *S. mansoni* but insufficient to recommend its use against this species. In *S. japonicum* infections in China, it has been used to produce an hepatic shift of worm pairs to the more central locations of the superior mesenteric vessels and portal venous radicals, after which furapromidium (see below) was given as a schistosomicide. This treatment has not been used in other areas of *S. japonicum* endemicity.

Some activity has been shown against hookworm, ascariasis, trichuriasis, creeping eruption and onchocerciasis (Cerf *et al.*, 1962; Salazar-Mallen *et al.*, 1969), but this is inconstant and metrifonate is not regarded as a drug of choice for these infections.

Metrifonate is an organophosphorous ester, one of a group of compounds with insecticidal properties dependent on enzymic inhibition of specific esterases in ganglionar synapses and neuro-muscular junctions. Originally, it was available under various names as a pesticide and anthelmintic for agricultural and veterinary use respectively, before its issue in pure form for therapeutic use in human *S. haematobium* infections.

Extensive toxicological studies in many animal species de-monstrated the essential safety of the compound but did confirm that, as with other organophosphorous drugs, inhibition of plasma and erythrocyte acetylcholinesterases occurred in vari-ous species at different dose levels.

In human urinary schistosomiasis, cholinesterase levels in red cells, whole blood and plasma were monitored (Plestina *et al.*, 1972). Cholinesterase activities were determined by a sensitive spectrophotometric technique (Ellman *et al.*, 1961; Vandekar *et al.*, 1968; Wilhelm, 1968).

A few hours after each dose of a three-dose regime of 7·5, 10·0 or 12·5 mg of metrifonate/kg of body weight given once every 14 days, plasma cholinesterase was almost completely inhibited, regardless of the amount given in this dose range, but ery-throcyte cholinesterase was inhibited, in a dose-dependent fashion, down to some 40–60% of the individual patient's pre-treatment activity. Inhibited plasma cholinesterase returned to normal activity fairly rapidly. After 14 days, plasma cholines-terase activities, having been completely inhibited within 24 h of each dose, were some 75% of the 'normal' activity for each individual patient. At 4 weeks after the last dose of a three-dose regime, activities were 'normal'. However, erythrocyte cholines-terase activities, considered the closest parallel monitoring measurement of brain cholinesterase, although inhibited to a lesser extent and at a slower rate than plasma cholinesterases, were also slower to recover. Activities were not regained within 14 days of a dose of metrifonate and the subsequent dose depressed red cell cholinesterase activity further to 35–50% of the level existing at the time of dosing. After the last dose of a three-dose treatment, erythrocyte cholinesterase activities did not return to 'normal' for times varying between 8 and 15 weeks.

Despite these inhibitions of erythrocyte and plasma cholinesterases, no correlation could be established between the degree of cholinesterase inhibition and any symptom after treatment. Thus, enzyme inhibition occurring after metrifonate treatment in man should be regarded as indicative of satisfactory absorption and biotransformation of the compound into 2,2-dichlorovinyl dimethyl phosphate (DDVP), the actual inhibitory substance, rather than evidence of drug toxicity.

Pharmacology
The pharmacology of metrifonate has been studied extensively in many experimental animal models and no undue physiopathological effects other than the anticholinesterase action could be found at dose levels comparable to those used in man. Absorption after oral administration of ^{32}P-labelled substance is very rapid. Using mass-fragmentography, it has been demonstrated recently that DDVP, a directly acting cholinesterase inhibitor, is formed non-enzymatically from metrifonate in body fluids and substrates in patients undergoing treatment (Nordgren *et al.*, 1980). The plasma curves of both metrifonate and DDVP do not correlate with those of enzyme inhibition in which action may be prolonged for days or weeks. It thus appears that metrifonate acts as a slow release formulation for DDVP which is formed in man as the result of a chemical transformation unrelated to enzymatic metabolism. This mechanism of inhibition is less prone to the phenomenon of 'ageing', although it does occur and may well be the explanation for the well-known prolonged enzyme inhibition observed after metrifonate treatment (Nordgren *et al.*, 1980).

Mode of action
The reasons either for the overwhelmingly monospecific activity of metrifonate against *S. haematobium*, or for its mode of action are unknown. The primary evidence for its clinical chemotherapeutic effect is the continued disappearance of eggs from the urine on repeated examinations for 12 months after treatment. In theory, this may be caused either by destruction of the adult worms or by their displacement from their usual location to an ectopic site from whence the eggs, even if laid, are unable to

reach the exterior. Thus the two basic theories of the mode of action may be termed the chemical and the mechanical.

It is known that the cholinesterase receptors present in *S. mansoni* are not identical to those present in man (Barker *et al.*, 1966). It appeared possible that the action of metrifonate was due to enzyme inhibition in adult worms, the enzymes and their receptors being affected in a similar fashion to the cholinesterases present in man. There are, however, gaps in this theory; no species difference between *S. haematobium* and *S. mansoni* was detected when determining the molar concentrations of metrifonate producing 50% inhibition of enzyme activities either in isolated enzyme preparations or following exposure of the intact worms to the drug *in vitro* (Bueding *et al.*, 1972). However, *S. haematobium* was more affected by acetylcholinesterase inhibition since, after metrifonate administration to infected hamsters, an hepatic shift of parasites was seen at a dose of metrifonate of 150 mg (0·6 mmol) per kg, which produced no shift in *S. mansoni*-infected animals although actual inhibition of acetylcholinesterase was comparable in both species. Hence, the difference in the chemotherapeutic activities of metrifonate in humans infected by *S. haematobium* and *S. mansoni* could not be explained by differences in the inhibitory potency of metrifonate on the enzymes catalysing the hydrolysis of acetylcholine in the two species.

Alternatively, it has been hypothesised that the adult schistosomes, under the paralysing influence of the drug, drift in the tributaries of the inferior vena caval system to the small arterioles of the lungs, where they become trapped, encased by leucocytes and die (Forsyth, 1965; Forsyth and Rashid, 1967). The reason advanced for the failure of metrifonate in *S. mansoni* infections was that since adult worms live within the draining area of the portal venous system, they can, on recovery from the action of metrifonate, and/or its metabolites (which are rapidly excreted), retrace a path down the portal system and return to their preferred sites of egg laying. Furthermore, in experimental infections in hamsters, metrifonate produced a strong but reversible paralysing effect on adult schistosomes and an apparently irreversible lung shift in a high proportion of treated animals (James *et al.*, 1972). (However, the vascular anatomy of the hamster differs from that of man and in this model the site of location of the adult schistosomes does not parallel the human situation.)

Clinical evidence neither supports nor confirms the 'mechanical' hypothesis—pulmonary complications which might be expected to occur as a result of a lung shift following metrifonate treatment have not been reported. The theory further fails to explain the phenomenon of clinical relapse in treated *S. haematobium* infections, unless it is postulated that 'relapses' are, in fact, maturing pre-infections. Although a lung shift has been described in a baboon infected with *S. haematobium* (James and Webbe, 1974), 92% of the worms found at *post mortem* in an untreated control animal were found in vessels round the large intestine, thus indicating an abnormal distribution of the parasite in this experimental infection. Hence, these results cannot be extrapolated directly to man. It was shown clinically that metrifonate exerted little effect on *S. mansoni* localised in mesenteric vessels but markedly reduced the numbers of *S. mansoni* eggs in the urine which originated from adults located in the vesical plexus (Omer and Teesdale, 1978). The true explanation of metrifonate action remains unclear. In fact these varying suggestions are compatible since the 'mechanical' explanation is merely a description of the physical events following metrifonate treatment and does not deal with the mode of action at a molecular level.

Clinical use
Early clinical studies were characterised by pronounced variation in both dose, ranging from 5 mg/kg to over 20 mg/kg, and in times of treatment, from 2 to 14 days.

Trials confirmed that the optimum individual dose was 7·5–10 mg/kg (Davis and Bailey, 1969) and a widely adopted schedule of 7·5 mg/kg given in three oral doses, at an interval of 14 days, became the 'standard' treatment regime. In fact, all investigations have shown that doses of 5 mg/kg are too low and that some strains of *S. haematobium*, particularly in Egypt, seem to respond best to a repeated dose of 10 mg/kg. Whether each individual dose is given at intervals of two or four weeks is immaterial (Davis and Bailey, 1969). On these regimes, cure rates, which are inversely proportional to pre-treatment urinary egg output, range from 60–90% in different population samples. Variable proportions of low-density infections are cured after one or two doses and relapses are uncommon.

Although a fixed dose schedule of three doses was commonly used, there is no reason, patient tolerance permitting, why four or more doses should not be given at appropriate intervals. Multiple monthly doses given to uninfected yet exposed children appeared to possess a prophylactic effect against the acquisition of *S. haematobium* infection (Jewsbury *et al.*, 1977).

Side-effects

In practically all reported trials at levels of 7·5–10 mg/kg per individual dose, tolerance has been extremely good. Since metrifonate, like other organophosphorous compounds, inactivates the enzyme destroying acetylcholine, thus allowing the chemical transmitter to persist, cholinergic symptoms would be anticipated during treatment. These symptoms include fatigue, muscular weakness, muscle tremor, sweating, fainting, abdominal colic, diarrhoea, nausea or vomiting and bronchospasm, all reflecting stimulation of cholinergic synapses in the autonomic nervous system, ganglionic and postganglionic sites in both parasympathetic and sympathetic divisions, the neuromuscular junction and several sites in the cardiovascular system. However, metrifonate provides an excellent example of the dictum that each anticholinesterase drug does not necessarily produce every theoretical effect, nor are such effects necessarily seen at a therapeutic dose.

The frequency of cholinergic side-effects is extremely low, their severity is mild and they disappear spontaneously in a few hours. One constant accompaniment of metrifonate treatment is depression of acetylcholinesterases in both plasma and erythrocytes but, as noted, this appears to be an inseparable pharmacological adjuvant rather than an adverse side-effect.

Even in the rare recorded examples of therapeutic errors where patients received single doses ranging from 30 mg/kg to 72 mg/kg, recovery from cholinergic symptoms, usually with the help of atropine, occurred in 24–48 hours (Bayer, 1972). Monitoring of hepatic, renal and haematological function has not revealed any changes of clinical significance. In short, metrifonate is a safe and effective drug for *S. haematobium* infections and has in fact been employed in large-scale chemotherapy in control projects in Egypt and Ghana.

Precautions

Since there is a possibility that potentiation of the effects of one organophosphorous (OP) compound by another may occur, and since seasonal use of OP compounds in agriculture is not uncommon, special care must be taken with occupational groups such as spraymen, unsupervised farmers or workers engaged in manufacture of OP insecticides. In these situations, pre-treatment estimation of blood cholinesterases would be a wise precaution. In normal clinical practice, this is unnecessary.

Should cholinergic symptoms arise, the parenteral administration of atropine sulphate, repeated if necessary, will block the muscarinic but not the nicotinic effects. Finally, the availability of pralidoximine iodide (2-PAM) as an enzyme reactivator for cases of profound enzyme inhibition is a welcome safeguard, but in practice PAM use has been restricted to acute organophosphorous intoxication and there are no records of its necessity during metrifonate treatment.

Furapromidium, a nitroheterocyclic compound similar to niridazole, is used only in China. In chronic cases of *S. japonicum* infection, a total dose of 60 mg/kg per day is given in three divided doses for periods varying between 14 and 20 days. Cure rates of 80% at 1 month, which fall at 6 and 9 months, are claimed. Side-effects include diarrhoea, nausea, vomiting, muscle spasms, occasional melaena and psychotic reactions. In some treatment centres, furapromidium is supplemented with metrifonate at a dose of 4 mg/kg in the early days of treatment. Metrifonate given thus has been administered by intramuscular injection or by rectal suppository (Anon, 1977). In a clinical study of the combined treatment in 180 patients reported recently, 88% completed the course of treatment but in the others treatment was either prolonged or abandoned or the total dose was reduced due to the severity of gastrointestinal side-effects. Major side-effects were muscular cramps (87%), dizziness (57%), abdominal pain (53%), diarrhoea (50%), bloody stools (24%). anorexia (18%), nausea (13%) and fatigue (12%). Follow-up at 6–8 months by five consecutive hatching tests revealed 72% 'cures' (Xu, 1980).

Drugs active against two species of parasite

Hycanthone mesylate (Etrenol® Winthrop)

The structural formula is shown in Fig. 9.3.

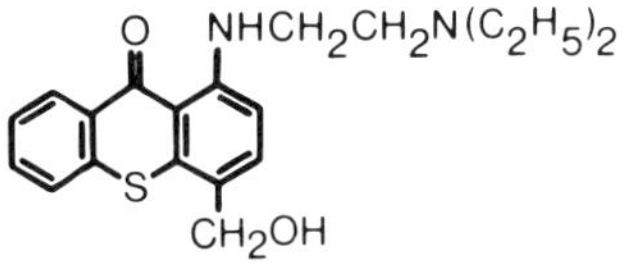

Fig. 9.3 Hycanthone.

A thioxanthone compound, 1-[2-(diethylamino)ethyl]amino]
-4-(hydroxymethyl)-thioxanthen-9-one, related to lucanthone,
the isolation of hycanthone arose from the discovery that a
mould, *Aspergillus sclerotiorum*, converted lucanthone biologically
into a mixture of new substances (Rossi *et al.*, 1965). The major
transformation product of this conversion was separated,
characterised and identified as an acid-sensitive hydroxymethyl
derivative, subsequently named hycanthone. Treatment of *S.
mansoni* infections in mice and hamsters showed that this
4-hydroxmethyl analogue of lucanthone possessed greater antischistosomal activity than lucanthone itself and it was thought
that the new compound was in fact the active metabolite of
lucanthone (Berberian *et al.*, 1967). The drug is active against *S.
haematobium* and *S. mansoni* but ineffective against *S. japonicum*
(Yarinsky *et al.*, 1972).

Pharmacology
After oral or intramuscular administration, hycanthone is
quickly absorbed, peak concentrations in the blood being
reached in 30 minutes; it has a rapid plasma clearance with a
half-life of about one hour, and in turn tissue clearance is
essentially complete in some 24 hours after dosage. About 60%
of an injected dose is excreted as hycanthone and different
conjugated metabolic products, mainly in the bile and faeces,
and some 10–15% is excreted via the urine. Some 5–10% of
injected hycanthone is excreted as unidentified forms. There
appears to be little qualitative species difference in the mode of
elimination of hycanthone. The highest tissue concentrations,
which are transient, are found in the liver and kidney. The
mechanism of action of hycanthone is not known (Senft, 1975).

Clinical use
Early clinical trials were conducted with both oral and parenteral formulations of hycanthone, but manufacture has been
restricted for some years to the parenteral form as troublesome
side-effects arose during oral treatment (Argento *et al.*, 1967;
Katz *et al.*, 1968; Clarke *et al.*, 1969). Hycanthone mesylate is
now supplied as a powder in vials of 200 mg base to be dissolved
in 2 ml sterile water for injection.

The importance of hycanthone lay in the fact that treatment
could be completed in one intramuscular injection. This opened
new prospects for population coverage in endemic areas. Num-

erous clinical trials standardised the dose as 3.0 ± 0.5 mg/kg of body weight and cure rates for both *S. mansoni* and *S. haematobium* varied between 50% and 90% in different samples (WHO, 1972). However, immediate side-effects were reported in all clinical trials and by 1972, 20 deaths occurring two to five days after treatment were recorded in over 300 000 patients treated (WHO, 1972). The great majority of these were due to acute hepatic necrosis. Although attempts to induce hepatic necrosis in the rhesus monkey and the dog failed, the cat was found to be extremely sensitive to hycanthone and severe jaundice and death frequently followed treatment. Although acute hepatic necrosis did occur in man, rigid case selection was considered to be a protective factor and it was thought that the hepatotoxicity was no bar to large-scale treatment (WHO, 1972). That this was a correct decision was substantiated by the report that, given care in patient selection, treatment and follow-up, no jaundice, liver necrosis or other serious side-effects was encountered in 2723 patients in St Lucia given hycanthone (Cook and Jordan, 1976).

The frequency of other side-effects caused clinicians to explore alternative dose regimes. These side-effects included vomiting, sometimes occurring in over 50% of treated patients in some trials, nausea, anorexia, abdominal pain, dizziness, headache and local pain at the injection site. It was observed in some trials that serum transaminase levels rose after hycanthone but returned to normal in one to three weeks. The vital importance of pre-treatment examinations to exclude patients at risk of liver damage was emphasised by the demonstration of direct hepatotoxicity of hycanthone (Andrade *et al.*, 1974). In eight patients dying after hycanthone treatment, centrilobular necrosis was demonstrated histologically with associated fatty change, diffuse mononuclear cell infiltration, swelling of hepatocytes and a fine vacuolisation of the cytoplasm. In one patient who became jaundiced after hycanthone treatment, liver biopsy revealed a cholestatic picture. When 14 patients with mild active schistosomiasis were subjected to liver biopsies and liver function tests before and 48 hours after hycanthone, the liver function tests remained within normal limits, but in every post-treatment liver biopsy there was present a diffuse microvesiculation of the endoplasmic reticulum of the hepatocytes.

Smaller doses were found to reduce the frequency and severity of side-effects yet retain a high degree of antischistosomal efficacy—in *S. haematobium* infections (Davis *et al.*, 1971), 2.5

mg/kg was optimal in retaining cure rates while minimising side-effects and for *S. mansoni* (Cook *et al.*, 1976) 1·5–2·0 mg/kg was considered an acceptable dose. Later investigations (Warren *et al.*, 1978) have used smaller dose ranges of 0·375–1·5 mg/kg and have claimed 96% reduction in egg output at four months with, however, only a 32% cure rate. The smaller doses gave cure rates of 1·8–7·5% and, in theory, carry a risk of inducing resistance.

The parasitological curative effect of hycanthone in man has never really been in doubt. Although it has been suggested that in experimental animals the hepatic shift of *S. mansoni* after hycanthone is not long lasting (Rogers and Bueding, 1971), this finding cannot necessarily be extrapolated to man. In 433 patients treated with 3 mg hycanthone per kg of body weight, the therapeutic effect remained virtually constant for two years (Cook *et al.*, 1974). Thus the claim that a significant number of *S. mansoni* return to the mesenteric vessels after treatment, or that reversible inhibition of egg laying occurs, could not be substantiated in clinical practice. What was clearly shown, additionally, was that hycanthone caused regression of hepato-splenomegaly due to *S. mansoni* infection.

Of more concern to clinical investigators was the increasing number of reports indicating that hycanthone produced changes in a variety of experimental test systems which were indicative of mutagenicity. While it was generally agreed that hycanthone was a mutagen in many submammalian test systems including *Salmonella*, *Neurospora*, yeast and *Drosophila*, extensive studies on the transmitted genetic effects of hycanthone in mammals showed no genetic effect (Russell, 1975).

These experimental findings, mysterious and confusing to the clinical physician, generated a series of meetings where full discussion of the findings was aired (WHO, 1972; US Japan Cooperative Science Program, 1975).

In addition to this controversy over the findings in experimental mutagenicity test systems, hycanthone was shown to be teratogenic in mice and rabbits (Moore, 1972; Sieber and Adamson, 1975).

Finally, hycanthone was reported to produce a significant increase in hepatic hyperplasia and induction of hepatocellular carcinomas in mice previously infected with *S. mansoni* (Haese *et al.*, 1973; Haese and Bueding, 1976). These findings were not confirmed by another study in which mice were infected with *S.*

mansoni by a different route and given different doses of hycanthone but in which there was a low survival rate (Yarinsky *et al.*, 1974).

Thus the data available from carcinogenicity tests do not allow a definite judgement on the tumorigenic potential of hycanthone. No epidemiological evidence exists to confirm or refute any suspicion of carcinogenicity production in man.

Conclusion

Hycanthone is a highly effective drug in the treatment of *S. mansoni* and *S. haematobium* infections when used by a physician with a full appreciation of its drawbacks. In many areas of endemicity it is unnecessary to use the recommended dose of 3 mg/kg, since a lower dose minimises side-effects yet retains an acceptable cure rate. In all cases not parasitologically cured, reduction of excretal egg output is of a very high order, implying that the majority of the body population of flukes has been killed.

Yet the drug has many disadvantages. Contraindications to its use are numerous and have been listed by the manufacturers. They include impaired liver function from any cause, hepatic disease from causes other than schistosomiasis, jaundice, a tender liver, a recent history suspicious of jaundice or hepatitis and the concurrent use of drugs known to affect liver function. Any significant pyrexial condition due to bacterial, viral or other causes must be investigated and treated before hycanthone is given. Advanced disease states and malnutrition are indications for a full clinical appraisal before hycanthone is contemplated. Early pregnancy is a bar to treatment. Advanced cases of *S. mansoni* should preferably be given another antischistosomal drug.

When the unresolved controversy on mutagenicity and carcinogenicity is added to this formidable list of contraindications, plus the fact that a true hycanthone resistance is known to occur (Katz *et al.*, 1973; Campos *et al.*, 1976), then it is scarcely surprising that the use of the drug has not attained the levels predicted a few years ago. Alternative effective compounds exist and, while hycanthone can be used with good expectations of cure in healthy young people or adults, the combined weight of its disadvantages, suspected or actual, have made physicians hypercautious about its therapeutic use.

Although several active chloroindazole analogues of hycanthone show antischistosomal activity in mice (Bueding *et al.*, 1973;

Bueding, 1975), some are also weakly mutagenic, as is lucanthone, and it seems doubtful whether they will be developed for clinical use.

Lucanthone hydrochloride (Nilodin®: Miracil D, Wellcome)

The parent compound of hycanthone, active when given by mouth, was widely used from 1948 to the mid-sixties. Like hycanthone, it was ineffective against *S. japonicum*, but when given as a short treatment course over three to six days, had moderate activity against both *S. haematobium* and *S. mansoni*.

Its great drawback was that it produced frequent, and often severe, anorexia, nausea, vomiting, abdominal discomfort and occasionally diarrhoea. Mental symptoms and states of confusion or mania were also rarely associated with its use. These side-effects proved to be the major limiting factor in its general acceptance and there are virtually no indications for its use nowadays.

Drugs effective against all species of schistosome

Praziquantel (Biltricide®, Bayer A.G.)

Praziquantel, a newly developed heterocyclic pyrazino-isoquinoline compound, is a 2-Cyclohexylcarbonyl-1,2,3,6,7,11b-hexahydro-4H,pyrazino[2,1-a]isoquinoline-4-one. It has the structural formula shown in Fig. 9.4.

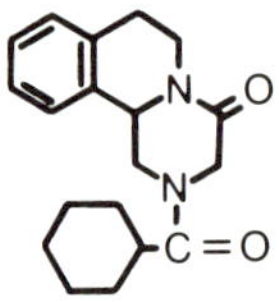

Fig. 9.4 Praziquantel.

The active substance is an hygroscopic, colourless, almost odourless crystalline powder with a bitter taste, which is stable under normal conditions but melts at 136–140°C with decomposition. It is very soluble in chloroform and dimethylsulphoxide, sparingly soluble in ethanol and very slightly soluble in water.

Preclinical studies

It is not structurally related to previously used antischistosomal drugs and, in wide-ranging experimental preclinical studies in many animal species, was highly effective against *S. japonicum, S.*

mansoni, S. haematobium, S. intercalatum and *S. mattheei* (Gönnert and Andrews, 1977; James *et al.*, 1977; Pellegrino *et al.*, 1977; Webbe and James, 1977), in addition to which it exhibited potent cestocidal properties (Thomas and Gönnert, 1977).

Mode of action

Praziquantel is active against schistosomes both *in vitro* and *in vivo*. In *in-vitro* experiments, schistosomes instantly become immobile and undergo contraction on contact with the drug. A serum concentration of $0.3\,\mu$g/ml is fully effective; one of $0.1\,\mu$g/ml is without effect. When schistosomes are kept in culture media containing a little protein, all concentrations of drug above $0.04\,\mu$g/ml are effective. It seems that the contraction of the schistosome musculature is due to an interference by praziquantel with inorganic ion transport mechanisms, resulting in a decreased influx of K^+ but an increase in influx of Ca^{2+} and Na^+ into the worms (Pax *et al.*, 1978).

In parallel with these biochemical studies, scanning and transmission electron microscopy of *S. mansoni* after *in-vitro* exposure to concentrations of praziquantel ranging from 0–$100\,\mu$g/ml for times varying from 5 to 60 minutes has shown that the drug causes vacuolisation of the schistosome tegument, finally leading to the disruption of the apical tegumental layer (Becker *et al.*, 1980). This appears to be a direct and primary effect of praziquantel, not only on schistosomes, but also on other parasites—cestodes—which are sensitive to the drug. Glucose uptake of schistosomes, and hence lactic acid production, is reduced by praziquantel and the worm compensates by breakdown of its endogenous glycogen store. Egg formation in the female is inhibited at concentrations as low as $0.001\,\mu$g/ml and totally inhibited at $0.01\,\mu$g/ml.

Pharmacology and toxicology

In the customary pharmacological screening tests, no significant actions of praziquantel were observed in therapeutic doses. When very high subtoxic doses were given to mice, rabbits and cats, sedation occurred with, in some experiments, transitory convulsions which were not related to barbiturate-like anaesthetic effect or to peripheral muscle relaxation. No effects were noted on the cardiovascular system, the peripheral nervous system, blood clotting, bone marrow function, metabolism or liver or renal function.

Acute studies, conducted in rats, mice and rabbits, showed that, in comparison with other antischistosomal drugs, praziquantel had a very low acute toxicity profile. Rats tolerated daily doses of up to 1 g/kg for 4 weeks and dogs tolerated daily dosages of up to 180 mg/kg for 13 weeks without organ damage. No effects were seen on the whole reproductive process in rats. Teratogenic effects were not observed in mice, rats and rabbits (Frohberg and Schulze-Schencking, 1981). A wide range of studies revealed no mutagenic activity of praziquantel in tissue-, host- and urine-mediated assays with *Salmonella typhimurium* TA98 and TA100 strains (Obermeir and Frohberg, 1977), in dominant lethal and micronucleus tests in mice and in spermatogonial tests in Chinese hamsters (Machemer and Lorke, 1978) and in a battery of investigations in *S. typhimurium*, *Schizosaccharomyces pombe*, *Saccharomyces cerevisiae*, *Drosophila melanogastes* and cultured V79 Chinese hamster cells, with or without a metabolic activation system where appropriate (Bartsch *et al.*, 1978).

Current carcinogenicity studies with oral doses of 100 mg and 250 mg praziquantel per kg, given once weekly to Syrian hamsters for 80 weeks and to rats for 104 weeks, have not revealed any carcinogenic potential to date (Frohberg and Schulze-Schencking, 1981).

In man, praziquantel is rapidly absorbed after oral dosage and, after a pronounced first-pass biotransformation process, metabolites are excreted mainly in the urine. In healthy volunteers, maximum serum concentrations are reached in 1–2 hours. By use of an isotope-measuring technique with ^{14}C-labelled praziquantel and a specific gas chromatographic assay, the elimination half-life of the drug from the serum was $1–1\frac{1}{2}$ hours and that for praziquantel plus metabolites was 4–5 hours. The renal elimination half-life for praziquantel plus metabolites was 4–6 hours and the cumulative renal excretion of praziquantel within 4 days was over 80% of the dose, 90% of which was eliminated on the first day (Buhring *et al.*, 1978; Leopold *et al.*, 1978).

Clinical experience

Co-operative multicentre clinical trials of tolerance to praziquantel and of its therapeutic effect against the three common species of schistosome infecting man were conducted jointly by the World Health Organization and the manufacturing company (Bayer AG, Federal Republic of Germany) in Africa,

Brazil, Japan and the Philippines. Double blind trials of tolerance were followed by clinical trials of efficacy using a standard trial design and agreed technical protocols, although parasitological methods of therapeutic assessment varied with the species of infecting parasite (Davis and Wegner, 1979; Davis *et al.*, 1979; Ishizaki *et al.*, 1979; Katz *et al.*, 1979; Santos *et al.*, 1979).

In all these trials, praziquantel was well tolerated, produced no changes of biological significance in a battery of haematological and biochemical monitoring tests or in serial electrocardiograms or electroencephalograms, and gave cure rates at six months of between 75% and 100% in the various samples of patients treated.

Virtually all trials to date have confirmed the absence of toxic effects of the drug on vital organs, systems and functions. Side-effects of treatment are generally mild and disappear within 24 hours. The most frequent symptoms reported are epigastric pain or diffuse abdominal discomfort, nausea, anorexia, loose stools or diarrhoea, dizziness, headache, pruritus or urticarial-type skin eruptions and fever. Predictably, the proportion of those complaining of side-effects varies with the ethnic origin of the patients. Abdominal pain has occurred in up to 50% of some series, but is generally mild and is only rarely accompanied by vomiting.

Another series of trials was initiated to explore a wider dosage range and the influence of the intensity of pre-treatment excretal egg output on cure rates. In a recent review of the results of the treatment of more than 1000 patients, the six-month cure rates for *S. haematobium* varied between 83% and 100%; for *S. mansoni*, 67% and 100%; for *S. japonicum*, between 71% and 100% (Wegner, 1979).

Chinese experience with praziquantel in the treatment of *S. japonicum* parallelled the initial findings in the Philippines. In 1276 cases treated with total doses ranging from 45–90 mg/kg body weight for one or two days, side-effects were mild and transient, although a few patients exhibited neuropsychiatric or cardiovascular symptoms, stools were negative for ova within 15 days and post-treatment hatching tests at 1, 3 and 6 months were negative in 91–98% of different samples of patients (Pyquiton Research Group, 1980).

In another detailed study of 502 patients using various doses, daily hatching tests showed that eggs disappeared from the stool at times varying between 7 and 18 days after treatment.

Follow-up of 501 patients at 6 months gave a cumulative negative rate of 99% (Pyquiton Coordination Group, 1980).

The results of many clinical trials in Africa against *S. mansoni*, *S. haematobium*, double infections and *S. intercalatum* amply confirmed the data from the earlier trials, and consistently high cure rates with good patient tolerance of the drug were features in all (Biltricide Symposium, 1980).

Conclusion

It is clear that praziquantel is a major therapeutic advance; it is well tolerated, has no significant effect on liver, renal, haematopoeitic or other body functions and is highly effective against all schistosomes parasitising man.

Although trials are continuing to establish optimal doses for the different species, the present recommended dose for *S. haematobium* is a single oral dose of 40 mg/kg; this will also be effective in many cases of light infections with *S. mansoni*, but heavy infections may require two doses, each of either 25 mg/kg or 30 mg/kg, given at an interval of four hours. For the treatment of *S. japonicum*, the present recommended regime is three doses, each of 20 mg/kg (total dose 60 mg praziquantel per kg body weight), given at intervals of four hours.

It is particularly noteworthy that advanced cases of *S. japonicum* or *S. mansoni* with ascites or portal hypertension have tolerated the drug well and this feature augurs well for the future treatment of late cases.

Praziquantel will undoubtedly become a drug of first choice for all schistosome infections in the future. It is dispensed under the trade name 'Biltricide®', (Bayer AG) in the form of tablets of 600 mg, which can be quartered easily.

Niridazole (Ambilhar®, Ciba-Geigy)

Niridazole is 1-(5-nitro-2-thiazolyl)-2-imidazolidinone; its structural formula is shown in Fig. 9.5.

The drug, formulated as orange-coloured tablets of either 500 mg or 100 mg, has been in widespread clinical use since 1964.

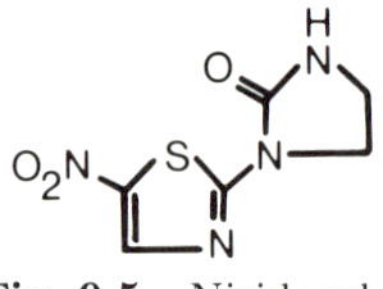

Fig. 9.5 Niridazole.

Pharmacology
Niridazole is given by mouth and is well but slowly absorbed from the gastrointestinal tract. It undergoes a first-pass metabolic transformation in the liver. Maximum blood concentrations are reached in six hours. After administration of a radiolabelled drug, serum radioactivity was higher when doses were given twice daily than when the same amount was given as a single dose. This indicated improved absorption of the drug and clinical trials have confirmed the desirability of giving the daily dose in two or three divided portions. Non-metabolised drug is schistosomicidal and is concentrated in the germinal cells of the schistosome and eggs. Metabolites are inactive and are bound to plasma albumin. Portal and intestinal blood that has not passed through the liver exhibit concentrations of non-metabolised drug much higher than those found in peripheral blood. Since, in hepatosplenic schistosomiasis due to *S. mansoni* or *S. japonicum*, portocaval and systemic vascular communications may permit the transfer of blood containing higher levels of non-metabolised drug to the systemic circulation, this fact is thought to be related to the production of neuropsychiatric side-effects seen during treatment of late cases of these infections. Excretion of the metabolites, while slow, is almost complete and divided equally between urine and faeces.

Clinical use
Niridazole has been widely used for the treatment of *S. haematobium*, *S. mansoni* and *S. japonicum*. Side-effects are more common in the treatment of *S. japonicum* and least frequent in *S. haematobium* infections. Claims that the concurrent administration of sedatives, tranquillisers or antihistamines is effective in diminishing the frequency of both major and minor side-effects do not withstand critical analysis. In general, children tolerate the drug much better than adults.

Many clinicians regard niridazole as a highly useful drug for the treatment of *S. haematobium* in children. At a total dose of 175 mg/kg of body weight, given either as 25 mg/kg per day for 7 days or as 35 mg/kg per day for 5 days, high cure rates of the order of 80–100% in different samples are usual (Davis, 1966; Fontanilles, 1969). In the treatment of the individual patient, it is preferable that the dose be given in two or three divided portions in the day.

Treatment of *S. mansoni* infections has not been as satisfactory and there is a wide range of reported cure rates from 30% to 70% in children and somewhat higher in adults (Fontanilles, 1969). The occurrence of side-effects, although frequently minor, has limited the enthusiasm for niridazole in *S. mansoni* infections.

In general, the treatment of *S. japonicum* infections with niridazole, whether in China, Japan (Kurata, 1973) or the Philippines (Pesigan *et al.*, 1966), has been disappointing. Side-effects have been of frequent occurrence, thus necessitating a lower total dose than is given in African schistosomiasis and cure rates have been only about 50%. Niridazole cannot be recommended as a primary drug for either *S. japonicum* or *S. mansoni* infection in the individual patient and, owing to the frequency of neuropsychiatric symptoms, the drug is contraindicated where portal systemic vascular shunts permit the by-pass of portal blood from the liver to the systemic circulation.

Niridazole is also contraindicated in patients with mental disturbance, frank mental illness, any form of epilepsy, patients receiving isoniazid and in severe heart disease.

Side-effects

A wide range of side-effects has been reported. While of frequent occurrence, the majority are not severe. However, the most important (fortunately rare) are those associated with the nervous system and these can be serious. Many different clinical syndromes have been recorded during or after niridazole treatment, including hyperexcitability, mania, agitation, confusion, depression, hallucinations, loss of consciousness and even generalised convulsions. Electro-encephalography before or during treatment was of no help in predicting the occurrence of these neuropsychiatric symptoms. In 810 documented cases of *S. mansoni* treated with niridazole, 5% of 730 with the intestinal form exhibited convulsions, loss of consciousness, hallucinations or agitation, while 21% of 80 patients with hepatosplenic schistosomiasis showed the same symptoms (Fontanilles, 1969).

Numerous other side-effects have been reported: anorexia, nausea, vomiting, abdominal pain, diarrhoea, headache, vertigo, skin rashes, a dark brown colour of the urine, an increased heart rate during treatment and non-specific flattening of the T waves in the electrocardiogram.

The proportions of patients developing one or more side-effects naturally vary markedly. In a tabulation describing the average incidence of minor side-effects during niridazole treatment of 444 cases of *S. mansoni*, headache, nausea and/or vomiting occurred in 70%, anorexia in 67%, weight loss in 65%, abdominal discomfort in 52%, dizziness in 52%, myalgia or anthralgia in 35%, palpitations and anxiety in 17% and skin rashes in 6% (Fontanilles, 1969).

While testicular damage and reduction of spermatozoa have occurred in experimental animals treated with niridazole, little is known of the effect on human gonads. Fertility has not been impaired in adult males or females, but spermograms and testicular biopsies have occasionally displayed a transitory reduction in the number of spermatozoa in the ejaculate (Fontanilles, 1969).

Conclusion

While niridazole occupies an important place in the history of chemotherapy of schistosomiasis, its use and popularity can be expected to decline in parallel with the increasing use of alternative effective, less toxic antischistosomal agents. The demonstration of mutagenicity in various test systems (Straus, 1974; Legator *et al.*, 1975; McCann *et al.*, 1975; Ong and de Serres, 1975; Shahin, 1975) and the fact that the compound is carcinogenic in mice and hamsters after oral administration (Urman *et al.*, 1975; Bulay *et al.*, 1977; International Agency for Research on Cancer, 1977) have induced a justifiable sense of uneasiness amongst clinicians, although there are no epidemiological studies linking niridazole and cancer in man. Investigations have shown that niridazole inhibits granuloma formation and suppresses delayed hypersensitivity in mice (Moore, 1972) and man (Webster *et al.*, 1975). Further advances in this field can be anticipated and the drug may well pass from the clinician to the experimental biologist as a source of new data.

Antimonial compounds

From 1918, when the use of tartar emetic in the treatment of *S. haematobium* infections began (Christopherson, 1918), the trivalent antimonials occupied pride of place in the therapy of human schistosomiasis, whether caused by *S. japonicum, S. mansoni* or *S. haematobium*, until the advent of new drugs in the last decade.

Pharmacology

Many antimonial compounds are available. All have a similar action. Given intravenously or intramuscularly, a high but transient blood level of antimony is produced and appreciable tissue levels can be detected in the liver, the thyroid gland and the heart. The continuous excretion of antimony during treatment, mainly by renal mechanisms, and the constant movement of antimony from blood to tissues, complicate attempts to achieve long-lasting high blood concentrations. Antimonial drugs are cumulative and, after treatment, excretion of the metal may take some weeks. In comparative trials of the commonest antimonial preparations, it was shown that in the treatment of *S. haematobium* infections in adults in Tanzania, antimony retention in the body was greater after intravenous antimony sodium tartrate and least after intravenous antimony sodium gluconate when these drugs were given in equimetallic dosage to comparable recipients. The degree of retention of antimony within the body correlated well with the incidence, the frequency and the severity of the side-effects of the individual preparations used (Davis, 1968).

While antimonial compounds have been used for the treatment of individual patients successfully for many years, the numerous variables which determine their effects at the site of action have always made their application difficult and have, in no small part, adversely affected their use in large-scale human chemotherapy. The efficiency of antimony as a therapeutic agent depends on its valency, on the type of bond linking the metal to the organic moiety and on the nature of the linkage element. Oxygen linkage of trivalent antimony to aliphatic or aromatic radicals appears to be necessary for antischistosomal activity. However, the final clinical effects of antimony are dependent on numerous factors, interaction of which is unpredictable. Friedheim (1973) stressed this and cited the dissociation constants of the antimonial drug, the antimony complexes formed *in vivo* with tissue constituents of both host and parasite and the differences in both absorption and elimination rates which cannot be extrapolated from one species to another. To add to this confused situation, the differences in antimonial content of the preparations available and the varying techniques of administration have all, in practice, combined to ensure that antimony treatment of schistosomiasis was essentially a pragmatic undertaking based on clinical experience rather than scientific logic. The basic mode of action of antimony is by inhibition of phosphofructokinase, an enzyme regulating schistosomal energy. Intrauterine eggs are damaged and there is controversy as to whether or not eggs already deposited in host tissues are also affected.

Clinical use

Although many preparations of organic trivalent antimony have been used in clinical practice, only two will be described since both possess a deserved therapeutic superiority.

Antimony sodium tartrate (AST), containing 38·5% of trivalent antimony, is given intravenously as an isotonic solution in distilled water. The British Pharmacopoeia preparation contains 60 mg in 1 ml. The initial dose is 30 mg AST by i.v. injection, increasing by 30 mg daily or on alternate days (dependent on patient tolerance) to a maximum single dose of 120 mg AST. The total dose given, which is frequently dictated by patient tolerance, is 1·5–2·0 g AST, approximately equivalent to 577·5–770 mg of antimony.

This treatment is highly effective against all three species of schistosomes, but the disadvantages of daily intravenous injections and the high frequency of side-effects, sometimes serious, restrict its utility to adults.

An alternative popular preparation is antimony dimercaptosuccinate ('Stibocaptate'; 'Astiban®'; TWSb) which contains 25–26% trivalent antimony. The total dose is 30–40 mg/kg and it is customarily administered as five intramuscular injections, each of 6–8 mg/kg every 2–4 days (although once weekly dosage is satisfactory). The maximum single dose should not exceed 500 mg and the total dose should not exceed 2·5 g. The total antimony content of the course varies with the body weight and the dose level selected. The drug is effective against all the three common species of schistosome and is to be preferred over AST if an antimonial has to be used in children. There must, however, be few instances where this is necessary since effective, better tolerated alternatives are nowadays available to treat any schistosome infection.

Other antimonial compounds, such as antimony potassium tartrate, sodium antimonyl gluconate (Triostam®)—both of which are given intravenously—sodium antimony bis-pyrocatechol-3,5-disulfonate (Stibophen B.P; neoantimosan; Fuadin®; Reprodal®; Fantorin®) lithium antimony thiomalate ('Anthiomaline®')—which are given intramuscularly—may be available regionally, but nowadays there are few if any indications for their use.

Side-effects

Frequent, sometimes severe, and occasionally fatal adverse effects have marked the use of antimonial drugs and have certainly played a major role in restricting their applications to large populations.

Those antimonials given intravenously can produce painful local perivenous inflammation if leakage of the injection occurs. Skin ulceration may supervene should a leak during injection take place.

Should vomiting, cough, substernal pain or syncope occur during the intravenous injection of an antimony compound, it should be abandoned at once.

Other adverse effects may be manifested at gastrointestinal, hepatic, musculoskeletal, dermatological or cardiovascular sites. They tend to increase in frequency as the therapeutic course progresses and frequently lead to incomplete treatments. Gastrointestinal symptoms are prominent and a bitter taste in the mouth, salivation, anorexia, nausea, vomiting and diarrhoea may be encountered. Epigastric discomfort associated with a tender liver is a danger sign and treatment should be stopped. Arthralgia and myalgia are irritants, and the combination of many different side-effects can induce misery and depression in patients. Many skin complications have been described but severe exfoliative dermatitis is rare.

Liver function tests almost always show abnormalities during antimony treatment and cardiotoxicity can be evidenced by syncope, by substernal pain or discomfort, by T wave inversion, lengthening of QT interval or partial branch block. The fatal cardiovascular events that have been described, cardiac dysrhythmias or the shock syndromes resembling anaphylaxis, are extremely rare.

As may be inferred, many contraindications to antimonial treatment exist. Physicians using these compounds were always understandably cautious in treating patients with schistosomiasis.

Conclusion

Despite a prominent place in chemotherapeutic history, the time has come to consign antimony to the museums. There are in existence alternative and better tolerated drugs for all types of human schistosomiasis. There are few if any indications for antimony in modern clinical practice.

Antischistosomal drugs currently under development

Two new antischistosomal compounds have undergone limited clinical trials.

Amoscanate (C9333-Go/CGP450; nithiocyaminum, Ciba-Geigy)

The structural formula is shown in Fig. 9.6.

$$O_2N-\!\!\langle\bigcirc\rangle\!\!-NH-\!\!\langle\bigcirc\rangle\!\!-NCS$$

Fig. 9.6 Amoscanate.

This new isothiocyanate anthelmintic exhibits marked activity under experimental conditions against the hookworms and all three species of schistosome pathogenic for man. It also appears to have macro- and microfilaricidal properties in appropriate test systems (Sen, 1976; Striebel, 1976; Saz *et al.*, 1977).

In man it has proven activity against *S. mansoni* and *S. japonicum*, but in the initial trials against *S. haematobium* there was no parasitological response, possibly owing to imperfect pharmaceutical formulation and consequently poor absorption (McMahon, 1977). New pharmaceutical formulations have resulted in enhanced effectiveness of the compound experimentally (Bueding *et al.*, 1976). Small particle-size suspensions tested for efficacy against *S. mansoni* and *S. haematobium* in primates in comparison with praziquantel have confirmed that, under these experimental conditions, amoscanate has high antischistosomal activity (Striebel and Stauffer, 1980).

There has been considerable experience of the use of the drug in China (where it is named nithiocyaminum) and by 1979, over 100 000 patients had been treated (Gang, 1979). Several dose regimes were tried and when a particle diameter size of 3–6 μ was used in the tablets and total oral doses of 6–7 mg/kg were given over three consecutive days, then in two trials 81% (108/133) and 84% (562/672) of patients followed in two different endemic areas at six months were egg negative (Gang, 1979). Side-effects of treatment were noted, among which were central nervous system reactions and a post-therapeutic jaundice of mixed cholestatic and hepatotoxic cause.

In 1949 cases of *S. japonicum*, six dosage regimes ranging from 3 mg/kg to 8 mg/kg in one to four days were tried and three formulations of nithiocyaminum were used. Jaundice developed one to two weeks after treatment in 21 of 1737 patients (1·21%) given a microcrystal formulation of the drug. The incidence of jaundice in those patients receiving a dose of 6 mg/kg or more was over twice as great as in those receiving 5 mg/kg or less. In an experimental pathological investigation, electron microscopy revealed that the drug caused injury of hepatic organelles and epithelial proliferation in the bile ducts (Sichuan Institute of Parasitic Diseases, 1980).

Intensive investigations and further toxicity studies with new formulations of this interesting compound are now in progress.

Oltipraz (R.P. 35.972. Rhone-Poulenc)

The structural formula is shown in Fig. 9.7.

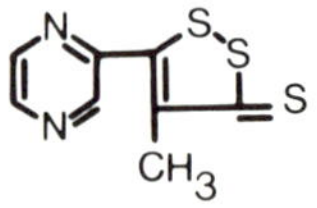

Fig. 9.7   Oltipraz.

This new antischistosomal compound was active by both oral and parenteral routes in mice infected with *S. mansoni* and its efficacy compared favourably with both niridazole and oxamniquine (Leroy *et al.*, 1978).

Initial clinical trials demonstrated its efficacy in both *S. haematobium* and *S. mansoni* infections at doses of 1·5 g per day for three days (Gentilini *et al.*, 1979).

Later studies confirmed that doses of 3 g or 4·5 g given in one day were effective in the treatment of *S. mansoni* and *S. haematobium* but side-effects, although mild, were frequent and consisted of nausea, vomiting abdominal pain, insomnia, headache, dizziness and weakness. No untoward effects were seen in laboratory monitoring of blood counts, serum creatinine, serum transaminases, alkaline phosphatases or in the ECG and EEG (Woehrle *et al.*, 1980).

Larger scale clinical trials involving 321 patients from Mali, Gabon, and immigrants in Paris have been reported recently (Gentilini *et al.*, 1980). In *S. haematobium* infections, a 92% cure rate was obtained in 86 patients who received total doses ranging from 2 g to 7·5 g over one to five days. In *S. intercalatum* infections, a cure rate of 87% in 72 patients receiving 1·25–4·59 g over three days was attained. All 47 patients with *S. mansoni* infections who received a total dose ranging from 3–5 g over two to five days were cured. Clinical and clinicopathological toleration was good.

Obviously, further dose-ranging studies will continue on this new antischistosomal compound and its future place in the chemotherapeutic spectrum will be determined by the ratio of patient tolerance to parasiticidal effect.

The choice of chemotherapy

The great majority of uncomplicated cases of schistosomiasis can, with modern drugs, be treated in the home, the out-patient clinic or the rural dispensary. Cases of *S. mansoni* or *S. japonicum* with complications of severe polyposis, portal hypertension, ascites or malnutrition still must be managed in hospital since chemotherapy is only one part of total patient care and the general medical management may be of equal or greater importance than specific chemotherapy, since the problems are mainly due to the structural or functional derangements resulting from long-standing infections.

For *S. haematobium* infections, metrifonate is cheap and well tolerated but has the disadvantage of necessitating repeated doses. Praziquantel is highly efficacious in a single oral dose. Standard niridazole and antimony therapy are second choices and experience with Oltipraz is as yet limited.

S. mansoni infections can be treated easily with oxamniquine, with good patient tolerance, and praziquantel is again an effective agent. One of the major therapeutic advances of recent years is in the provision of highly effective yet well-tolerated drugs which can be used to treat complicated cases of late *S. mansoni* infection such as advanced hepatosplenic schistosomiasis (Farid *et al.*, 1980) or diffuse colonic polyposis (Farid *et al.*, 1976), conditions which until only a few years ago posed difficult problems in management. As with *S. haematobium* infections, niridazole or antimony can be used if no alternatives are available, but care must be taken and troublesome side-effects anticipated.

Double infections with *S. mansoni* and *S. haematobium*, of frequent occurrence in the Egyptian Delta, the Sudan and many areas of sub-Saharan Africa, can be given praziquantel, effective against both parasites and well tolerated, or combined oxamniquine and metrifonate treatment. A third alternative in otherwise healthy adults would be hycanthone and, finally, niridazole or antimonials are available.

In *S. japonicum* infections, the treatment of which was always unsatisfactory, praziquantel is the treatment of choice. It is too early to assess the future role of amoscanate but there is little doubt of its efficacy. Finally, niridazole and antimonials can be used although with care and in the dual knowledge of rather poor cure rates and the occurrence of troublesome side-effects.

For the treatment of *S. intercalatum* or other more exotic species infections, praziquantel will be the primary drug.

The assessment of the effects of chemotherapy

It is important that physicians, whether in tropical or temperate areas, should bear in mind that at least two sources of variation in bio-availability which are directly under their control can occur in the range of antischistosomal drugs, those of storage conditions and age of preparation. Both of these factors must be checked at regular intervals to avoid the use of unsuitably stored or out-of-date drugs.

Tablets of metrifonate ('Bilarcil'®) are estimated to have a shelf-life of two years in warm climates, i.e. storage temperature of approximately 25°C, and of four years in moderate climates, i.e. storage temperature of approximately 20°C. In general, metrifonate tablets must be moisture-proof packed, stored in a cool place, preferably a refrigerator at 4°C, and the contents of opened tins should be used as soon as possible. Storage at high temperatures may cause discolouration of the tablets which are then no longer suitable for treatment.

The shelf-life of oxamniquine capsules ('Mansil'®, 'Vansil'®) is five years and that of the syrup, three years. Storage conditions should be those used normally for pharmaceutical products and no special recommendations are made.

The lacquered 600-mg tablets of praziquantel ('Biltricide'®), whether packed in tins or glass containers, have a shelf-life of three years in hot humid climates and four years in temperate zones. If packed in PVC press-out dispensers, it is probably wise to allow a shelf-life of two years in hot humid areas, three years in hot dry climates and four years in temperate zones.

Niridazole ('Ambilhar') tablets have a shelf-life of five years. The tablets should be protected from light but no other special storage conditions are necessary.

Hycanthone ('Etrenol'), presented as a powder in 2-ml glass vials, has a shelf-life of 60 months (five years) without any unusual storage conditions other than protecting the lyophilised product from moisture.

Antimony sodium tartrate (BP) and antimony potassium tartrate (BP) should be stored in the powder form in airtight containers. Both are available as an injection preparation which could be sterilised by autoclaving, steaming or filtration without an increase in toxicity. Injection stored at room temperature, at 4°C or at 40°C showed no increase in toxicity for at least 12 months. (Somers & Whittet, 1958).

Stibocaptate ('Astiban'®) is available as a powder for preparing injections in ampoules of 500 mg. Solutions in water are unstable and should be used within 24 h of preparation.

Stibophen (BP) must be stored in airtight neutral-glass containers, protected from light, and contact with iron compounds should be avoided. It is possible that stibophen could undergo molecular dissociation with enhanced toxicity after long storage and therefore stocks should be rotated after a year.

The assessment of the effects of chemotherapy

The results of chemotherapy can be assessed by various means:

(i)   clinical evaluation;
(ii) direct parasitological examination;
(iii) indirect parasitological examination;
(iv) ancillary examinations to indicate regression of lesions.

Clinical assessment is made from repeated follow-up of the patient, the history, the improvement of symptoms (particularly the loss of haematuria and disappearance of urinary complaints in *S. haematobium* infections), the gain in weight and diminution of bowel symptoms if present in *S. mansoni* or *S. japonicum* infections, and the regressing physical signs due to a shrinkage in size of hepatosplenomegaly. Diminution of hepatosplenomegaly, when solely due to *S. mansoni* or *S. japonicum*, as a result of treatment with a number of antischistosomal agents, is well documented and can be striking. Other physical signs, such as ascites or gastrointestinal bleeding in advanced cases with gastro-oesophageal varices, may not regress or may regress only slightly.

Direct parasitological examinations of patients after antischistosomal treatment are essential, for opinions on the curative values of schistosomicides are of necessity based on measurements of the presence or absence of eggs in the excreta or in rectal biopsy material—measurements which may or may not use quantitative techniques. The concept of clinical cure, which may merely indicate clinical improvement co-existing with continuing egg deposition and excretion after treatment, is not susceptible to objective measurement (WHO, 1966). Similarly, serological tests are not indicative of the exact parasitological status of the patient after treatment.

It should be noted that even techniques of egg isolation in excreta are basically themselves indirect indicators of cure. Cessation of egg excretion after chemotherapy does not necessarily indicate death of adult schistosomes which, under the influence of chemotherapeutic agents, may have been stimulated to desert their normal venous habitats for longer or shorter periods. Yet, faced with these imperfections, a considerable body of evidence derived from clinical and laboratory experiences with numerous antischistosomal drugs has indicated that multiple post-treatment parasitological examinations of excreta and/or rectal biopsy material for eggs give the only currently realistic basis for the evaluation of antischistosomal effect. Two qualifications are essential for this reliance to be valid. The parasitological technique used for egg isolation should be known to be sensitive and emphasis should be placed on the ability of the technique to demonstrate viable eggs, since dead eggs may be shed and excreted for months after antischistosomal treatment and their excretion is not incompatible with parasitological cure (WHO, 1953; Davis, 1968; Weber *et al.*, 1969).

To the clinician, faced with the management and follow-up of an individual patient, a discussion on the importance of ensuring accurate estimates of parasitological cure may appear academic since he will be aware that continued excretion of small numbers of viable eggs after treatment is compatible with a symptom-free existence. He will, therefore, be satisfied to base his prognosis on the results of regular follow-up examinations of stools or urine, using a good concentration technique in a qualitative manner. To those physicians engaged in clinical research, in comparative evaluations of drugs or in operational chemotherapy in field control programmes, accurate estimates of the potential of an antischistosomal drug under widely varying conditions, in different populations and against different strains of the same species of parasite are essential.

Direct parasitological examination of excreta should be performed after chemotherapy at regular intervals for at least one year and only when all examinations are negative for eggs, either by a proven microscopic technique or by hatching, should 'cure' be claimed.

In general, four categories of response to treatment are recognised during direct parasitological follow-up of treated patients using quantitative techniques of examination.

1. Patients may be 'cured'. In practice, this means that viable eggs have never been isolated from excreta or from rectal biopsy material over an arbitrarily defined period.

2. The egg output after treatment may remain unchanged, indicating a therapeutic failure.

3. In some patients, excretal egg output may fall to 10% of its pre-treatment level. If long lasting, this is interpreted as evidence of the death of a high proportion of the pre-treatment population of female flukes in the body. If short lived, the reduction merely points to a transient migration of flukes from their sites of oviposition and their subsequent return.

4. Finally, in a few patients, excretal egg output may actually rise during the period of follow-up.

This limited categorisation of post-treatment parasitological responses has been adopted because current techniques of investigation and quantitation are too crude to allow finer subdivisions (Davis, 1972).

Difficulties in post-chemotherapeutic assessment may be encountered because several basic biological questions remain unanswered. Optimum times of follow-up after treatment are undecided because neither the incubation periods of the parasites in man nor the natural variation of life span of female flukes are known accurately, although numerous estimates have appeared in the literature (see Chapter 10). A pre-infection—that is, an infection acquired in the few weeks immediately preceding treatment—may confuse therapeutic assessment since maturing forms of the parasite might be unaffected by drugs which are lethal to the adult parasites. Unaffected larval forms may mature and produce viable eggs in the immediate post-treatment period. A re-infection acquired immediately after treatment might result in viable egg production a few months later. Combinations of such events can still further complicate therapeutic assessment. Immunity in schistosomiasis is of a relatively low order and, whereas its effects can be appreciated in the population spectrum of age-specific *S. haematobium* infections, this applies less in other species infections and, in any individual, its protective effects can be overcome relatively easily by a large quantum of infection.

In endemic areas it is customary to conduct repeated parasitological follow-up examinations for some six months before deciding on the outcome of treatment. By that time, 80–90% of therapeautic failures will have become manifest by the passage of viable eggs in the excreta (Davis, 1966, 1968). In endemic areas with constant exposure to infection, some compromise is necessary to be able to make a logical evaluation of the efficacy of antischistosomal drugs. The production of viable eggs in the first six months after treatment can reasonably be regarded as a therapeutic failure, although a maturation of a pre-infection could theoretically produce the same sequence. The production of viable eggs in the excreta one year after treatment in a patient previously free of eggs for six months can reasonably be regarded as a re-infection.

Naturally, in areas where the risks of pre-infection and re-infection are absent, parasitological and therapeutic assessment is accordingly much easier. Despite undoubted advances in parasitological technology, supplementary techniques for the assessment of cure are needed.

Indirect parasitological assessment, by means of serological techniques, has proved disappointing in the assessment of a patient's state after chemotherapy. All of the current techniques measure antibody. It is anticipated that antibodies, after an initial increase, will fall in titre after successful chemotherapy and this can be demonstrated in a variety of ways. There are, however, rarely any population measurements of antibody profiles using these serological techniques to enable investigators to appreciate cut-off points, below which it might be said that a patient is probably free of active schistosomal infections. Neither complement fixation nor circumoval precipitin reactions were satisfactory in assessing post-chemotherapeutic states in *S. japonicum* infections in humans (Tanaka, 1976). Although much more sensitive serological tests are coming into use for survey work, e.g. radio-immunoassay with purified egg antigen (Pelley *et al.*, 1977) or ELISA using a crude *S. mansoni* egg antigen (McLaren *et al.*, 1979), their performance as assessors of the post-chemotherapeutic state in man is unknown. In the follow-up of patients given Oltipraz where quantitative immunofluorescence, passive haemagglutination and counter immunoelectrophoresis were all used, results were disappointing since rather variable findings were recorded in the post-treatment sero-immunologic test reactions (Gentilini *et al.*, 1980).

It must be concluded that the current techniques of serological assessment of cure are far from satisfactory.

Ancillary clinicopathological measurements, radiology and endoscopy are of great value in assessing the reversibility of macroscopic lesions after specific chemotherapy. The disappearance of bladder granulomas after treatment, the relief of ureteral obstructions and the resolution of hydro-ureter and hydronephrosis have been documented. Impressive improvements in renal function may occur and resolution of colonic polyposis can be followed by fibre-optic colonoscopy. The subject has been well reviewed recently (Farid *et al.*, 1976). Any of these investigations may be indicated in an individual patient.

Surgical treatment

In the great majority of patients, specific antischistosomal chemotherapy is the only treatment needed. Intractable symptoms resulting from long-standing bladder and ureteric damage or the presence of a carcinoma of the bladder would of course require appropriate genito-urinary surgery.

In advanced cases of *S. mansoni* or *S. japonicum* infections with hepatosplenomegaly, worms have been removed from the body by inserting a filter into the portal vein during splenectomy and utilising an extracorporeal shunt. An antimonial is given intravenously, causing the schistosomes to be swept into the portal venous system where they are collected on the filter (Goldsmith *et al.*, 1967). This highly specialised technique is practised at only a few centres, is by no means suitable for all patients and is of greatly restricted application in population terms. It can be considered in the individual patient.

Bleeding gastro-oesophageal varices in *S. mansoni* or *S. japonicum* infections are managed by conventional methods. Liver cell function in these cases remains relatively good since most of the pathology is localised in the portal tracts and hepatic coma is less frequent than in patients with classical portal cirrhosis.

Prognosis

The prognosis of uncomplicated schistosomal infections is very good, providing that specific chemotherapy is given. The advent of well-tolerated, highly effective new drugs has given physicians flexibility and opportunities to alleviate many chronic complications which were, in the past, therapeutic nightmares. Improved functional and structural changes can be anticipated in damaged organs.

REFERENCES

Abaza, H. H., Hammouda, N., Abd Rabbo, H. and Shafei, A. Z. (1978). *Trans. R. Soc. Trop. Med. Hyg.* **72,** 602.

Andrade, Z. A., dos Santos, H. A., Borojevic, R. and Grimaud, J. A. (1974). *Revta Inst. Med. Trop. S. Paulo* **16,** 160.

Anon (1977). *Am. J. Trop. Med. Hyg.* **26,** 427.

Argento, C. A., Nerves, P. F., Galvao, F. A., Penna, D. R. and da Silva, J. R. (1967). *Revta Soc. Bras. Med. Trop.* **1,** 37.

Barker, L. R., Bueding, E. and Timms, A. R. (1966). *Br. J. Pharmac.* **26,** 656.

Bartsch, H., Kuroki, T., Malaveille, C., Loprieno, N., Barale, R., Abbondandolo, A., Bonalti, S., Rainaldi, G., Voge, E. and Davis, A. (1978). *Mutat. Res.* **58,** 133.

Bassily, S., Farid, Z., Higashi, G. I. and Watten, R. H. (1978). *Am. J. Trop. Med. Hyg.* **27,** 1284.

Bayer, A. G. (1972). Manufacturer's literature on metrifonate.

Becker, B., Mehlhorn, H., Andrews, P., Thomas, H. and Eckert, J. (1980). *Ztschr. Parasitkde* **63,** 113.

Berberian, D. A., Freele, H., Rosi, D., Dennis, E. W. and Archer, S. (1967). *Am. J. Trop. Med. Hyg.* **16,** 487.

Biltricide Symposium (1980). *Summary of proceedings*, 2nd edn., English version. Bayer, A. G.

Bueding, E. (1975). *J. Toxicol. Envir. Hlth* **1,** 329.

Bueding, E., Batzinger, R. and Petterson, G. (1976). *Experientia* **32,** 604.

Bueding, E., Fisher, J. and Bruce, J. (1973). *J. Pharmac. Exp. Ther.* **186,** 402.

Bueding, E., Liu, Ch. and Rogers, S. H. (1972). *Br. J. Pharmac.* **46,** 480.

Buhring, K. U., Diekmann, H. W., Muller, H., Garbe, A. and Nowak, H. (1978). *Eur. J. Drug Metab. Pharmacokin,* 179.

Bulay, O., Urman, H., Clayson, D. B. and Shubik, P. (1977). *J. Nat. Cancer Inst.* **69,** 1625.

Campos, R., Moreira, A. A. B., Sette, Jr. H., Chamone, D. A. F. and da Silva, L. C. (1976). *Trans. R. Soc. Trop. Med. Hyg.* **70,** 261.

Cerf, J., Lebrun, A. and Dierickx, J. (1962). *Am. J. Trop. Med. Hyg.* **11,** 514.

Christopherson, J. B. (1918). *Lancet* **ii,** 325.

Clarke, V. de V., Blair, D. M. and Weber, M. C. (1969). *Cent. Afr. J. Med.* **15,** 1.

Clarke, V. de V., Blair, D. M., Weber, M. C. and Garnett, P. A. (1976). *S. Afr. Med. J.* **50,** 1867.

Cook, J. A. and Jordan, P. (1976). *Ann. Trop. Med. Parasit.* **70,** 109.

Cook, J. A., Jordan, P. and Armitage, P. (1976). *Am. J. Trop. Med. Hyg.* **25,** 602.

Cook, J. A., Woodstock, L. and Jordan, P. (1974). *Am. J. Trop. Med. Hyg.* **23,** 910.

Davis, A. (1966). *Bull. Wld Hlth Org.* **35,** 827.

Davis, A. (1968). *Bull. Wld Hlth Org.* **38,** 197.

Davis, A. (1972). In *Medicine in a Tropical Environment*, p. 56. Eds A. G. Shaper, J. W. Kibukamusoke and M. S. R. Hutt. British Medical Association, London.

Davis, A. and Bailey, D. R. (1969). *Bull. Wld Hlth Org.* **41,** 209.

Davis, A., Bailey, D. R. and Desai, P. (1971). SCHISTO/WP/71, quoted in WHO (1972), *Bol. de la Oficina Sanitaria Panamericana VI*, p. 84. WHO, Washington.

Davis, A., Biles, J. E. and Ulrich, A. M. (1979). *Bull. Wld Hlth Org.* **57,** 773.

Davis, A. and Wegner, D. H. G. (1979). *Bull. Wld Hlth Org.* **57,** 767.

Ellman, G. L., Courtney, K. D., Andres, V. and Featherstone, R. M. (1961). *Biochem. Pharmac.* **7,** 88.

Farid, Z., Higashi, G. I., Bassily, S., Trabolsi, B. and Watten, R. H. (1980). *Trans. R. Soc. Trop. Med. Hyg.* **74,** 400.

Farid, Z., Higashi, G. I. and Hassan, A. (1976). *J. Trop. Med. Hyg.* **79,** 164.

Fontanilles, F. (1969). *Ann. N.Y. Acad. Sci.* **160,** 811.

Forsyth, D. M. (1965). *Lancet* **i,** 354.

Forsyth, D. M. and Rashid, C. (1967). *Lancet* **ii,** 909.

Foster, R. (1973). *Revta Inst. Med. Trop. S. Paulo* **15** (Suppl. 1), 1.

Foster, R. and Cheetham, B. L. (1973). *Trans. R. Soc. Trop. Med. Hyg.* **67,** 674.

Foster, R., Cheetham, B. L. and King, D. F. (1973). *Trans. R. Soc. Trop. Med. Hyg.* **67,** 685.

Friedheim, E. A. H. (1973). In *International Encyclopaedia of Pharmacology and Therapeutics*, Vol. 1. Section 64, p. 29. Eds R. Cavier and F. Hawkins. Pergamon Press, Elmsford NY.

Frohberg, H. and Schulze-Schencking, M. (1981). *Arzneimittel Forschung (Drug Research)* **31** (1), 555.

Gang, Chen Ming (1979). WHO Regional Office for the Western Pacific. Regional Steering Committee for the working group on *Schistosoma japonicum*. Unpublished.

Gentilini, M., Brucker, G., Danis, M., Niel, G. and Charmot, G. (1979). *Bulletin de la Société de Pathologie exotique* **72,** 466.

Gentilini, M., Duflo, B., Richard-Lenoble, D., Brücker, G., Danis, M., Niel, G. and Meunier, Y. (1980). *Acta tropica* **37,** 271.

Goldsmith, E. I., Luz, F. F. C., Prata, A. and Kean, B. H. (1967). *J. Am. Med. Ass.* **199,** 235.

Gönnert, R. and Andrews, P. (1977). *Ztschr. Parasitkde* **52,** 129.

Guimaraes, R. X., Tchakerian, A., de Souza Dias, L. C., de Almeida, F. M. R., Vilela, M. P., Cabeca, M. and Takeda, A. K. (1979). *Revta Ass. Med. Bras.* **25,** 48.

Haese, W. H. and Bueding, E. (1976). *J. Pharmac. Exp. Ther.* **197,** 703.

Haese, W. H., Smith, D. L. and Bueding, E. (1973). *J. Pharmac. Exp. Ther.* **186,** 430.

Higashi, G. I. and Farid, Z. (1979). *Br. Med. J.* **2,** 830.

International Agency for Research on Cancer (1977). *IARC Monographs on the Evaluation of Carcinogenic Risk of Chemicals to Man.* **13,** 123.

Ishizaki, T., Kamo, E. and Boehme, K. (1979). *Bull. Wld Hlth Org.* **57,** 787.

James, C. and Webbe, G. (1974). *Trans. R. Soc. Trop. Med. Hyg.* **68,** 413.

James, C., Webbe, G. and Nelson, G. S. (1977). *Ztschr. Parasitkde* **52,** 179.

James, C., Webbe, G. and Preston, J. M. (1972). *Ann. Trop. Med. Parasit.* **66,** 467.

Jewsbury, J. M., Cook, M. J. and Weber, M. C. (1977). *Ann. Trop. Med. Parasit.* **71,** 67.

Kale, O. O. and Lucas, A. O. (1978). *Revta Inst. Med. Trop. S. Paulo* **20,** 55.

Katz, N., Dias, E. P., Aravjo, N. and Souza, C. P. (1973). *Revta Soc. Bras. Med. Trop.* **7,** 381.

Katz, N., Grinbaum, E., Chaves, A., Zicker, F. and Pellegrino, J. (1976). *Revta Inst. Med. Trop. S. Paulo* **18,** 371.

Katz, N., Pellegrino, J., Ferreira, M. T., Oliveira, C. A. and Dias, C. B. (1968). *Am. J. Trop. Med. Hyg.* **17,** 743.

Katz, N., Rocha, R. S. and Chaves, A. (1979). *Bull. Wld Hlth Org.* **57,** 781.

Katz, N., Zicker, F. and Pereira, J. P. (1977). *Am. J. Trop. Med. Hyg.* **26,** 234.

Kaye, B. and Woolhouse, N. M. (1976). *Ann. Trop. Med. Parasit.* **70,** 323.

Kurata, M. (1973). *Jap. J. Trop. Med. Hyg.* **1,** 135.

Lambertucci, J. R., Pedroso, E. R. P., de Souza, D. W. C., de Lima, D. P., Neves, J., Salazar, H. M., Marinho, R. P., da Costa Rocha, M. O., Coelho, P. M. Z., de Lima Costa, M. F. F. and Creco, D. B. (1980). *Am. J. Trop. Med. Hyg.* **29,** 50.

Legator, M. S., Connor, T. H. and Stoeckel, M. (1975). *Science* **188,** 1118.

Leopold, G., Ungethum, W., Groll, E., Diekmann, H. W., Nowak, H. and Wegner, D. H. G. (1978). *Eur. J. Clin. Pharmac.* **14,** 281.

Leroy, J. P., Barreau, M., Cotrel, C., Jeanmart, C., Messer, M. and Benazet, F. (1978). In *Current Chemotherapy*, p. 148. Proceedings of 10th International Congress of Chemotherapy. American Society for Microbiology, Washington DC.

McCann, J., Choi, E., Yamasaki, E. and Ames, B. N. (1975). *Proc. Natn. Acad. Sci. U.S.A.* **72,** 5135.

McLaren, M., Long, E. G., Goodgame, R. W. and Lillywhite, J. E. (1979). *Trans. R. Soc. Trop. Med. Hyg.* **73,** 636.

McMahon, J. E. (1976). *Ann. Trop. Med. Parasit.* **70,** 121.

McMahon, J. E. (1977). WHO/FIL/77.148. WHO/SCHISTO/77.45.

Machemer, L. and Lorke, D. (1978). *Arch. Toxicol.* **39,** 187.

Mahmoud, A. A. F. and Warren, K. S. (1974). *J. Immunol.* **112,** 222.

Moore, J. A. (1972). *Nature* **236,** 107.

Nordgren, I., Holmstedt, B., Bengtsson, E. and Finkel, Y. (1980). *Am. J. Trop. Med. Hyg.* **29,** 426.

Obermeir, J. and Frohberg, H. (1977). *Arch. Toxicol.* **38,** 149.

Omer, A. H. S. (1978). *Br. Med. J.* **2,** 163.

Omer, A. H. S. and Teesdale, C. H. (1978). *Ann. Trop. Med. Parasit.* **72,** 67.

Ong, T.-M. and de Serres, F. J. (1975). *J. Toxicol. Envir. Hlth* **1,** 271.

Pax, R., Bennet, J. L. and Fetterer, R. (1978). *Naunyu-Schmildebergs. Arch. Pharmacol.* **304,** 309.

Pellegrino, J., Lima-Costa, F. F., Carlos, M. A. and Mello, R. T. (1977). *Ztschr. Parasitkde* **52,** 151.

Pelley, R. P., Warren, K. S. and Jordan, P. (1977). *Lancet* **ii,** 781.

Pesigan, T. P., Banzon, T. C. and Zabala, R. G. (1966). *Acta Trop. Suppl.* **9,** 224.

Pfizer Inc. manufacturers' data 1978. Sandwich, Kent.

Pitchford, R. J. and Lewis, M. (1978). *S. Afr. Med. J.* **53,** 677.

Plestina, R., Davis, A. and Bailey, D. R. (1972). *Bull. Wld Hlth Org.* **46,** 747.

Pyquiton Coordination Group, Zhejiang Province (1980). *Natn. Med. J. China* **60,** 142.

Pyquiton Research Group. National Schistosomiasis Research Committee (1980). *Natn. Med. J. China* **60,** 129.

Rogers, S. H. and Bueding, E. (1971). *Science* **172,** 1057.

Rosi, D., Peruzotti, G., Dennis, E. W., Berberian, D. A., Freele, R. and Archer, S. (1965). *Nature* **208,** 1005.

Russell, W. L. (1975). *J. Toxicol. Envir. Hlth* **1,** 301.

Saif, M., Gaber, A., Hassanein, Y. S. and Khameis, S. (1978). *J. Egypt Med. Ass.* **61,** 427.

Salazar-Mallen, M., Gonzalez-Barranco, D. and Mitrani-Levy, D. (1969). *Lancet* **i,** 427.

Santos, A. T., Blas, B. L., Nosenas, J. S., Portillo, G. P., Ortega, O. M., Hayashi, M. and Boehme, K. (1979). *Bull. Wld Hlth Org.* **57,** 793.

Saz, H. J., Dunbar, G. A. and Bueding, E. (1977). *Am. J. Trop. Med. Hyg.* **26,** 574.

Sen, H. G. (1976). *Acta Trop.* **33,** 101.

Senft, A. W. (1975). *J. Toxicol. Env. Hlth* **1,** 335.

Shahin, M. M. (1975). *Mutat. Res.* **30,** 191.

Sichuan Institute of Parasitic Diseases (1980). *Chinese J. Intern. Med.* **19,** 132.

Sieber, S. M. and Adamson, R. H. (1975). *J. Toxicol. Envir. Hlth* **1,** 309.

Silva, L. C., da Sette, H., Jr., Chamore, D. A. F., Alquezar, A. S., Punskas, J. A. and Raia, S. (1974). *Revta Inst. Med. Trop. S. Paulo* **16,** 103.

Somers, G. F. & Whittet, T. D. (1958). *Pharm. J.,* **ii,** 494.

Striebel, H. P. (1976). *Experientia,* **32,** 457.

Striebel, H. P. and Stauffer, P. (1980). *Joint Meeting of the Royal Society of Tropical Medicine and Hygiene and Schweizerische Gesellschaft für Tropenmedizin und Parasitologie, Basle, 12–15 March 1980.* Abstract No. 18.

Straus, D. S. (1974). *Genetics* **78,** 823.

Tanaka, H. (1976). *S.E. Asian J. Trop. Med. Publ. Hlth* **7,** 176.

Thomas, H. and Gönnert, R. (1977). *Ztschr. Parasitkde* **52,** 117.

Urman, H. K., Bulay, O., Clayson, D. B. and Shubik, P. (1975). *Cancer Letters* **1,** 69.

US Japan Cooperative Science Program 1974 (1975). *J. Toxicol. Envir. Hlth* **1,** 175.

Vandekar, M., Hedayat, S., Plestina, R. and Ahmandy, G. (1968). *Bull. Wld Hlth Org.* **38,** 609.

Warren, K. S., Arap Siongok, T. K., Ouma, J. H. and Houser, H. B. (1978). *Lancet* **i,** 352.

Webbe, G. and James, C. (1977). *Ztschr. Parasitkde* **52,** 169.

Weber, M. C., Blair, D. M. and Clarke, V. de V. (1969). *Cent. Afr. J. Med.* **15,** 82.

Webster, L. T. Jr., Butterworth, A. E., Mahmoud, A. A. F., Mugola, E. N. and Warren, K. S. (1975). *New Engl. J. Med.* **292,** 1144.

Wegner, D. H. G. (1979). The treatment of human schistosomiasis with BILTRICIDE (Praziquantel, EMBAY 8440). In *14th Joint Conference on Parasitic Disease,* Aug. 12–15, 1979. USA-Japan Cooperative Medical Science Program, New Orleans.

Wilhelm, K. (1968). *Arh. Hig. Rada.* **19,** 199.

Woehrle, R., Tran Mauh Sung, R. and Garin, J. P. (1980). *Current Chemother. Infect. Dis.* **22,** 1109.

WHO (1953). *Wld Hlth Org. Techn. Rep. Ser.* **65,** 40.

WHO (1966). *Wld Hlth Org. Techn. Rep. Ser.* **317,** 30, 36.
WHO (1972). WHO Reports on Schistosomicidal Drugs. *Bol. de la Officina Sanitaria Panamericana* **VI,** 82.
Xu, R. K. (1980). *Chinese J. Internal Med.* **19,** 63.
Yarinsky, A., Drobeck, H. P., Freele, H., Wiland, J. and Gumaer, K. J. (1974). *Toxicol. Appl. Pharmac.* **27,** 169.
Yarinsky, A., Hernandez, P., Ferrari, R. A. and Freele, H. W. (1972). *Jap. J. Parasit.* **21,** 101.

10 Epidemiology

Peter Jordan and Gerald Webbe (with assistance from Michael Goddard)

The epidemiology of schistosomiasis involves a vertebrate definitive and a molluscan intermediate host and their common presence in an environment in which transmission can take place. The parasites require the internal environments of the two hosts in order to complete the respective sexual and asexual phases of the life-cycle, while the free-living larval stages present in a common external environment provide the essential links in the chain of infection. The dynamics of transmission are, therefore, necessarily complicated and subject to considerable variations due to the many factors which may influence the common environment and, in turn, behaviour patterns of the definitive host and the bionomics of the intermediate host. The different factors which indirectly or directly influence the variations in transmission patterns may also have a profound effect upon the pathology of infection in the final host.

Intermediate hosts are found in many different geographical areas, though there are situations where, despite their presence, transmission does not occur for climatic and other reasons. In other situations infected persons may be present but owing to local water characteristics the snail intermediate hosts cannot exist. Apart from such unusual situations, schistosomiasis is widespread in the Tropics, transmission of one species or another being possible in water bodies as variable as Lake Victoria and collections of rainwater in borrow pits, the River Nile and small streams, in swamps and paddy fields.

Transmission occurs in areas of high and low rainfall and, in the latter, dry conditions may force snails to aestivate in the dried mud, leading to wet season transmission.

On the other hand, in some areas snails may be flushed out in the rainy season, leading to dry season transmission. Seasonal transmission may also result from extreme changes in temperature. Although snails survive within a wide temperature range, it is of interest that *Biomphalaria* spp. are rarely found along the hot coastal areas of tropical Africa and little or no transmission of *S. mansoni* occurs there. It has been suggested that this is due to the temperature being too high for successful colonisation of the waters. Natural water bodies and man-made habitats may provide suitable breeding sites for snails and the increased use of irrigation and other water conservation methods, by providing additional snail habitats and by attracting man to them, has increased the danger of transmission in many tropical areas. In rural areas of the Tropics, conditions are frequently such that the waters which support the snail intermediate host of schistosomiasis are those upon which the local population depend for water for domestic, recreational and in some cases occupational requirements.

The epidemiology of schistosomiasis involves study of community contact with, and usage of, water which leads to infection; it involves a study of the incidence of new infections (to measure the level of transmission), and the prevalence and intensity of infection in the definitive host (or hosts) as an indication of the potential level of contamination of the environment with schistosome eggs. These factors are related to the social, economic and cultural patterns of the human population and influence the free-living stage of the parasite and its complex relationship with the intermediate snail host.

Epidemiology also involves a study of the occurrence of schistosomal disease in the community and particularly the relationship of disease to prevalence and intensity of infection.

WATER-CONTACT STUDIES

Transmission of schistosomiasis depends on communities having contact with infected surface water, though the possibility of piped water being infected should not be overlooked.

Transmission from water carried into towns from rural areas has been reported and sentinel mice have been infected when exposed in stored water in houses (Polderman, 1974).

The value of water contact studies is being increasingly appreciated, but the objective of a study should be clearly defined as this affects the scope, design and degree of sophistication of the investigation.

While water-contact studies are considered useful for a variety of reasons, the ethics—in relation to invasion of privacy—can be questioned. In association with parasitological and biological studies they aid epidemiological research and may lead to a better understanding of questions relating to the stability or otherwise of egg excretion levels in different age groups, the cause of the declining prevalence rates in adults, the development and role of immunology. Detailed studies may also provide data for use in predictive models.

With studies of the snail intermediate host, water-contact investigations can indicate when and where transmission occurs—knowledge critical for the rational planning of focal snail control.

Studies indicate the most common reasons for contact, and their relative importance in relation to transmission (infection and contamination). This could lead to appropriate alternative facilities (such as laundries, shower units) being provided to reduce contact. Where this is done (see Chapter 11) further studies can indicate whether they are being utilised.

Workers in Puerto Rico appear to have been the first to attempt to correlate water contact with prevalence of *S. mansoni* (Pimental *et al.*, 1961). The number of contacts was established by questionnaire and a direct relationship was shown between the admitted number of contacts per day and the prevalence of infection as based on stool examination. In Egypt, studies were made by observation, and data on domestic, recreational and religious activities were recorded. It was recognised that water contact involves exposure and, very often, contamination (Farooq and Mallah, 1966). While observations can provide data on exposure, they are unlikely to give accurate information on contamination.

Although later studies have become more sophisticated in design, the Egyptian study included the essential elements to be noted—age and sex of individuals, activity, and factors it is assumed are important in leading to infection. These factors are the extent of body exposure, the number of contacts, their duration and time of day, although results of laboratory experiments with animals suggest other factors may be involved.

In aquaria in the laboratory, penetration of the skin of mice can take place very rapidly, particularly with high cercarial concentrations—16% of mice became infected when exposed to 160 *S. mansoni* cercariae for only 60 s (Upatham and Sturrock,

1973). Prolonged exposure for 16 min to one cercariae per mouse resulted in a low 5% infection rate, but it is possible that the skin reaction to the first penetrating cercaria may protect against the penetration of other cercariae (Stirewalt, 1953). With short exposures to heavy infections such a protective mechanism (if it occurs) would probably not operate.

In flowing water, infection rates and worm burdens increased in direct proportion to cercarial concentration and exposure times (Upatham, 1974a and 1974b).

S. mansoni cercariae that fail to penetrate during exposure die on drying skin (Warren and Peters, 1967). However, hamsters exposed to *S. japonicum* cercariae with short periods of drying between exposures showed a greater maturation rate of worms than occurred with longer single exposures terminated by drying (Pan *et al.*, 1954).

As the relevance of these animal findings to human infection is unknown, frequency of contact, duration of exposure and time of day must still be regarded as of importance.

Studies have now been made in Puerto Rico (Jobin and Ruiz-Tiben, 1968), Ethiopia (Polderman, 1974), Zimbabwe (Husting, 1965 and 1970), St Lucia (Dalton, 1976) and Ghana (Dalton and Pole, 1978) and many other studies were reported recently at a WHO workshop to discuss the subject. These studies confirm the broad classification of domestic, recreational, religious and occupational reasons for contact and, while religious and occupational contacts will vary in different endemic areas, the main domestic and recreational contacts are similar (Table 10.1).

Table 10.1 Data from different water contact studies showing that observed domestic and recreational contacts account for between 57% and 70% of contacts.

	Egypt	St Lucia	Zimbabwe*	Ghana*
	Washing utensils, clothes; bathing; playing	Washing clothes; bathing; swimming (playing)	Washing utensils; carrying; swimming	Domestic; recreational
Percentage of contacts	57	66	70	58
Percentage of time	76	95	50+	54

* Females only.

Contacts with water for specific purposes may occur at selected sites, so that water for drinking may be obtained at one site while clothes are washed at another; bathing may take place at different sites and the sexes may be segregated. Sites for the washing of clothes are often central points for gossip and communication and are invariably as conveniently located as possible. Points of contact may be large or small, diffuse on a vegetation-free shoreline or river bank, or small and localised at a site only made accessible by the clearance of aquatic vegetation (Fig. 10.1).

Domestic contacts

In St Lucia, the typical daily pattern commences with children being sent early in the day to collect water for use at home. They are exposed to minimal risk of infection since cercariae of *S. mansoni* are not shed in large numbers until later in the day, and further, usually only hands and perhaps feet get wet and then for only a brief period (Dalton, 1976).

In areas where a community standpipe is available, this early morning contact of children is not observed but, later in the day, young children accompany their mothers to the rivers to wash clothes and are at a higher risk of becoming infected while playing in the water for an hour or more and, at times, being completely immersed.

Amongst children, contact is principally for bathing (with a high degree of exposure) and playing, but the duration and proportion of total time exposed in these activities declines with age (Table 10.2; Fig. 10.2)

The pattern of exposure at this time of life, with repeated exposure to infection, probably determines the future disease manifestations.

Amongst adult females, the total time in contact increases with age; over 90% of contact time involves washing with minimal exposure but the risk of infection is increased as washing is usually carried out at the peak cercarial shedding time (Rowan, 1958; Webbe and Jordan, 1966). Bathing carries an increased risk as it involves total immersion—but probably not for long and the risk of infection may be reduced when soap is used as it has a strong cercaricidal action. Natural soaps—such as Endod—may have a similar action.

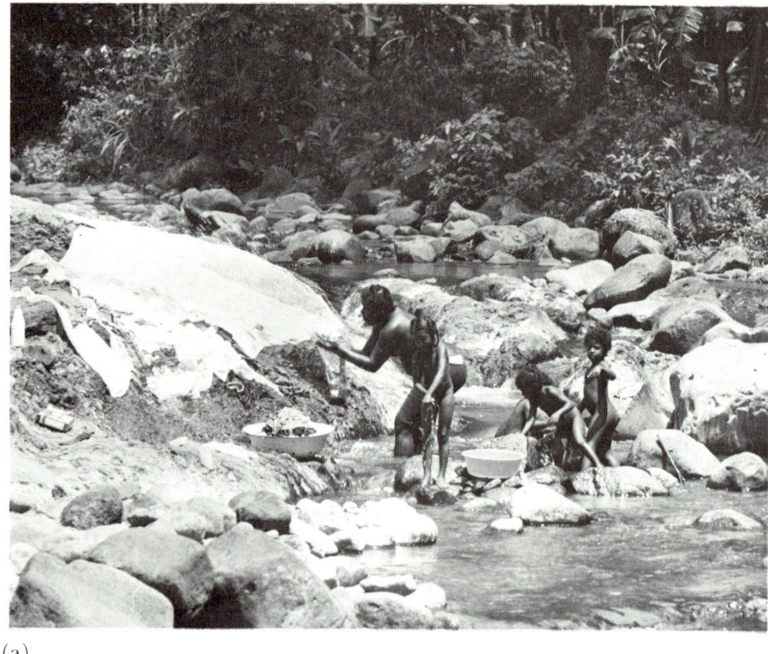

(a)

Fig. 10.1 Domestic water contact: (a) in a natural stream in St Lucia; (b) on an open beach on Lake Volta; (c) on an irrigation canal in Egypt.

(b)

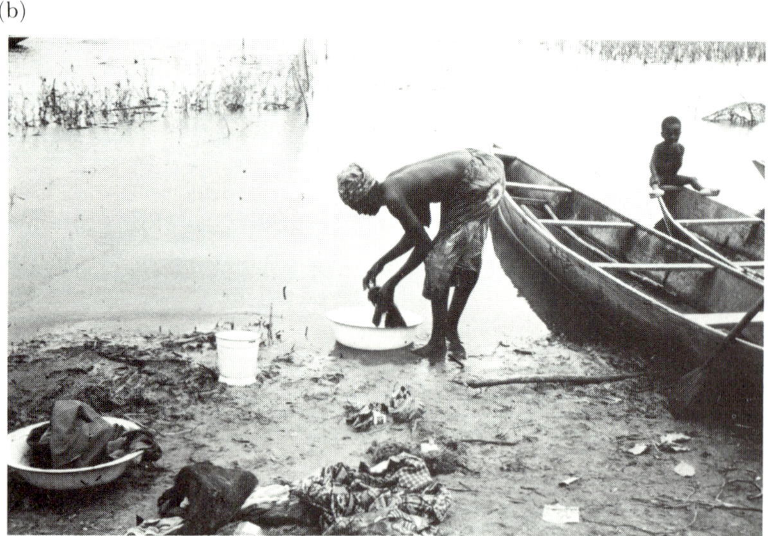

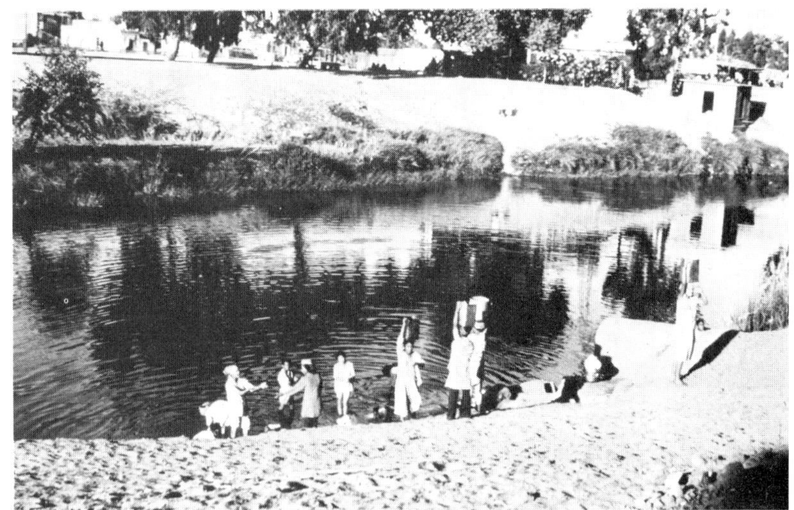

(c)

In the study from which the above results were obtained, the duration of observed water contact of individual women and children showed a log distribution, with 289 (77%) of the 377 contacts being for less than 1 h, 60 (16%) for up to 2 h, 16 (4%) to 3 h, 8 (2%) to 4 h, 2 (0·5%) for 5 h, and 2 (0·5%) for 6 h or more.

Because the surface area of adults (male St Lucians, 1·8 m²; females, 1·6 m²) is far greater than that of children (5–9 years old, 0·8 m²) the risk of adults being infected or re-infected during similar water activity (e.g. bathing with total immersion) is presumably greater. This presupposes that there is no preferential attraction of cercariae to the skin of young or old persons.

However, while observing cercarial penetration of human skin it was noted that walls of wrinkles were preferred penetration sites (Stirewalt, 1956) but it is not known whether cercariae are attracted to the wrinkled skin of the elderly. On the other hand, it has been shown that young mice are more susceptible to infection than older ones and that the loss of cercariae in the skin after penetration is proportional to the age of the mouse (Ghandour and Webbe, 1973).

Table 10.2 Showing how, with age, the pattern of water contact changes. (Data from an unpublished study in St Lucia when 377 females were observed at seven contact sites. Observation design was based on a random block. Sites were observed daily from 6 a.m.–6 p.m. for one week every month for seven months. Fording excluded; village standpipes available.)

Age group (years)	Total individuals	Observed contacts	Mean time/ individual (min)	Mean time (min) per N individuals observed					
				N washing		N bathing		N play/casual	
0–4	40	108	16	2	29	22	6	29	15
5–9	88	292	19	23	29	32	10	60	12
10–14	78	341	38	36	64	37	11	32	8
15–19	48	230	54	33	71	23	9	10	5
20–29	43	145	44	29	60	14	7	10	6
30–39	33	204	89	29	98	12	6	5	2
40–49	25	91	51	18	68	5	6	5	2
50–59	13	50	47	9	63	1	30	5	5
60+	9	19	24	6	36	—	—	3	1

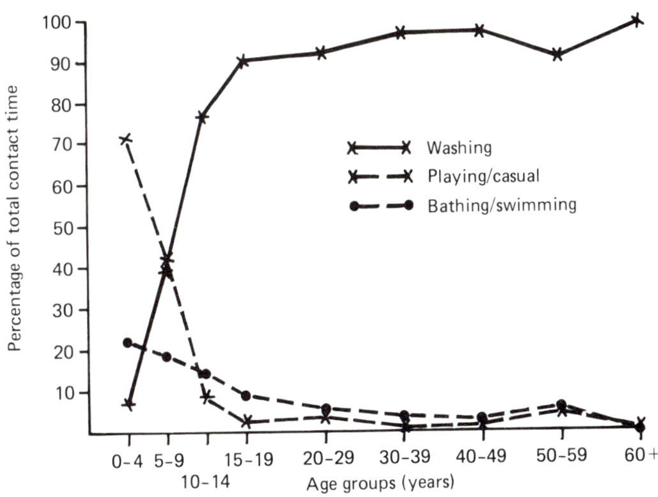

Fig. 10.2 Showing that the proportion of the total time spent in contact with water for different purposes varies with age (St Lucia).

Contact for religious reasons

Religious practices can be important reasons for water contact, as in the ritual washing, five times a day before prayers, required of male Muslims (Farooq and Mallah, 1966). Infected snails have been found in water containers specially provided for this function (Kuntz, 1952a).

In the Malumfashi District of Nigeria, the imposition of strict Muslim principles starts at an early age, resulting in girls having minimal contact with water. As a result, their peak of *S. haematobium* prevalence was only 15% compared with 60% amongst boys (Pugh and Gilles, 1978).

In Ethiopia, Christians of all ages and both sexes were seen to have more contact with water than Muslims (Polderman, 1974).

Occupational contacts

The pattern of domestic and recreational contacts can show daily, weekly and monthly cycles, be associated with seasons and may be interrelated with occupation (Dalton, 1976). Thus, while basic contacts such as water carrying may not change, days for washing may be dictated by the need to plant, harvest and market different crops, and by religious duties, etc.

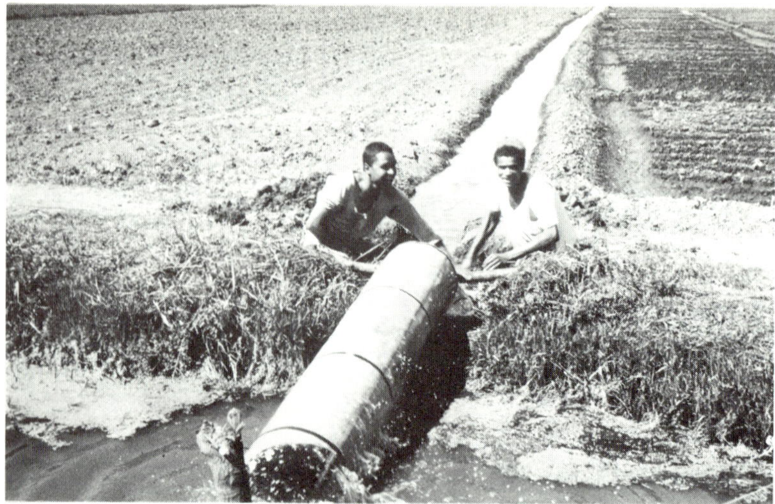

Fig. 10.3 Occupational hazard in the case of an Archimedes screw used to transfer water potentially infested with cercariae from a small irrigation canal into another section of cultivated area in a *S. haematobium* endemic district in Egypt.

The risk from occupational contacts will vary. In St Lucia, persons fording shallow rivers carrying banana stems are minimally exposed, while Sudanese canal cleaners are almost totally immersed for many hours a day and are at very high risk of becoming infected. Ghanaian fishermen risk infection when entering or leaving their boats on the edge of Lake Volta, but when fishing are probably minimally exposed. Ethiopian professional water carriers experience frequent contact with minimal exposure (Polderman, 1974).

Canals of irrigation schemes pose two problems—frequently they are the source of domestic water for the worker and his family, and workers may come in contact with the water in the course of their agricultural field work (Fig. 10.3). However, in the stirred up muddy water in irrigated fields, the infectivity of cercariae might be reduced.

The surface area of the body (Diem and Lentner, 1970) can be derived from the formula:

$$\text{Log S} = \text{W} \times 0 \cdot 425 + \text{Log H} \times 0 \cdot 725 + 1 \cdot 8564$$

where S = surface area in cm^2; W = weight in kg; H = height in cm.

The surface areas of different parts of the body that might be in contact with water are:

both ankles	7%	both wrists	6%
to knees	19%	to elbows	12%
to thighs	37%	to shoulders	20%
to waist	42%	to neck	88%

While the chance of infection is probably dependent on various factors—including those discussed above (extent of body exposed, number and duration of contacts and the time of day)—the concentration of cercariae in the water is of course vital to the issue and this is variable.

However, in spite of the vast numbers of cercariae produced by an infected snail, it seems likely that only a small fraction complete the life-cycle and it has been calculated from Egyptian data that from the age of 5 years onwards, man acquires only 0·83 and 1·46 *S. mansoni* and *S. haematobium* worms, respectively, per year (Hairston, 1965a and 1965b).

INDICES OF HUMAN INFECTION

Transmission over a given time period is measured by the number of new infections occurring amongst uninfected children. This is expressed as a percentage to give the *incidence* rate.

The *prevalence* of infection is the percentage of the population, or an age group, found to be infected at a given point in time and depends on past incidence and the rate of loss of infections.

Quantitatively, the level of infection in the community is indicated by the *intensity of infection*, or the worm burden of a group of persons. This is measured indirectly by the number of schistosome ova being excreted.

These indices are best obtained by demonstrating eggs in stool or urine, thus establishing the presence of an active infection. (See also immuno-epidemiology.)

Incidence rate

This is a measure of the level of transmission over a given time period.

In endemic areas, virtually all children are eventually infected—initially, perhaps with a single-sex infection (i.e. only male

Table 10.3 Incidence (%) of new infections amongst children who were negative on examination in 1969 and who were re-examined in 1970.

Age (years) at 1969	Number negative in 1969	Number positive in 1970	Percentage	Incidence	
0	22	3	13·6		
1	26	5	19·2	10/78	13%
2	30	2	6·6		
3	33	6	18·2		
4	30	9	30·0	22/88	25%
5	25	7	28·0		
6	20	7	35·0		
7	12	7	58·3	14/32	44%
8	17	8	47·1		
9	18	11	61·1	27/47	57%
10	12	8	66·7		

or female worms) but later with worms of the opposite sex. The sexes mate so that eggs are excreted. A child thus found to have become infected or positive (having previously been uninfected or negative) is said to have 'converted'. The annual number of children converting expressed as a percentage of the total uninfected, but at risk of being infected, represents the incidence of new infections between examinations and is the only true measure of the level of transmission.

Incidence is usually measured over a 12-month period to allow for seasonal variation in transmission.

There is often confusion over this investigation, particularly if annual incidence data are collected over a number of years—as they may be prior to control.

An initial survey must be made of children in an appropriate age group—such as 0–7, 0–10 or 2–10 years (as it may be difficult to obtain samples of excreta from the very young). Uninfected children from this survey are re-examined in 12 months. For clarity when reporting, it should be stated at which survey children are of a stated age—i.e. children 0–10 years at the first of two surveys. The children are re-examined when they are aged 1–11 years old.

Incidence is generally low in the younger age groups but, with increasing contact with water, the risk of infection increases with age and incidence rises (Table 10.3).

If a second measure of incidence is required, i.e. after a third examination, those children who have converted (become infected at the second examination) and children who are then 11 years old are dropped from the study; but to maintain the 0–10 age group, newborn children are now added as well as any other uninfected children between the ages of 0 and 10 years. Children missing from the second examination are dropped.

A difficulty in incidence determinations is the possibility that the initial negative parasitological result may be a false negative—a light infection (with few eggs being excreted) having been undetected. A subsequent apparent 'conversion' might thus be false. True negatives are more likely amongst very young children who have had little exposure; conversely, older children are more likely to give false negatives. (For this reason adults who, in endemic areas, have probably all been infected at some time, are not considered suitable for incidence studies.)

While study of the very young is thus parasitologically preferable, incidence amongst them is likely to be low and, as referred to above, problems arise in obtaining excreta samples—particularly urine.

However, in areas where high prevalence rates are found early in the first decade of life, as was the situation in the Lake Volta epidemic of *S. haematobium*, and is the case in Uganda (see Fig. 10.3), the very young may have to be used for determining incidence as there may be no uninfected older children. With successful control, however, more negative older children will be found and can be brought into post-control incidence studies to show continued successful control. As incidence increases with age, in the analysis of data, attention must be given to the age composition of the pre- and post-control groups of children. If they differ, suitable statistical methods must be employed for comparing the two.

In areas of high transmission when the conventional method of calculating incidence may not be possible owing to there being insufficient uninfected children, use can be made of the 'cumulative prevalence', from which an incidence rate can be estimated.

The method also enables incomplete data to be utilised for a 'cohort study'. The hypothetical results from three surveys from six individuals indicate the basis of the calculations (Table 10.4).

One assumption is made: that a person once infected remains infected, so that a person infected at survey 1 (I.J.) is assumed positive at surveys 2 and 3 (but may not be examined), and

Table 10.4 Hypothetical results from three surveys from six persons. (In brackets, assumed result if person had been examined.)

Subject	Survey 1	Survey 2	Survey 3
A.B.	−ve	+ve	(+ve)
C.D.	−ve	−ve	+ve
E.F.	−ve	−ve	−ve
G.H.	(−ve)	−ve	−ve
I.J.	+ve	+ve	(+ve)
K.L.	(−ve)	−ve	+ve
	1 +ve	2 +ve	4 +ve

Table 10.5 Cumulative prevalence and estimated incidence between Surveys S1 and S2, and S2 and S3. (Actual data from Lake Volta by courtesy of the late Dr D. Scott.)

Age (years) at Survey 1	Numbers examined	Number positive at S1	S2	S3	Age (years) at Survey 3
0	5	0	0	0	2
1	8	0	0	0	3
2	10	2	2	4	4
3	18	5	9	12	5
4	20	10	12	12	6
5	9	6	8	9	7
6	15	9	11	12	8
7	10	7	7	7	9
Total	95	39	49	56	
Total number negative		56	46	39	
Prevalence (%)		41·1	51·6	58·9	
Estimated incidence between surveys			10/56	7/46	
			17·9%	15·2%	

persons uninfected at survey 3 (G.H.) would have been uninfected at surveys 1 and 2 if they had been examined.

Using the technique with data from the Lake Volta project, the results shown in Table 10.5 were obtained.

Incidence data based on the apparent rate of re-infection after treatment may be unreliable as it is usually impossible to differentiate between an unsuccessful treatment and a re-infection.

Loss of infection

Although records indicate that adult worms can live for up to about 30 years (Wallerstein, 1949; Berberian *et al.*, 1953), recent evidence suggests that such reports are of the extreme range of longevity and that the *mean* life span is likely to be between 3 and 8 years (Hairston, 1962; Warren *et al.*, 1974; Goddard and Jordan, 1980).

Thus, as some worms will die in less than 3 years, children may change from excreting eggs one year to being apparently negative the next—such findings indicating a 'reversion' or loss of infection.

Young children with light infections and excreting few eggs, that may be undetected on re-examination, will be considered negative and therefore false reversions. This is less likely with the heavier infections of older children.

In communities in endemic areas, over a given period some children will acquire infections and others will lose an infection, but where uncontrolled transmission is taking place there will be more new infections than lost ones, i.e. the ratio of conversions to reversions will be more than 1. At the end of the year in a cohort of children followed, there will thus be an increase in the number of children infected, the children then being a year older than when first examined.

By adding to the incidence data in Table 10.3, findings from children who were positive in 1969 and who were negative in 1970 or who remained positive, the change in status of infection in the cohort can be seen.

Table 10.6 Change in status of infection in a cohort of children examined in 1969 and again in 1970 (in an area of active *S. mansoni* transmission).

Age (years) in 1969	Number examined both years	Number positive in 1969*	Conversions†	Reversions*	Number positive in 1970*
0–2	97	19 (20)	10 (13)	11 (58)	18 (19)
3–5	127	39 (31)	22 (25)	9 (23)	52 (41)
6–7	66	34 (51)	14 (44)	8 (24)	40 (61)
8–10	103	56 (54)	27 (57)	6 (11)	77 (75)
0–10	393	148 (38)	73 (30)	34 (23)	187 (48)

* Numbers in parentheses are percentages.
† Numbers in parentheses indicate percentage incidence.
NB Conversion/reversions: 73/34 = 2·2:1.

It is apparent that there were 73 conversions and 34 reversions (ratio 73:34 = 2·2) and the percentage infected increased from 38% to 48% (the age of the group changed from 0–10 to 1–11 years).

If prevalence or the percentage infected in 1969 and 1970 amongst the 1–10 year olds is considered, i.e. amongst the age group common to both surveys, there is seen to have been little change from the 1969 rate of 39·2% (144 of 367) to 44·0% (158 of 359) in 1970. Also from the table, the increasing incidence with age of children will be noted, and the decreasing rate of reversion.

Intensity of infection

Intensity of infection relates to the worm burden of infected individuals or groups of people. Data on the actual number of *S. mansoni* worms harboured by infected subjects have been obtained from extracorporeal filtration studies (Goldsmith *et al.*, 1967) and from the detailed autopsy studies carried out in Brazil and Egypt (Cheever, 1968; Cheever *et al.*, 1977). These show that the number of *S. mansoni* worms present is related to the level of faecal egg excretion. Extracorporeal studies in *S. haematobium* infections failed (Goldsmith and Kean, 1969), but data on the excretion of *S. haematobium* eggs were collected preoperatively from patients who were to undergo cystectomy for bladder cancer, and were related to postoperative findings of the number of adult worms in the dissected tissues; the relationship with viable eggs was questionably significant but a better correlation was obtained when living and dead eggs were considered (Cheever, 1975).

These results support the concept of using egg output as an indication of intensity of infection—in recent years recognised as important in the development of schistosomal disease.

Eggs are randomly distributed in faecal specimens (Martin and Beaver, 1968; Woodstock *et al.*, 1972) and although there is day-to-day variation in the output of *S. mansoni* eggs in the stool, this is no greater than amongst eggs of other intestinal helminths. In individuals, a single stool or urine examination may not give an accurate level of infection and more reliable data will be obtained if multiple (usually three) specimens are quantitatively examined; amongst groups of people, the mean egg output of an age group or other specified segment of the population gives useful epidemiological information.

Distribution of egg output

In different age groups and in the whole population, a few people appear heavily infected and excrete large numbers of eggs, but the majority excrete lower numbers. However, in areas of high prevalence a greater proportion of people are heavily infected and at greater risk of developing severe schistosomal disease.

The log-normal distribution of egg output has lead to a variety of methods of recording quantitative results. The arithmetic and geometric means and the mean log are all used; in some series, results are given for infected persons only and in others a mean includes the uninfected. However results are presented, what they represent must be clearly stated.

With the log-normal distribution of eggs, a log transformation and the reporting of the mean log, or the geometric mean is preferable as it provides a better indication of the central tendency of egg distribution than the arithmetic mean. The mean log tends to be used for *S. haematobium* studies and the geometric mean for *S. mansoni* egg output, but these may be considered complex and not easily calculated without mechanical assistance. (In calculating the geometric mean of infected and uninfected persons, 1 must be added to all counts including zero counts.)

The arithmetic mean may be easier for field workers to calculate and for this reason its use should not be discouraged.

In addition to the variety of ways of expressing results, different techniques have been used for visually portraying them. These usually involve categorising counts with or without the use of histograms, but categories used by different workers vary considerably, thus again making comparisons difficult.

A technique which readily shows the proportion of counts above different levels is useful (Fig. 10.4; Bradley, 1965).

The log-normal distribution of egg output in a community reflects the worm burden; amongst asymptomatic *S. mansoni* autopsy subjects, 51% harboured less than 10 worm pairs and only 7% had more than 80 (Cheever, 1968). The mean number of worm pairs per infected person in Egypt was calculated as 1·5. Hairston calculated figures of 2·8 and between 2·2 and 5·2 worm pairs for *S. haematobium* and *S. japonicum* respectively (quoted in Cheever, 1968).

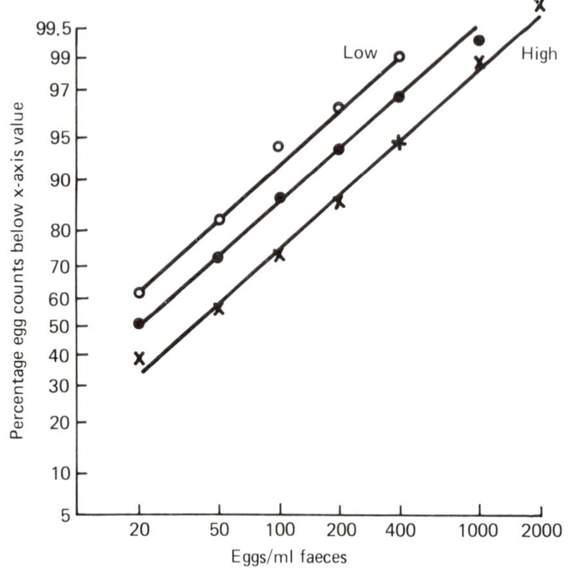

Fig. 10.4 *S. mansoni* data from St Lucia showing percentage distribution of eggs/ml faeces in populations in low, moderate and high areas of endemicity (cf. Table 10.8).

Variations in prevalence and intensity of infection

Prevalence and intensity of infection are directly related and usually show similar patterns of variation with age; both increase generally to the 10–20 year age group, followed by a decline in adults. A slight increase may occur in the elderly (Fig. 10.5). Variations of this general pattern occur, with peak rates being found in younger age groups in areas of high transmission and varying degrees of decline in older age groups, depending usually on the extent of contact with water and with the species of parasite.

Thus, in a fishing community in the West Nile region of Uganda, high rates of *S. mansoni* infection were found before the age of 10 years and, amongst adults, prevalence was virtually 100% in both sexes. Intensity of infection was exceptionally high, but was higher amongst fishermen than females and showed a greater fall than in the women (Fig. 10.6; Ongom, 1970; Ongom and Bradley, 1972).

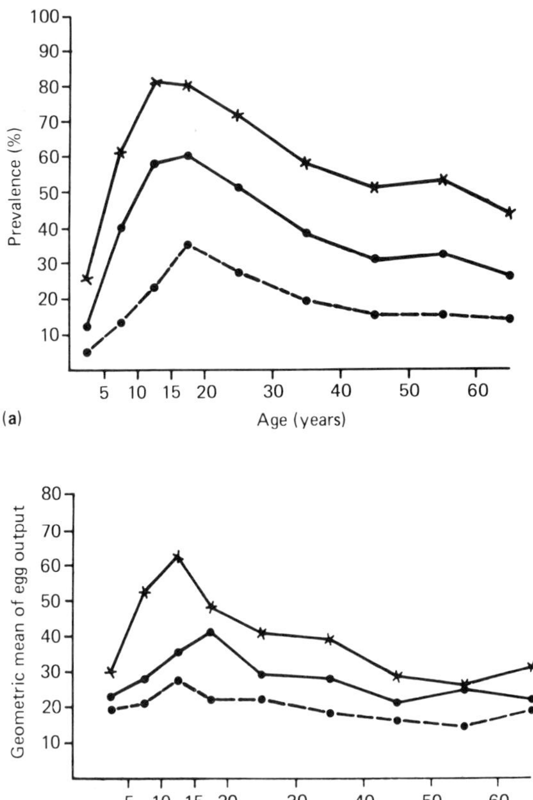

Fig. 10.5 *S. mansoni* data from St Lucia: (a) age-specific prevalence data from villages in areas of high, moderate and low endemicity; and (b) the corresponding geometric mean of egg output amongst those infected.

In a less heavily infected fishing community on the shores of Lake Victoria, prevalence and intensity of infection were again higher in the females but in neither sex was there a consistent decline in either parameter of infection (Smith *et al.*, 1979).

These findings contrast with the pattern amongst fishing communities on the shores of Lake Volta, where *S. haematobium* is endemic. After peaks of prevalence and intensity in the 10–14 year age groups, prevalence rates amongst adults decline, but more rapidly amongst females than males (Fig. 10.7). Intensity of infection shows a dramatic decrease in egg output in both sexes. This marked fall in egg output of *S. haematobium* has been

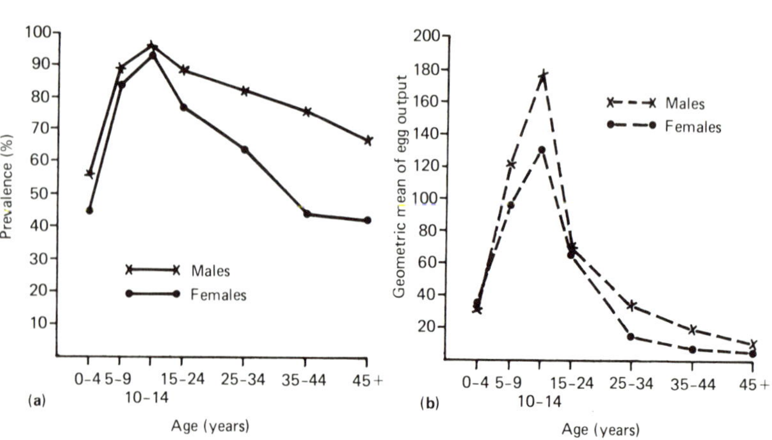

Fig. 10.6 *S. mansoni* data from West Nile, Uganda: showing (a) high rates of prevalence in children and adults; (b) infection intensity higher and falling more amongst men than women. (Data from Ongom, 1970.)

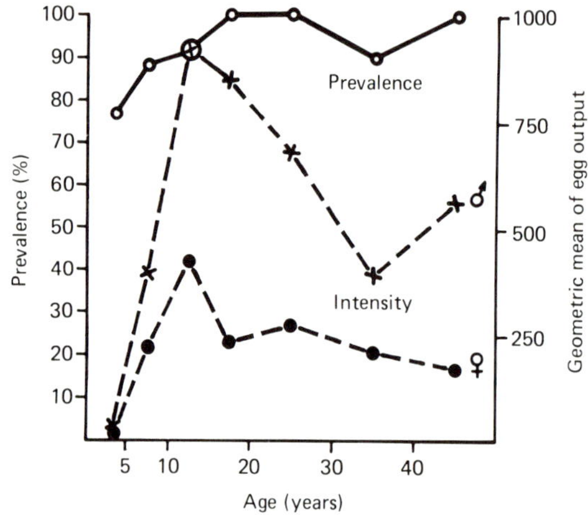

Fig. 10.7 *S. haematobium* data from Lake Volta, Ghana: showing high rates of prevalence in children and declining rates (females more than males) in adults but dramatic decline in intensity of infection in both sexes. (Data by courtesy of Dr David Scott.)

reported from many areas including Sierre Leone (Gerber, 1952), Zimbabwe (Clarke, 1966), Gambia (Wilkins, 1977) and Egypt (Wilkins and El-Sawy, 1977).

Declining rates in the older age groups are generally associated less with *S. mansoni* than with *S. haematobium*, in which the decline in intensity of infection is more marked than the decline in prevalence.

The reasons for the changing rates of prevalence and infection intensity amongst adults remain uncertain, but accumulating evidence suggests different mechanisms may be involved, viz. an immune mechanism particularly involving *S. haematobium*, and reduced water contact. In support of the former and suggesting immunity takes 15 or more years to develop, is the finding that amongst a population of uninfected adults who immigrated into an *S. mansoni* endemic area, irrespective of age, a peak prevalence was found after 15–19 years of residence; those who had been there longer showed declining rates (Kloetzel, 1967; Kloetzel and Da Silva, 1967). The peak thus appeared to be associated with duration of exposure to infection and not with reduced contact.

Other reasons put forward have been a lowered fecundity in old female worms and, although Cheever (1968) found no evidence of this, it has been demonstrated in experimental animals (Cheever and Duvall, 1974; Cheever *et al.*, 1974; Damian *et al.*, 1976; Webbe *et al.*, 1976). In *S. haematobium* infections, fibrosis of the bladder tissue and calcification of retained eggs may hinder the passage of other eggs through the bladder walls. However, in *S. mansoni* infections there is less accumulation of eggs in the tissues and colonic fibrosis is not marked (Cheever *et al.*, 1978), but the age prevalence and intensity patterns still show a decline, though not as marked as in *S. haematobium*.

Owing to the focal nature of transmission in many areas, neighbouring villages may show different rates of prevalence depending on the distance they are from common transmission sites. Thus, while villages on a lake shore may show high rates of infection, in those a little inland lower rates are invariably found owing to the population having less frequent contact with water.

The stability of egg output

The output of *S. haematobium* eggs by children has been the subject of detailed longitudinal studies in Tanzania and the Gambia (Bradley and McCullough, 1973; McCullough and Bradley, 1973; Wilkins and Scott, 1978).

In the Tanzania studies, it was shown that intensity of infection increased steadily to the age of 10 years and then declined, but prevalence continued to increase to the age of 14 years. Infected 9-

to 11-year-old children with excretion egg counts ranging from low to high were followed for three years. Egg counts from individual children remained relatively steady, a finding thought to provide evidence of concomitant immunity to superinfection. Alternative interpretations of the data, a change in the patterns of transmission or a change in exposure, were suggested (Jordan *et al.*, 1974). The possibility that the worm burden is in a dynamic stage of equilibrium (with equal rates of losing and acquiring infections) was rejected as being unlikely but, in the Gambia, young children showed seasonal changes in egg output with cycles of superinfection in the transmission season followed in a few months by a fall in egg output. Such changes were less marked amongst older children, however, possibly reflecting increasing resistance or decreased water contact or both.

The interpretation of egg output studies of this nature is difficult. Biological investigations are necessary to monitor seasonal and annual variation in snail densities and infection rates and the water-contact pattern of individuals needs clarification to facilitate rational interpretation of findings. In the Gambia studies, seasonal changes in urine concentration were investigated but these were not considered to be responsible for the findings.

Relationship of infection in different areas

Although different quantitative methods had been used in investigations in Brazil, St Lucia and Tanzania, there was evidence of a direct relationship between prevalence and intensity of infection in the different endemic areas (Jordan, 1972).

More recently, this has been confirmed in a limited number of studies using exactly the same techniques in different areas. Thus, using a modified Kato technique in two villages in Kenya—with high (Siongok *et al.*, 1976) and low (Smith *et al.*, 1979) rates of infection—and in a moderately infected St Lucia village, prevalence rates of *S. mansoni* were 82% (Kenya), 62% (St Lucia) and 43% (Kenya), with corresponding arithmetic means of egg output 499/g, 311/g and 199/g. Similarly, in an area of the Gambia where 100% prevalence was maintained in the population from about the age of 8 to 18 years, a very high proportion of subjects were excreting more than 1000 *S. haematobium* eggs per 10 ml urine. Using the same technique in Egypt, prevalence was lower and a smaller proportion of subjects were excreting more than 1000 eggs/10 ml of urine (Fig. 10.8;

Wilkins, 1977; Wilkins and El-Sawy, 1977). Comparable clinico-pathological data from the two areas are not available.

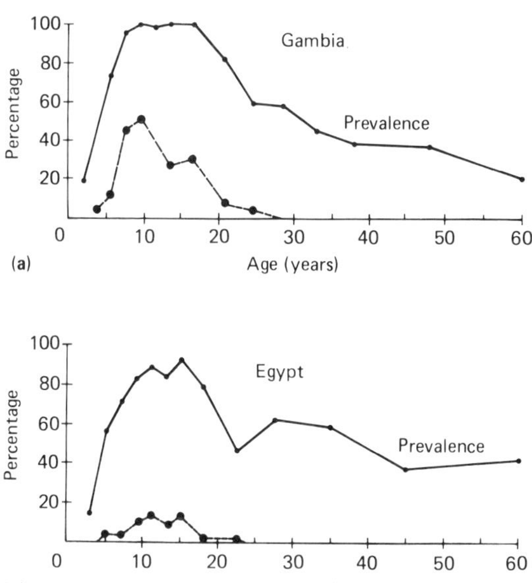

Fig. 10.8 *S. haematobium* data from (a) the Gambia, and (b) Egypt: a comparison of prevalence and intensity of infection determined by identical techniques. In the Gambia, with a very high prevalence (●——●), the percentage of persons with egg counts over 1000/ml urine (●······●) is much greater than in Egypt, where prevalence is lower in the younger age groups. (Data from Wilkins, 1977; Wilkins and El Sawy, 1977.)

IMMUNO-EPIDEMIOLOGY

Sensitive and specific immunodiagnostic tests, while not presently available (Memoranda, 1974), would have advantages over parasitological examinations in epidemiological studies for a variety of reasons.

When acceptable antigens are available they may provide data on prevalence and incidence and perhaps levels of infection.

There were high hopes that the intradermal test would be of use but in spite of its simplicity, because of its now accepted lack of sensitivity and specificity it has been used only in investigational research studies rather than for practical epidemiology. The island-wide immediate skin test surveys in Puerto Rico

(Kagan *et al.*, 1966) are exceptions to this, but a recent survey there showed that sensitivity was as low as 36% for infected children under 14 years old and only 73–79% for adults (Hiatt *et al.*, 1978); similar results were obtained in St Lucia (Warren *et al.*, 1973) while in the uninfected population on the neighbouring island of St Vincent, 26% gave positive reactions. It is of little use in areas where mixed human infections are common and where non-human schistosomes occur (i.e. Africa). The test does not become negative when the schistosome infection dies out, so that high positivity rates are recorded amongst adults when parasitological rates are low.

The immediate intradermal test overestimates prevalence when rates are low, and underestimates it when rates are high (Hiatt *et al.*, 1978).

In addition to the lack of specificity and sensitivity in many serological tests, the need for intravenous blood is a further constraint to their widespread use in epidemiology. The finding that the FAT (Anderson and Cheever, 1972) and the ELISA and RIA (Long and Pelley, personal communication) can be performed on finger-prick blood collected on filter papers is an important advance. Although the development of antigens for the latter two tests is still in the experimental stage, owing to the complexity of the necessary apparatus for the RIA, it is unlikely that this test will be of use in endemic areas; but automated equipment allows for rapid processing of large numbers of specimens which on filter paper could easily be sent to central well-equipped laboratories.

In a recent community study of the RIA and ELISA, the former gave better results (Long *et al.*, 1981). Both tests gave higher rates of prevalence in the older age groups than was obtained by stool examination, but rates were falling far more than is generally seen with intradermal testing. With expected improvements of antigen for the ELISA, and less complicated equipment than the RIA requires, this test appears to have a promising future—sensitivity was 82–99·5% (depending on intensity of infection) using a crude *S. mansoni* egg antigen (McLaren *et al.*, 1979). Using reconstituted freeze-dried antigens and buffers, the test has been used under field conditions (Polderman, 1974). Although efforts are being made to improve the test for *S. mansoni*, an antigen for *S. haematobium* is at a less advanced stage owing to it being more difficult to maintain the infection in laboratory animals.

Table 10.7 Calculation of index of potential contamination (IPC). (High transmission area of Fig. 10.4.)

Age group	Population structure (%)	Prevalence (%)	Eggs/ml faeces	Eggs/day in 1 ml faeces of all infected persons per 100 population	Relative contribution (%)	IPC	Relative IPC (%)
	(1)	(2)	(3)	$(2 \times 3 = 4)$	(5)	$(4 \times 1/100 = 6)$	(7)
0–4	19·2	25	68	1700	3·3	326	5·3
5–9	18·5	61	150	9150	18·0	1693	27·6
10–14	14·0	81	149	12069	23·8	1690	27·5
15–19	10·0	80	104	8320	16·4	832	13·6
20–29	12·3	71	74	5254	10·4	646	10·5
30–39	8·0	58	76	4408	8·9	353	5·8
40–49	7·7	51	61	3111	6·1	240	3·9
50–59	5·0	53	55	2915	5·7	148	2·4
60+	5·4	44	87	3828	7·5	207	3·4
Overall	100	58	100	50755		6135	

POTENTIAL CONTAMINATION OF THE ENVIRONMENT

Of major importance in transmission is the level of contamination of the environment with schistosome eggs which potentially can hatch and infect snails. A measure of this can be obtained (Jordan, 1963; Farooq and Samaan, 1967) from the prevalence and egg output of a community. As these indices of infection vary with age, some groups contribute more than others to contamination and 5-to 14-year-old children were calculated to be potentially responsible for 41·8% of contamination in St Lucia (Table 10.7, column 5).

In developing countries, children form a high proportion of the population and when this is considered their importance in transmission is emphasised. Thus, when the age structure of the population is considered, the 5–14 year age group is responsible for 55·1% of contamination (Table 10.7, column 7).

Table 10.8 Cumulative percentage of persons with different levels of egg excretion and their contribution to contamination (from areas shown in Fig. 8.4).

Level of egg excretion (eggs/ml)	Level of endemicity Low (352)*		Moderate (1146)*		High (1626)*	
	Infected persons (%)	Contamination (%)	Infected persons (%)	Contamination (%)	Infected persons (%)	Contamination (%)
<50	83·2	38·0	72	22·4	57	11·1
−100	94·3	60·0	87	39·2	73	22·8
−400	99·7	91·0	97·5	69·7	94·8	60·5
−500	100	100	98·4	76·4	96·2	66·2
−1000	—	—	99·3	85·6	98·8	82·7
−2000	—	—	100	100	99·7	92·6
−3000	—	—	—	—	100	100

* Number of infected persons.

In areas of lower transmission, older children and young adults are responsible for the bulk of contamination.

In addition to investigating the relative contribution of different age groups to pollution of the environment, the theoretical contribution made by individuals with different levels of egg excretion to the total load of environmental contamination can be calculated.

Table 10.8 shows, for areas of low, moderate and high prevalence, the proportion of persons with egg excretion rates above specific levels and the contribution they make to the total contamination.

As intensity of infection and prevalence are directly related, the daily egg output in areas of high prevalence is disproportionately greater than in areas with lower rates (Table 10.9).

Table 10.9 Showing the relationship between prevalence, intensity of infection and eggs available to contaminate the environment daily. (Data from the three endemic areas of Figs 10.4 and 10.5.)

Area	Prevalence (%)	Eggs/ml faeces*	Eggs/day in 1 ml faeces of all infected persons per 100 population	Estimated daily egg output of infected persons per 100 population†
	(1)	(2)	3 (1 × 2)	(3 × 100)
A	17	38	646	64 600
B	38	66	2508	250 800
C	58	110	6380	638 000

* Arithmetic mean of egg output (infected faeces).
† Based on approximation of 1 ml equivalent to 1 g and output 100 g/day.
The relationship between prevalence and egg output should be noted. Although prevalence C is a little more than three times that of A, daily contamination is ten times greater.

Contamination

While groups and individuals who contribute significantly to contaminating the environment can be identified, there is little information on the relative importance of the routes by which infected faeces get into snail-infested waters. Obvious routes are defaecation directly into water, i.e. from latrines built over rivers or canals, particularly in the Far East, from bridges over rivers (common in St Lucia), or, more rarely, while swimming or bathing. In areas of extremely low rainfall it seems possible that direct faecal contamination of water occurs. In many areas faeces are frequently seen on rocks in rivers or on river banks, and the greatest amount of contamination is probably from faecal matter deposited behind bushes or in tall grass or river banks and subsequently washed into streams. There is evidence that infection rates of sentinel snails increase with the onset of rains—wash-in of the faeces deposited probably being responsible (Christie and Upatham, 1977). However, exposure of faeces containing schistosome eggs to direct or indirect sunlight will decrease the longevity of the eggs (Maldonado *et al.*, 1949). In spite of an accumulation of faecal material adjacent to a river, during the dry season it is perhaps only the infected material deposited a short time before the onset of, and during, the rains that is important in infection of the snail.

The washing of faecally contaminated clothing (Chernin and Antolics, 1973) and cleansing of the perianal area (Radke *et al.*, 1961) may add small numbers of schistosome eggs to the water. These habits, especially the latter which is practised amongst Muslim males after defaecation, may be important in transmission because of their frequency and non-dependence on the rainy season.

Contamination of snail habitats with *S. haematobium* eggs is due essentially to infected persons urinating directly into water. Reasons for this may be of interest but are not relevant to the present discussion.

While faecal and urinary contamination are the main source of *S. mansoni* and *S. haematobium* eggs respectively, the finding of these eggs in urine and faeces respectively is not unusual (Blair and Husting, 1965).

The numerous animal definitive hosts of *S. japonicum* and, of less importance, those of *S. mansoni*, add to the contamination of snail habitats with eggs of these worms. Their importance in the transmission model and control of *S. japonicum* has been discussed (Hairston, 1962).

Overflowing latrines may facilitate the spread of the parasites (Maldonado *et al.*, 1949) and in some situations treated sewage may be the source of contamination. In Puerto Rico it was found that 83% of *S. mansoni* eggs were removed by primary sedimentation and decantation and 99·7% by trickling filter and activated sludge plants (Rowan, 1964). In spite of these high rates of egg removal, it was estimated that, from the activated sludge plant investigated, over 130 million *S. mansoni* eggs or miracidia per year were discharged. The epidemiological effect of this was unknown.

While the total egg load available for contaminating the environment is important in transmission, the eggs must be hatchable. In a comprehensive investigation, hatching rates of

S. mansoni eggs varied between 17% and 64%, decreasing with age of patient and increasing with intensity of infection (Upatham, 1976; Upatham *et al.*, 1976).

The rate of hatching depends partly on the consistency of the stool. Thus, eggs in soft and hard stools, respectively, hatched 24–48 h and 32–128 h after being in water. In flowing water, hard infected stools could thus be carried a considerable distance (Upatham, 1972a).

Experimental findings indicate that, when released at the surface, miracidia could locate *B. glabrata* at depths of 1·22 m (4 ft) (Upatham, 1972a) and were recorded as moving over 100 cm horizontally (Upatham, 1972b). The miracidia tend to concentrate at the edges of containers and probably natural snail habitats.

Before successfully locating a suitable snail intermediate host, miracidia may be eaten by fish or carnivorous invertebrates or plants (Gibson and Warren, 1970; Chernin and Perlstein, 1971). They are also removed from the habitat by other aquatic biota (snails insusceptible to infection), such a sponge effect being a possible side-benefit of biological control through snails as predators or competitors.

DISEASE IN THE COMMUNITY

The various stages of schistosomal disease are shown in Table 10.10. Stages 1 and 2 are rarely recognised in endemic areas. Nevertheless, Stage 2, characterised by fever with symptoms as varied as 'flu-like' or 'typhoid-like', may be recognised when control breaks down (Clark *et al.*, 1970) and should be considered as a possible diagnosis in travellers from endemic areas (Most and Levine, 1963); cardiac, cerebral (Zilberg *et al.*, 1967) and spinal cord (Neves *et al.*, 1973) abnormalities have also been reported in this stage.

Stages 3 and, particularly, 4 are of major concern and are now receiving greater attention at the community level.

While excreted schistosome eggs are responsible for maintaining the life-cycle of the parasite, the reaction to those retained in the tissues of the definitive host is responsible for schistosomal disease. It is not known what proportion of eggs is retained, but in view of the vast numbers found at autopsy, it may be as high as 50%—more than 10 million *S. haematobium* eggs were found in the bladders of 30- and 40-year-old autopsy subjects in Egypt (Smith *et*

Table 10.10 A classification of the course of schistosomiasis based on parasitological, clinical and pathological aspects. (From WHO, 1967.)

Stage	Parasitological	Clinical	Pathological
1. Stage of invasion	A. Penetration	Cercarial skin reaction, if present	Papular dermatitis
	B. Migration	Fever, cough, if present	Inflammatory reactions in lungs and liver
2. Stage of development	Completion of maturation and early oviposition with migration to definitive sites	Acute febrile illness, not always recognised or present	Hyperallergic reactions, generalised and local, to products of eggs and/or young schistosome
3. Stage of established infection	Intensive oviposition, accompanied by a corresponding egg excretion	Stage of early chronic disease, characterised, for instance, by haematuria or intestinal and other digestive manifestations	Local inflammatory reactions to ova resulting in granuloma formation. Fibrosis is not a predominant feature
4. Stage of late infection	Prolonged infection, (often with reduced or discontinued egg extrusion)	Stage of chronic disease, e.g. cor pulmonale, fistula, obstructive uropathy, renal failure, and portal hypertension	Progressive formation of fibrous tissue, varying with intensity of infection and possibly other factors with sequelae according to the organs involved

al., 1975), and it has been estimated that a third of *S. mansoni* eggs produced in the body of man reach the liver (Cheever, 1969).

S. haematobium adult worms tend to remain in one place for long periods, leading to localised massive egg accumulations (Warren, 1969; Sadun *et al.*, 1970; Warren and Domingo, 1976), which calcify (as do those of *S. japonicum*), in contrast to *S. mansoni* eggs which are less often laid in clusters and which more often undergo degeneration (Winslow, 1967).

S. haematobium

At the community level, few studies have been undertaken linking prevalence of *disease* and prevalence and intensity of *infection*.

Investigations in mainland Tanzania and on Zanzibar are unique in this respect; using intravenous pyelography, a high frequency of severe urological disease was demonstrated in apparently healthy school children infected with *S. haematobium* (Forsyth and Bradley, 1964).

Significant differences were found in the frequency of pathological findings in different areas; they were generally related to levels of infection.

In these studies and others in Ghana (Wolfe and Quartey, 1967), the number of calcified bladders was about the same as the number of hydronephroses and about half the total with pathological IVP findings (Table 10.11).

Table 10.11 Parasitological findings and urological complications amongst Zanzibar school children in two groups of villages. (Data from Forsyth and Macdonald, 1966.)

	'Good areas' (%)	'Bad areas' (%)
Prevalence	30	98
Percentage egg loads >500/10 ml	22	67
Pathological IVPs	17	45
Calcified bladder	5	21
Deformed ureters	11	42
Hydronephrosis	8	19
Non-functioning kidney	1	—

Calcified bladders and ureteral deformity occurred with similar frequency in boys and girls, but hydronephrosis was less common in the latter—a finding noted in similar investigations in north-west Tanzania (Forsyth and Macdonald, 1965). It was suggested that this may be due to a physiological difference in the intrinsic mechanism of emptying the bladder shown on micturating cystography. It is probable that the female ureteric orifice affected by *S. haematobium* suffers less functional damage than that in the male.

A more extensive and two-year longitudinal study (Forsyth, 1969) confirmed and extended many of the earlier findings. Lesions in the urinary tract can occur in school children at an early age and amongst males there is evidence of their frequency increasing to middle age. Thereafter, the prevalence of calcified bladder and deformed ureter shows some evidence of declining but hydronephrosis and non-functioning kidney do not, although improvements may occur in some individuals.

Particularly amongst children, the reactions causing ureteric deformity, obstruction and hydronephrosis are reversible with treatment (Lucas *et al.*, 1966; Macdonald and Forsyth, 1968), but deterioration occurs on re-infection (Young *et al.*, 1973). Spontaneous improvement comes from endogenous desensitisation, resulting in smaller granulomas with less oedema (Domingo and Warren, 1968). Thus resolution of deformed ureters was noted, and amongst those with hydronephrosis resolution was observed in 15/37 (41%) of children and 12/48 (25%) of adults. Although improvement was noted in 12 adults, 4 of the 48 adults developed radiologically non-functional kidneys and a further 2 died. None of the 25 patients with radiologically non-functioning kidneys showed recovery and 3 died within two years.

Complete or partial resolution of bladder calcification occurred in 4 of 5 persons found cured five years post-treatment (Young *et al.*, 1973). In another 5, not cured, the severity of radiological changes had increased. However, there is evidence that years of slow but steady excretion of calcified ova may lead to decalcification (Blair *et al.*, 1969; Forsyth and Hughes, 1973; Cheever, Torky and Shirbiney, 1975).

Calcification of the bladder cannot be incriminated as necessarily predisposing to hydronephrosis, since it developed in 4% (of 99) and 3·4% (of 586) of persons with and without bladder calcification respectively. However, in about 50% of persons with calcification, other urinary tract abnormalities were found.

From these studies it was concluded that *S. haematobium* infection is a serious public health problem in Zanzibar, not primarily as a cause of morbidity but as a cause of death, usually due to renal failure precipitated by acute infection, particularly acute pyelonephritis. 'The observed overall annual death rate in the community of 11 per 1000 was much higher than the official estimate of 4·7 per 1000 for the whole of Zanzibar; both rates excluding neonatal rates.'

As a result of quantitative post-mortem studies in Egypt, it was found that 'the mortality attributable to severe urinary schistosomiasis was high and the findings strongly suggest that high prevalence of severe infections with *S. haematobium* is a significant threat to public health' (Smith *et al.*, 1974).

These opinions are based on studies in areas of high prevalence; in areas where this is lower, the disease is of less importance—as in Ibadan (Nigeria), where the intensities of infection, morbidity and mortality are relatively low (Edington *et al.*, 1970). In South Africa, hydronephrosis of schistosomal origin was found in only 5 of 7000 African autopsies and in only 3 was it the cause of death (Powell *et al.*, 1968).

East African studies in areas of different endemicity attempted to quantify the relationship between indices of *infection* and *disease* (Fig. 10.9; Forsyth and Bradley, 1966), but further studies are needed.

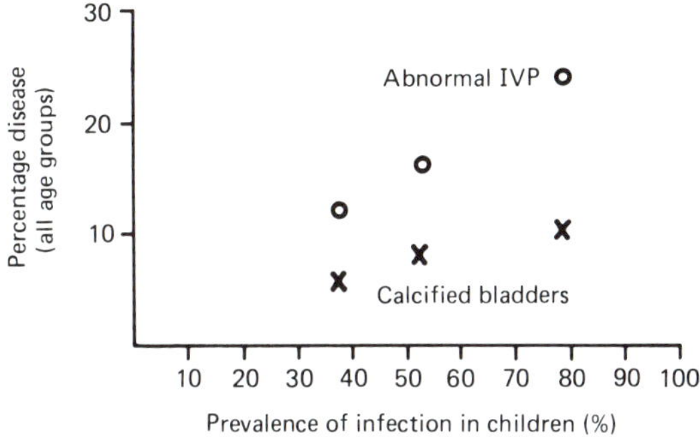

Fig. 10.9   Correlation between prevalence of *S. haematobium* and disease in areas of different endemicity. (Data from Forsyth and Bradley, 1966.)

Intravenous pyelography is not generally suitable for a community study, though plain x-ray of the pelvis might be feasible and would indicate the likely prevalence of severe kidney disease; combined with parasitological studies, disease rates and levels of infection could be related. It might thus be possible to identify priority areas for control and enable rational objectives to be set.

S. mansoni

As has been stressed elsewhere, *S. mansoni* infection is frequently symptom free. This was confirmed in a controlled study of morbidity amongst 138 infected children in St Lucia (Cook *et al.*, 1974). Quantitative data on their egg output was available from the previous four years and, based on this, children were categorised according to their mean egg count—10–75 eggs/ml, 100–300 and over 400 eggs/ml. Uninfected children formed a control group. *Ascaris, Trichuris* and hookworm infections were common in all groups, but no difference in abdominal symptoms (pain, cramp, diarrhoea etc.) or admission of weakness between the groups was found and no difference in anthropological data. Amongst Saudi Arabian recruits, however, abdominal pain and fatigue were associated with the level of infection (Gremillion *et al.*, 1978). In Saudi Arabia, a community study in Ethiopia (Hiatt, 1976), and a Puerto Rican enquiry (Cline *et al.*, 1977), blood in the stools was significantly associated with *S. mansoni*.

In the St Lucian study, livers (more than 2·5 cm below the costal margin) were palpable in 26% of the heavy–moderately infected group (more than 100 eggs/ml) compared with 12% and 9% respectively in the light (10–75 eggs/ml) and uninfected group (Fig. 10.10). The correlation between hepatomegaly and intensity of infection has been noted in community studies elsewhere (Kloetzel, 1963; Lehman *et al.*, 1976; Siongok *et al.*, 1976).

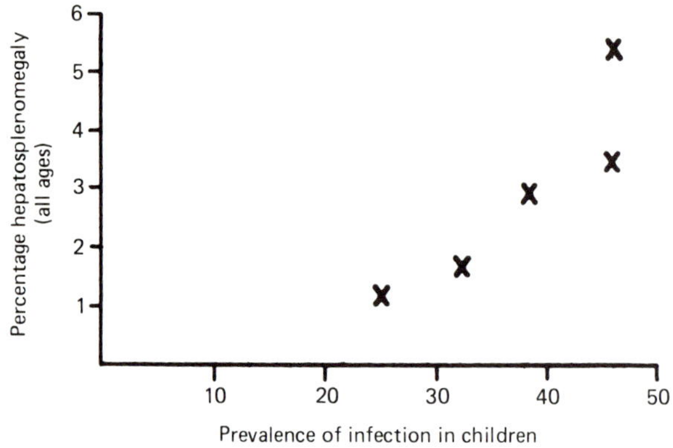

Fig. 10.10 St Lucian data: variation in hepatosplenomegaly rate in infected persons with prevalence of *S. mansoni* in children.

Results of studies in different endemic areas are rarely strictly comparable, owing to the use of different parasitological techniques and methods of reporting results, but the same general pattern is evident—high rates of hepatosplenic disease being associated with high intensities of infection. In north-east Brazil, a 19% hepatosplenomegaly rate was associated with a total population geometric mean of over 100 eggs/ml faeces (Bell technique) (Lehman *et al.*, 1976). At the other extreme is the 3% hepatosplenomegaly rate (arithmetic mean of 499 eggs/g by modified Kato method) in Machakos, Kenya (Siongok *et al.*, 1976) and the Ethiopian result (Hiatt, 1976) of less than 1% in areas with a geometric mean of just over 100 eggs/g by modified Kato. Similarly, a hepatosplenic rate of less than 1% was found in Puerto Rico amongst communities where the geometric mean was 13 eggs/g stool (modified formol–ether concentration technique) (Cline *et al.*, 1977).

(From the above studies the problems of true comparisons due to different parasitological techniques and methods of reporting quite apart from different standards of clinical examination are apparent.)

In comparable quantitative post-mortem studies in Brazil and Egypt, the patterns of disease were similar, and the intensity of *S. mansoni* associated with Symmer's fibrosis the same, with 37% and 36% of cases from the two countries harbouring more than 160 worm pairs (Kamel *et al.*, 1978).

Hepatosplenomegaly is uncommon before the age of 10 years, most cases being found between 10 and 20 years of age, with the prevalence falling in the older age groups (Kloetzel, 1962), although the rate was found to increase amongst adults in another study (Barbosa, 1975). The degree of splenic enlargement varies, but in a series of 159 cases about 50% were between two and four fingers below the costal margin, with about 25% being smaller or larger; above the age of 30 years, spleen sizes tend to be smaller.

In spite of the development in heavily infected communities of hepatosplenic disease (frequently accompanied by portal hypertension), many persons are unaware of their condition. Factors affecting prognosis are unclear—it does not appear to be related to the size of the spleen—and the factors that precipitate episodes of haematemesis are unknown. Longitudinal studies in Brazil have thrown some light on the outcome of these cases and such studies should be encouraged.

In a seven-year study of over 600 infected persons in a town in north-east Brazil (27% of children excreting *S. mansoni* ova), 3 persons died of schistosomiasis, representing an annual death rate of 44·8 per 100 000. Although different physicians made the examinations in 1959 and 1966, there was definite evidence to indicate a gradual progression of the disease (Barbosa and Voss, 1969). In a 10-year follow-up of 112 infected persons, 2 had died of haematemesis and 7 of 91 developed hepatosplenic disease; splenic enlargement regressed in 3 of 8 cases (Katz and Brener, 1966). Although spontaneous regression of true schistosomal splenomegaly is not universally accepted (Kloetzel, 1967), it can occur with chemotherapy. In another study of 159 subjects with schistosomal splenomegaly followed 3·6 years, 6 died of liver failure and 4 from haematemesis (Kloetzel, 1964).

While schistosomal hepatosplenomegaly is associated with intensity of infection, as shown by epidemiological (Kloetzel, 1963), clinical (Cook *et al.*, 1974) and autopsy (Cheever, 1968) investigations, some individuals with light infections are found with severe disease, and some harbour heavy infections causing, apparently, little harm.

These findings may be related to the duration of infection, but the age at which infection first occurs (and the intensity of the first infection) may be important; it seems reasonable to expect the effect of a given number of *S. mansoni* ova in the 300-g liver of a 1-year-old child would be more serious than in a 1500-g liver of an adult. Other factors which might predispose to late-stage disease have also been investigated.

No association was found between splenomegaly and alpha-1-antitrypsin deficiency (Goodgame and Bartholomew, 1978) but predominance of A group patients has been found amongst those with severe hepatosplenic disease (Khattab *et al.*, 1968; Camus *et al.*, 1977; Pereira *et al.*, 1979).

The role of malnutrition in the development of the hepatic changes is little understood, but it has been suggested that deficiencies in the diet of Egyptian peasants may make them more susceptible to 'toxic factors' produced by the schistosome infection or from other sources; furthermore, niacin and iron deficiencies have been reported as common amongst agricultural workers (Hamilton *et al.*, 1959). A protein-deficient diet has also been suggested as being of importance in the aetiology of hepatosplenic schistosomiasis (Gelfand, 1950) and, in mice, protein, calorie, thiamine and vitamin C deficiencies inhibited the granulomatous response to *S. mansoni* (Akpon and Warren, 1975).

Natural heterologous immunity or zooprophylaxis in human infections (Nelson, 1974) may account for observed differences in pathogenicity of infection in different parts of the world. It could also affect prevalence and intensity of infection; furthermore, cross-immunity between *S. haematobium* and *S. mansoni* may occur in man—as in experimental infections in the baboon (Webbe *et al.*, 1979) and mice (Michael *et al.*, 1979). In mainland Tanzania, observed 'mixed infections' were significantly fewer than expected, based on the infection rate in stools and urines from the same individuals (Forsyth and Bradley, 1966); but in autopsy material, mixed infections were more common than expected in Egypt, and if any cross-protection was induced, it was insufficient to prevent the establishment of severe double infections (Smith *et al.*, 1974). In mixed infections, *S. haematobium* infections were heavier when co-existing with *S. mansoni* than in cases of *S. haematobium* alone (Kamel *et al.*, 1978).

In a group of 28 children with hepatomegaly (13 with splenic enlargement), HLA A_1 and B_5 antigens were found to be related to hepatosplenomegaly (Salam *et al.*, 1979), but no correlation between HLA antigens and hepatosplenomegaly could be found in an extensive investigation in St Lucia (Goodgame, personal communication).

Splenomegaly is reported to be more common in Caucasians than Negroes in Brazil in spite of similar prevalence and intensity of infection in the groups (Prata and Schroeder, 1967; Bina *et al.*, 1978); and in St Lucia, those of East Indian (Asian) stock were significantly more liable to develop hepatospleno-megaly than Negroes (Goodgame, personal communication). These findings may be related to the finding that schistosomal hepatosplenomegaly in Africa south of the Sahara appears to be unusual and *S. mansoni* is generally considered to result in few serious complications (Gelfand, 1950; Manson-Bahr, 1958). The situation is very different north of the Sahara, with severe disease being common in Egypt and the Sudan.

Geographic strains of parasite have been reported with dif-fering capacities to induce liver reactions in animals (Saoud, 1965a and 1965b). Thus Brazilian and Puerto Rican strains appear most virulent; the Egyptian strain caused the least severe liver reactions; and the Tanzanian strain produced the fewest eggs (Warren, 1967). In Rhesus monkeys, the East African strain of *S. mansoni* was less pathogenic than the Egyptian or South American strain (Nelson and Saoud, 1968). However, other workers believe animal experiments are of little value in evaluating differences in man of geographic strains of *S. mansoni* (Anderson and Cheever, 1972; Powers and Cheever, 1972).

Scholastic and economic effects

In numerous studies in Africa, schistosomiasis has not been

shown to be a health handicap nor to affect scholastic ability in Black or Arab school children (Usborne, 1954; Clarke and Blair, 1966; Walker, 1977). However, school teachers not infrequently remark on the improvement in the children's concentration after treatment, and some support of this opinion was obtained when children treated for *S. haematobium* were found to improve their class positions more than uninfected or untreated groups (Jordan and Randall, 1962).

White children in South Africa suffer undoubted disability when infected—tiredness and reduced scholastic ability being pronounced, but reversible with treatment (Kieser, 1947); infected Nigerian children suffered fatigue and physical exhaustion after short bouts of exercise (Okpala, 1961).

Efforts have been made to assess the economic burden of schistosomiasis on different communities: in Egypt the disease has been estimated to cost $560 million annually (Farooq, 1967) and in Japan it was estimated that $2·5 million worth of wages were lost each year.

Amongst irrigation workers infected with *S. mansoni* in East Africa, no difference in productivity was found compared with uninfected groups. However, absenteeism was greater amongst them and infected labourers reported sick (for causes other than schistosomiasis) more frequently. Financially it was estimated that treatment in hospital and increased absenteeism cost approximately £6000 per year. It was further estimated that £3500 per year for molluscicidal control of snails and treatment of new labour should save the Company £2500 per annum (Foster, 1967).

In St Lucia, infected plantation workers appeared to have a lowered productivity, leading to their earnings being 15–30% below those of uninfected persons (Weisbrod and Helminiak, 1978). This is supported by recent work in the Sudan which showed the physical working capacity of heavily infected canal cleaners to be severely affected. An 18% difference in maximum aerobic power output between canal workers and villagers was found, but no difference between uninfected and lightly infected individuals (Awad El Karim *et al.*, 1980).

This study showed for the first time definite evidence of reduced physical working ability, but 'studies of labourers' inevitably mean the investigation of the relatively fit and active members of the community; those who may be more seriously ill are excluded (Collins *et al.*, 1976).

ANIMAL RESERVOIRS OF HUMAN SCHISTOSOMES

Animal reservoirs of human schistosomes assume their greatest importance in relation to the epidemiology of *S. japonicum*. In recent years, *S. mansoni* has been found in a number of wild animals, but their importance has yet to be clarified. Infection of animals with *S. haematobium* seems at the present time to be of little importance.

The status of the schistosomes in relation to infection in man and animals varies with the schistosome species. In the case of *S. japonicum*, the 'infection is naturally transmitted between man and other vertebrates; the infection being maintained by either man or animals'. It has been suggested that this relationship is an amphixenosis as compared with a zoo-anthroponosis—'the infections of vertebrates naturally acquired from man where the maintenance host is man, and animals are incidental hosts'. *S. mansoni* in Africa is generally considered to fall into this classification of a zoonosis, although recent work suggests that in South America, at least, it might in fact be in the same classification as *S. japonicum* (Nelson, 1960).

S. mansoni

No detailed studies of the epidemiological significance of animal infections with *S. mansoni* have been made, and information on the subject is largely restricted to reports of various animals having been found infected.

It is of interest that the first report of *S. mansoni* in an animal host came from St Kitts in the West Indies when *Cercopithecus sabaeus* were found infected (Cameron, 1928). Although at the time the disease was a problem in the island (Jones, 1932), it is no longer so. Nothing is now known about the monkey infections in St Kitts.

Examination of monkeys and baboons in various parts of Africa generally showed little evidence of schistosome infection until a high infection rate of *S. mansoni* was found in baboons (*Papio doguera*) in Kenya (Miller, 1959 and 1960), Tanzania (Fenwick, 1969), and subsequently 35 baboons of 64 from different parts of East Africa were found infected, while the vervet monkey (*Cercopithecus aethiops johnstoni*) and Sykes' monkeys (*C. mitis*) were not. *P. anubis* has been found naturally infected in Ethiopia as well as the grivet monkey (*C. aethiops*)

(Fuller *et al.*, 1979). Rodents were first found infected in the wild in Egypt when a gerbil was found with *S. mansoni* (Kuntz, 1952a and 1952b). Extensive surveys of wild rat populations were made in South Africa and *Otomys* and *Mastomys* were found naturally infected (Pitchford, 1959), but in Kenya only a single male of a *S. mansoni*-type worm was found amongst a variety of rodents (Nelson, 1960).

In the Congo, *Dasymys*, *Pelemys*, *Lophuromys* and *Oenomys* were found with *S. mansoni var rodentorum* (Schwetz, 1956) but it seems likely that these were in fact *S. mansoni* in rats (Teesdale and Nelson, 1958; Nelson, 1960; Pitchford and Visser, 1962).

While it is doubtful whether rodents play any part in the epidemiology of *S. mansoni* in Africa, high rates of infection have been found in rodents, in opossums and the peccary in South America. In areas where the human prevalence of infection was high, 8·5% of rats were found to be infected. *Nectomys squamipes*, *Holochilus sciureus* and *Oxmycterus angularis* are probably the most important (Amorin *et al.*, 1954). *Rattus frugivorus* were examined in the Pernambuco district of Brazil and 16 of 27 were found infected (Barbosa *et al.*, 1953); and in Minas Gerais, infections were found in a variety of wild animals. A 60% prevalence rate was found in the prea (*Cavia aperea aperea*) in Bahia, but this is probably not an important reservoir of infection since mature eggs are not excreted in the faeces (Barreto *et al.*, 1964). On the other hand, miracidia released from decomposing animals in water can infect snails (Pitchford and Visser, 1962) and dead prea in water might therefore be of some interest epidemiologically.

In Guadeloupe, *Rattus rattus* and *R. norvegicus* have been found naturally infected with *S. mansoni*, but their role in transmission is considered to be negligible (Theron *et al.*, 1978).

Cattle have been found with natural *S. mansoni* infections, but not all excrete eggs in the faeces (Barbosa *et al.*, 1962). The giant anteater and the squirrel monkey from Surinam have also been found naturally infected (Rijpstra and Swellengrebel, 1962; Swellengrebel and Rijpstra, 1965). Dogs were found lightly infected in Kenya.

S. haematobium

Wild animals have rarely been found infected with *S. haematobium* and although infections have been seen in the baboon, *P.*

doguera, *C. mitis* and the vervet monkey *C. aethiops* in East Africa (Nelson, 1960), in *P. rhodesiae* (Purvis *et al.*, 1965), in Otomys rats in South Africa (Pitchford, 1959), the domestic pig in Nigeria (Hill and Onabamiro, 1960) and the chimpanzee (*Pansatyrus*) in Sierra Leone (Paoli, 1965), it seems likely that these are no more than incidental infections which can be of little importance.

DYNAMICS OF SNAIL POPULATION

Snail population properties, such as density, dispersion, age and perhaps sex structure, reproduction and survival rates, and the intrinsic rate of natural increase ('*r*'), are profoundly affected by environmental factors. The oviposition, larval development and juvenile stages of the molluscan hosts are influenced by relatively narrow limits of such factors which are linked with climatic and seasonal cycles, and most of the snail intermediate hosts of schistosomes, therefore, have relatively unstable populations. The multiple quantitative effects of seasonal rainfall cycles, temperature and related factors have been discussed (see Chapter 2) in relation to specific snail intermediate hosts, but clearly it is essential, for the purpose of a complete epidemiological investigation, to obtain an accurate quantitative assessment of the snail population density, its possible fluctuations and other characteristics, as a basis for determining the transmission patterns in a given situation, or in evaluating applied control measures.

Sampling

Numerous sampling methods used in estimating snail populations have been described and evaluated (Ansari, 1973), and it is emphasised that the technique and method used should always be determined by the objectives of the study, by the nature of the habitat, by the facilities and personnel available and by the circumstances under which the study is made—and obviously it is impossible to devise uniform methodology applicable to all situations for such quantitative estimates.

Most snail populations are 'clumped', and calculations suggest that the negative binomial might adequately describe their distribution (Pesigan *et al.*, 1958; Yeo, 1962). A sample may be inaccurate in several ways but the simplest and most acceptable error is the missing of a constant proportion of snails present (Hairston, 1961). Greater confidence in the estimate of the mean number of snails per sample is obtained by increasing the number of samples, a large number of small samples being preferable to a small number of large samples—in most habitats no less than 30 samples are necessary for the data to be replicable with confidence, and 50–100 would be preferable. According to local conditions, some 5 to 20 habitats should be selected for population studies, representing a complete variety of situations in which snails occur, and at least two of each type of habitat should be studied, thus avoiding interpretations based upon atypical events. As infection rates in the snails must also be determined, habitats should embrace a range of degrees of probable human water contact (Ansari, 1973). Each should be sampled systematically at monthly intervals for at least one year. The tendency for snails to be aggregated in what are apparently uniform habitats often causes the average density of snail samples to have very wide confidence limits. It may be difficult, therefore, to demonstrate the statistical significance of differences that appear superficially to be very large, and the only method of narrowing the confidence limits is by increasing the number of samples. Many species of snails may double their populations in two to three weeks under optimum conditions (Dazo *et al.*, 1966) and this should be considered in deciding the pattern and frequency of sampling for epidemiological purposes.

The under-collection of small sizes of snails may also pose problems and result in wrong interpretation of the period for the most favourable breeding conditions or of the maximum density of a particular snail population. Up to 95% of the youngest age category and snails a month or more old may be missed to a substantial degree. Such information may be of considerable importance to the timing for snail control measures.

The habitats of the snail intermediate hosts are very diversified in character and their sampling, therefore, calls for a clear concept of the information sought, while taking into account the period for which the observations will be carried out (Webbe, 1965a). In large and regular habitats such as irrigation canals, reliable 'absolute data' can be obtained over a long period using direct and 'exhaustive' techniques, without apparently destroying the biological balance of the habitat (Pesigan *et al.*, 1958; Crossland, 1962; Sturrock, 1973a and 1975; Tanaka *et al.*, 1978).

'Relative population densities' may also be obtained using 'fractional sampling techniques' and these have been reviewed (Southwood, 1966). Population trends but not absolute density changes may be compared between ponds, lakes, streams and canals, provided that the collection processes are standardised to ensure the recovery of a constant proportion of the population (Olivier and Schneiderman, 1956; Webbe, 1962a and 1965a; Sturrock, 1973a).

Thus, having established the distribution of the relevant snail hosts in as wide a range of habitats as possible, it is possible to determine the characteristics of the snail population which are most important for a study of the dynamics of transmission—-namely, population density, the age and perhaps sex structure of the population, the reproduction and survival rates.

Only recently have methods used in the field of population ecology been adapted for use in the study of animal populations (Hairston, 1962 and 1965a; Slobodkin, 1962). These are basically demographic and require a knowledge of age-specific rates of survival and reproduction, from which an ecological life-table and the 'intrinsic rate of natural increase' can be derived (Jordan and Webbe, 1969).

Measurement of size is the only method of determining the age of snails in the field and, in order to estimate their ability to survive under natural conditions, one must know the age distribution of a population at any given time. Some workers measure snail samples using selective standards so that only two or three size categories are obtained, and such data may be useful in roughly indicating population trends. The measurement of snail shells, however, must be carried out with care and, if possible, to the nearest 0·1 mm if data suitable for conversion from size to age are required. Samples of *O. quadrasi* have been stuck on to cellulose tape, aperture up, and measured to the nearest 0·1 mm, using a dissecting microscope with an ocular micrometer (Pesigan *et al.*, 1958). This method is likely to be inconvenient if larger snails are involved or if one requires to return material to the field. In the case of bulinid snails, the height of the shell is the largest dimension parallel to the axis, and can be conveniently measured to the nearest 0·1 mm using callipers with a vernier attachment. Similarly, the maximum diameter of *Biomphalaria* can be conveniently measured and is the dimension which shows the biggest proportional increase as the result of growth. A radiographic method of measurement is available in which snails are photographed on radiographic film or plate; direct measurement of the image can then be accurately made. It also has the advantage that a permanent record of an entire sample is obtained. It is particularly useful for measurement of *Biomphalaria*, but is not practicable in the case of bulinid shells, which have to be placed aperture up and which may not present the main axis parallel to the plane of the film (Webbe, 1965b). In order that size may be used for the determination of age, an accurate growth curve must be obtained which, in turn, depends upon large complete samples and, of course, upon reliable sampling at suitable intervals (Webbe, 1962a; Shiff, 1964a; Sturrock, 1973b).

From successive size–frequency histograms of periodic samples and the growth rate data which may be derived from them, accurate calculations of the survival of adult snails can be made for each interval between sampling. The average daily mortality rate in a given habitat is then calculated using the exponential expression

$$l_x = e^{-xd}$$

where l_x = the proportion of snails surviving to age x
       x = the number of days between sampling
       d = the exponential daily mortality rate.

A knowledge of the adult mortality rate permits calculation of the length of life of an average adult snail. Survival data are normally required for the female population only, but when dealing with hermaphroditic animals, every individual is capable of egg production and the whole population must be considered for the collection of data.

The maintenance of different population structures independently of density must depend upon different survival rates, both for young and for adult snails, and both must be involved since equal survival rates for adults and different rates for young, or vice versa, would result in a direct relationship between population structure and density, which is clearly not the case (Pesigan *et al.*, 1958). It was found that population structures, like density, varied from place to place (Webbe, 1962a), with quite large changes occurring from time to time, and that the appreciable differences in the mortality rates of adult snails among the populations studied were large enough to effect the considerable changes in population density and structure which were apparent at different times.

Differences in the survival rates of young snails and in reproduction must influence population structure and density, but data on survival of young snails and the egg-laying capacity of adults cannot be determined under field conditions with the accuracy of adult mortality rates. An index of a combination of the two can be obtained, however, by dividing the number of mature snails at one sampling into the number of young at the next. The number of young is determined by reference to the growth-rate data, which give the maximum size that a young snail could reach if the egg was laid on the day that the mature snails were counted. The ratio thus obtained is divided by the number of days between sampling to obtain a mean reproductive index.

In calculating the reproductive index (Webbe, 1962a), it was found necessary to take a minimum interval of four weeks between samplings and different intervals for the two groups of population studies, because of the small numbers of 'very young' snails recognisable as offspring, which were collected for shorter intervals. This underlines the importance of sampling procedure and of obtaining large complete samples whenever possible. It was also found that the reproduction indices of the different populations varied considerably for individual intervals between samplings, but that the average daily reproduction indices of different populations for the entire periods of sampling were broadly similar. The reproduction indices appeared to be related to the average daily mortality rates, though not always to density.

In a study of the population dynamics of *B. glabrata* in St Lucia (Sturrock, 1973b), life-tables were drawn up (Jordan and Webbe, 1969). This method has been criticised (Hairston, 1971) because constant rather than age-specific values were used for birth and death rates. Direct observation of egg production, however, is not possible with any accuracy under field conditions and the 'reproduction index' is likely to be the only available estimate of birth rates. It was pointed out that it probably underestimates the true rate as it takes no account of mortality among eggs or hatchlings less than 2 weeks old, but that this drawback may not be too serious because snails which are just sexually mature and which play a significant role in determining the value of 'r' produce fewer eggs than older snails which, however, have a more uniform pattern of egg production (Sturrock, 1973b). Similarly, a constant daily mortality rate estimate was considered acceptable for the age-bands upon which it was based (5- to 7-week-old snails) and taking into consideration the average survival time of *B. glabrata* (12 weeks).

The life-table

Egg production per snail—fecundity—designated m_x, is given by a schedule of births or fertile eggs laid per unit of time by each female of age x. Only female births are normally required, but when dealing with hermaphrodites the whole population must be considered.

An ecological life-table has two principal features: survivorship, designated l_x, and fecundity, designated m_x. The proportion of snails surviving to each successive age x is entered in an l_x column; the average number of eggs laid per snail during each successive time interval is entered in an m_x column; the proportional contribution of each age group to the next—the 'net reproduction rate'—is designated R_o.

$$\Sigma l_x m_x = R_o$$

and if the population is neither increasing nor decreasing, the net reproductive rate will be 1·0. Under different conditions, the mean time per generation varies considerably, and since the net reproductive rate (R_o) is based on the generation and not on absolute time, it cannot be used to compare the effects of different extrinsic factors (Shiff, 1964a).

Any population behaving according to a given set of life-table data with age-specific survival and reproduction rates is considered to have a stable age distribution or equilibrium population structure, towards which the actual age distribution is tending. This stable age distribution is an intrinsic constant of the population and it provides a basis for evaluating actual age distributions as they may occur. Therefore, when the environment of the population is unlimited and other organisms do not exert a limiting effect, there is an excess of habitat space and food, and the age distribution is stable, and the population rate per individual (the specific growth rate) becomes constant for the prevailing physical conditions. This specific maximum growth rate is the intrinsic rate of natural increase 'r', a population parameter based upon the survival and fecundity of the species under particular environmental conditions. It can be calculated through use of the theorem of stable age distribution by trial and error substitution in the following formula (Slobod-kin, 1962):

$$\Sigma l_x m_x e^{-rx} = 1{\cdot}0$$

When conditions are optimum, 'r' is maximum and represents the maximum intrinsic rate of increase of the population, also called the 'biotic potential'. When conditions are not optimum, the mortality rate increases and 'r' assumes a value between the 'biotic potential' and zero. The difference between maximum 'r' and the actually observed value of 'r' expresses the environmental resistance of the population in the given environment. Changes in the environment result in a decrease of the population rate as population density approaches an upper limit, which is known as the 'saturation level' or 'carrying capacity'. When this is reached, population density tends to fluctuate above and below this level, and these fluctuations may depend upon changes in the physical environment or upon interactions within the population; they may be seasonal or periodic, and both extrinsic factors (rainfall, temperature) and intrinsic ones (birth rate, mortality) influence all of them, but one particular factor is usually the major cause (Webbe, 1962a). Thus the parameter will alter in relation to changing environmental conditions, and can be used to measure the reaction of a species to any particular environmental factor or the reaction of different populations to a particular set of conditions per unit of time. It also reflects the natural stability of a population, and the selective advantage of a high value of 'r' is apparent where a population goes through marked fluctuations, since it allows a population to recover rapidly with a return of favourable conditions—as in the case of *B. globosus* (Shiff, 1964a). Under more stable conditions, a slower rate of increase may be of greater advantage to a species, as in the case of *O.h. quadrasi* in the Philippines (Pesigan *et al.*, 1958).

In addition to errors incurred during the collection and measurement of snails, others may, of course, arise from the basic assumption required for life-table analysis—namely, that a particular habitat should have unlimited resources and a stable environment; and that the snail population should have a stable age structure. These conditions are rarely found in the field, particularly if seasonal changes occur, and some degree of migration in and out of the habitat may also occur. In view of these factors, it is considered that a number of estimates of 'r' should be obtained before the values can be accepted with any confidence and that added confidence may be given if individual values can be shown to describe the observed data.

A mathematical model of a population of aquatic snails has been written in Fortran II for an IBM 1620 digital computer (Jobin and Michelson, 1967) which required information on the snail species including age-specific survival rate, age-specific birth rate, a fecundity factor, the relationship of fecundity to temperature, the volume of the 'crowding zone' and information on the habitat (volume, temperature, shoreline, food). A three-year prediction of a snail population was calculated from these data and, in order to verify the model, its predictions were compared with the data of a snail population in a small pond (Shiff, 1964a, 1964b and 1964c). It was considered that the basic structure of this model was sound since there was general agreement of the predicted and observed population data. Such a model may have practical value in conjunction with field observations related to control measures.

Transmission patterns

Cyclic reproduction and population changes cause fluctuations in the transmission potential of snail intermediate hosts and considerable differences in the numbers of infected snails occur seasonally in different endemic regions, with relatively low infection rates usually accounting for high incidence and prevalence of infection in the human population. Definition of the foci and timescale of transmission in a given area and of the pattern and degree of cercarial production, and the factors which influence it, is essential for a proper understanding of the epidemiology of the infection and for planning cost-effective control measures.

At any given time the proportion of snails infected with schistosomes depends upon a complex interaction of different factors including: the distribution and behaviour of definitive hosts; the relative susceptibility to infection of a particular snail intermediate host; and climatic factors such as temperature and rainfall.

The use of 'percentage cercarial infection rate' and, in particular, the generally observed very low rate (1–2%) as an index of transmission, have been criticised (Hoffman *et al.*, 1979) because the absolute number of infected snails and, therefore, the risk of transmission, can remain reasonably constant during marked fluctuations in the total snail population—differential growth and death rates of infected snail populations are some of the factors influencing this.

The different factors which may influence the infection of the snail intermediate host have been discussed (see Chapter 3), but quantitative estimates of the degree of pollution in natural habitats in terms of viable ova or miracidia are very difficult to obtain and there is little information on the degree of contamination relative to a particular density level of the snail intermediate host population necessary to produce transmission.

However, there have been considerable advances made in studies of the larval stages of schistosomes using laboratory bred snails as 'sentinels' in different habitats to estimate contamination and the inoculation rate of snails (Upatham, 1972a, 1972b, 1973a, 1973b, 1976). The inoculation rates of naturally infected snails have also been calculated from their infection rates (Sturrock and Webbe, 1971) and the results were found to be similar to those obtained from exposures of sentinel snails. Subsequently it was noted that selective mortality due to infection which occurs among snails has measurable consequences in relation to 'catalytic curve' analyses which should not be ignored (Figs. 10.11 and 10.12; Sturrock *et al.*, 1975).

It has been suggested that in any transmission site there will be a 'time–concentration' factor affecting miracidial density (Wright, 1967). Schistosomes produce large numbers of eggs,

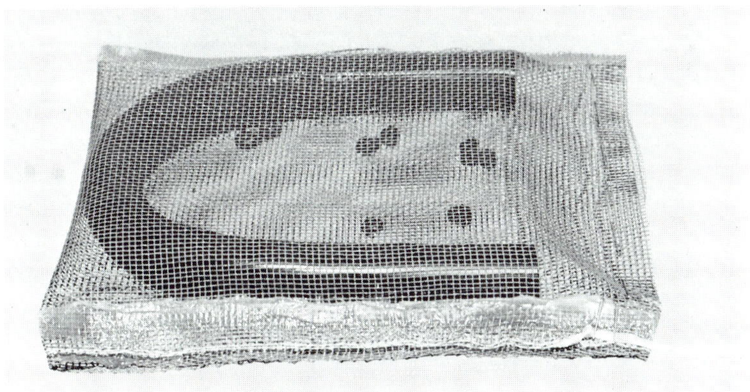

Fig. 10.11   Sentinel snails, *B. glabrata*, in cage made of glass-reinforced plastic mosquito screen over a PVC electricity conduit.

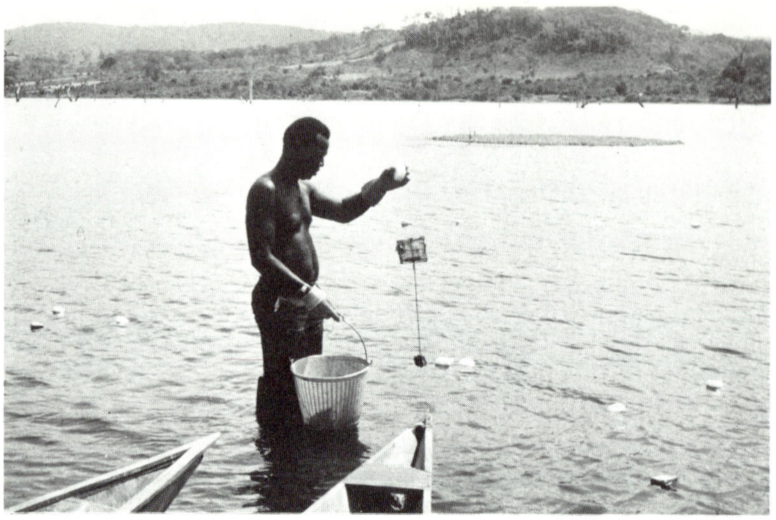

Fig. 10.12 Placing sentinel snails in bags and attached to floats in Lake Volta for estimating contamination, defining focality of transmission and evaluating intervention methods.

but only a fraction of the miracidia which hatch ultimately infect snail hosts, and a considerable wastage of both eggs and miracidia takes place.

Neither infected nor uninfected snails are randomly distributed and it is essential that any sampling programme should cover the entire area under consideration, so that a large number of small samples is obtained from many different foci over a prolonged period, in order to provide precise information on the distribution and frequency of infected snails.

Field samples can be examined for infection using a crushing technique, the tissues then being examined microscopically 'for daughter sporocysts and cercariae'. Alternatively, all snails collected may be exposed to artificial light in 3 in × 1 in (7·5 × 2·5 cm) specimen tubes containing a small quantity of water for four to five hours, consequent shedding of cercariae being observed. This permits measurement of all snails in the samples and their return to their respective habitats if it is deemed necessary. It is considered that under certain conditions this procedure is imperative if meaningful data on snail population density and structure and cercarial infection rates are to be obtained (Fig. 10.13).

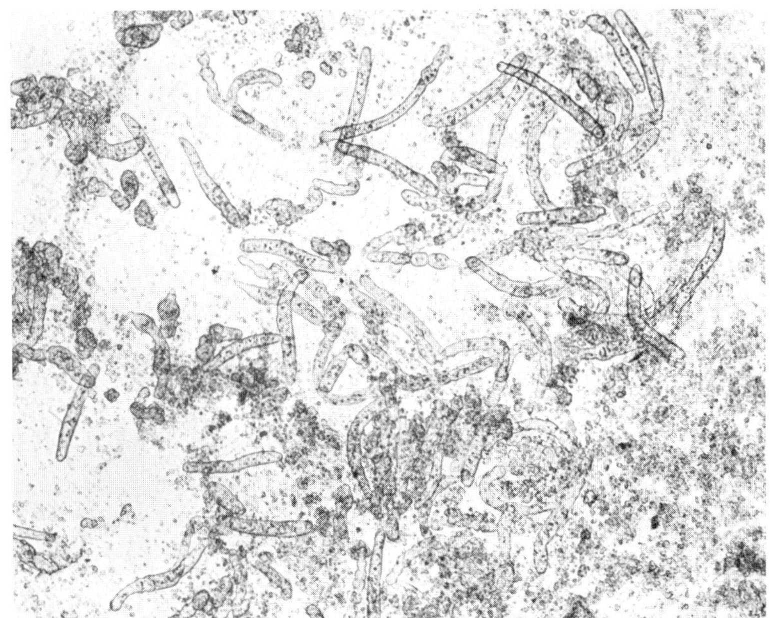

Fig. 10.13 Sporocysts in the head-foot region of *B. glabrata* 12 days after exposure as a sentinel snail.

In order to obtain accurate information on the proportion of snails infected in a particular area (containing a variety of locations and at all seasons), it is necessary to examine adequate numbers. Cercarial infection rates are often low (0·5–2%) and it may, therefore, be necessary to supplement the quantitative sampling procedures in different habitats with other collecting methods. Thus, if only 1–2% of the snails are infected, it will be necessary to examine 500–1000 snails in order to retain the 95% confidence limits within a factor of 2 of the observed rate (Ansari, 1973).

While the proportion of infected snails found in many endemic areas is relatively low (approximately 1%), this may vary from one type of habitat to another and seasonally.

In an area south of Lake Victoria, Tanzania, *B. (P.) nasutus productus* is present in small circumscribed pools, seepages, rice-bunds and temporary collections of water, usually of seasonal duration only. The main transmission period in the area studied lasts for four to five months, corresponding to the end of the main rains and the period immediately afterwards. Most snails infected with *S. haematobium* were found in June, July and

August with maximum monthly infection rates of 12·5%, 7·7% and 12·6% respectively. However, high cercarial infection rates were found in individual foci, and more than 50% of samples of more than 200 snails were frequently found infected at this time of year (Webbe, 1962a). Considerable fluctuations in the numbers of *B. pfeifferi* with *S. mansoni* cercarial infections were found in Tanzania, where large numbers of infected snails were sometimes collected even when watercourses were in flood, the highest infection rates being recorded, however, during the dry season (Webbe, 1962b); the highest infection rates in *B. sudanica* in swampy conditions were also recorded in the dry season when population numbers were high, but the highest infection rates in *B. choanomphala*, present in the body of Lake Victoria, were found in October to January (the short rainy season) when snail densities were lowest (Magendantz, 1972).

The production of cercariae by infected snails is also demonstrably different seasonally, and many factors including temperature, rainfall and human water-contact behaviour patterns may influence this. In the Middle East, cercarial infection rates are characteristically low, but generally increase during warmer, sunnier weather. The highest average rate of infection in *B. truncatus* in four years was 0·76% and the lowest 0·05%, the peak of infection being reached in the early and later summer months (El Gindy and Rushdi, 1962). In the Nile Delta, cercarial incubation periods are as short as three weeks in the summer and cercarial output is the highest, more than 90% of schistosome transmission taking place between June and September (Chu and Dawood, 1970). It was found that the June–September transmission potential is 88·24% of the cercarial abundance for the whole year and the October–November transmission potential is 7·70%. Cercarial infection rates in *B. alexandrina* of 4·26% and 5·96% were recorded during the months of August and September, respectively. The effect of lower temperature on the pre-patent period may affect transmission, which has been shown to decrease during the coldest months. This has been shown in Iran in the case of *S. haematobium* (Chu *et al.*, 1966) and in South Africa and Zimbabwe for *S. mansoni* and *S. haematobium* (Pitchford and Visser, 1965; Shiff *et al.*, 1975).

During the past 10 years there have been many interesting studies carried out which have added considerably to knowledge of the transmission of schistosomiasis in different endemic areas,

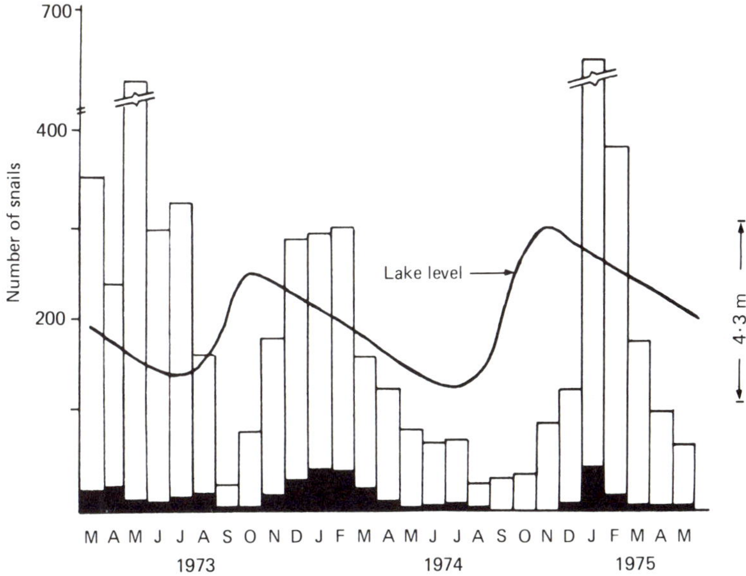

Fig. 10.14 Numbers of snails (*B. truncatus rohlfsi*) collected (open columns) and numbers of infected snails (black columns) per month in relation to the level of Lake Volta; first eight villages studied. (After Klumpp and Chu, 1977.)

highlighting particular features of seasonality and focality. These include studies in north-east Brazil (Coutinho *et al.*, 1973); in St Lucia, where snail population numbers and transmission cycles are largely determined by rainfall, and where snails from marshes and ponds are washed into rivers and streams during the wet season, to multiply in the dry season and cause most of the transmission (Sturrock, 1973b); in Zambia, where seasonal patterns of transmission of *S. haematobium* are associated with high and low veldt areas; and in the man-made Lake Kariba, in which transmission of *S. haematobium* and *S. mansoni* is of recent origin (Hira, 1969, 1972 and 1975); in Ethiopia, where transmission of both *S. haematobium* and *S. mansoni* occurs in some valleys in the mountain region in the dry season, *B. rueppelli* being found in streams in the hills around the valleys (Polderman, 1974) and *B. abyssinicus*, transmitting *S. haematobium*, being found in swamps in the valley bottoms where temperatures are higher (Kloos and Lemma, 1977); in Lake Volta, Ghana (Fig. 10.14), where the essential seasonality and focality of transmission of *S. haematobium* by

B. truncatus rohlfsi have been established in relation to annual lake-level drawn-down and associated vegetation changes in human water-contact sites (Chu and Vanderberg, 1976; Klumpp and Chu, 1977; Chu, 1978; Chu and Klumpp, 1978); in central Sulawesi, where *O.h. lindoensis* has been found widely but focally distributed in the Lindu and Napu Valleys and where, in discrete habitats in the dry season, it is responsible for transmitting *S. japonicum* (Carney *et al.*, 1974 and 1975; Sudomo and Carney, 1974; Hadidjaja and Sudomo, 1976); in the Mekong River focus, where on Khong Island, Laos, it is considered that transmission may be intermittent in time and place, but that *S. mekongi* is being mainly transmitted (during the dry season) by *Tricula aperta* in pools from the end of March to the beginning of the rains in mid-June, when the snails are present in the largest numbers (Kitkoon *et al.*, 1973; Kitkoon and Schneider, 1976). In the Philippines high infection rates in snails occur following the rains which wash faeces containing schistosome ova into snail habitats (Iwanaga *et al.*, 1977), but heavy rains also flush snails away, and most transmission probably occurs at the end of the rains and at the beginning of the dry season.

Cercariometry

Seasonal fluctuation in the density of a snail population and of its concomitant schistosome infection, together with changes in cercarial output, must exert a considerable epidemiological effect in relation to human exposure. Many factors influence the production and periodicity of output of cercariae and their behaviour and, thereby, the probability of infection of the definitive host. The behaviour of the host (human water-contact patterns) and the nature of the habitat will, of course, modify the role of some of these influences (Dalton, 1976; Dalton and Pole, 1978).

It is clear that there is a need for information on cercarial populations in the field in order to quantify the relationship between contamination and the infectivity of a particular focus of transmission and, therefore, the risk of infection. Different methods of cercariometry have been developed, including filtration, the use of 'phototaxic response equipment' and of 'continuous flow centrifugation', but the efficacy of recovery using these methods may be seriously impaired by particulate or colloidal turbidity in many foci and the differentiation of closely related species of cercariae is difficult. The efficiency of direct filtration techniques* has, however, been improved (Sandt, 1973a; Sandt, 1973b), and the technique was used in epidemiological studies in St Lucia and Ghana. It has also recently been shown that isoenzyme analysis may be used to distinguish the cercariae of different schistosome species, even when they emerge from the same species of snail (Mahon and Shiff, 1978).

Another method which has been used, with some success, to detect cercarial populations is that of exposure to sentinel rodents in natural waters (Pesigan *et al.*, 1958; Pitchford and Visser, 1962; Webbe, 1962b, 1965b and 1966; Sturrock, 1973b; Polderman, 1974; Upatham, 1976). This method may fail to detect cercariae at very low density level, and these may be of epidemiological significance, but it does permit a differentiation of different species of schistosomes. Low mouse infection rates obtained by such exposures may reflect low cercarial concentrations in the field, but the non-random, clumped distribution of adult *S. mansoni* in groups of infected mice is consistent with periodic, localised and high concentrations of cercariae in natural waters (Crofton, 1971). This technique is too costly for general widespread use, particularly since it yields only limited quantitative data, and such data can now be obtained more cheaply, rapidly and reliably by cercariometric techniques and direct snail sampling. (Sturrock, 1973b).

The daily pattern of output of cercariae will have considerable bearing on human exposure, since cercariae are predominant in certain habitats for only limited periods. It is apparent from evidence obtained in Africa, Puerto Rico and Brazil (see Chapter 3) that cercariae of *S. mansoni* and *S. haematobium* will be present for some hours at midday, but most of these may be swept away in watercourses by mid-afternoon. The velocity of a watercourse determines the time of maximum cercarial density, and other factors may also affect the numbers of cercariae and their infectivity. While the morphological identity of cercariae may be intact after travelling appreciable distances in flowing turbulent water, their viability is apparently reduced—610 m downstream from the point of introduction into a concrete-lined drain (Radke *et al.*, 1961), but in a natural stream cercariae were not detected more than 195 m from the source (Upatham,

---

* A further filtration technique using a new type of monofilament polyamide filter, Nytrel-Ti, has recently been described (Theron, 1979).

1974a). Cercariae were found to be infective to mice at a distance of approximately 100 m, while other studies showed that dispersion in a natural situation was approximately 400 m (Pitchford and Visser, 1960). It was established that cercariae are resistant to a high degree of turbulence, since cercariae which had traversed a 10-m waterfall were still infective to mice (Upatham, 1973c). In the case of impounded waters, cercariae of *S. mansoni* will be present during most of the 24 h, as will the cercariae of *S. haematobium* in such situations. The cercariae of *S. japonicum* are most abundant during the early part of the night.

The longevity and infectivity of cercariae will depend upon their energy reserves and the environmental factors which affect these. The survival patterns of both *S. mansoni* and *S. japonicum* are apparently similar during the first 24 h of their existence, but their infectivity decreases after about 12 h, their viability being seriously impaired at temperatures above 35°C and by ultra-violet light.

Where levels of cercariae have been investigated, they seem to be low; in St Lucia they have varied from 0·04–7·64 cercariae/l (mean 2·5) (Sandt, 1973a); less frequently, levels of 21/l being found (Upatham, 1976). In Puerto Rico a peak of 23 cercariae/l was found about midday (Rowan, 1958).

But even with high densities, few cercariae successfully penetrate the skin and mature in the definitive host, though the factors involved in this are not known. Thus in field experiments, between 1·2% and 6·9% and 0·1% and 0·2% of cercariae in static and flowing habitats, respectively, successfully infected mice (Upatham, 1974a). In ideal laboratory conditions, only 8% of 2000 cercariae used to infect a chimpanzee matured (Sadun *et al.*, 1966).

MATHEMATICAL MODELS

Attempts to use mathematical models to describe the distribution or spread of schistosomiasis in a population of snails or humans have only been studied during the past two decades. Models involving snails only are discussed below, followed by those which describe the prevalence of infection in humans and, lastly, models for the whole transmission cycle including the intensity of infection in man are examined.

Models of snail population dynamics and the transmission of

infection in snails originated primarily to determine efficient means of mollusciciding. The fecundity of snails as a function of snail density, available food and other factors, has been examined (Jobin and Michelson, 1967), and the effects of infection on age structure (Coutinho and Coutinho, 1968). From standing populations of snails, estimates of snail survival were obtained (Sturrock and Webbe, 1971; Sturrock *et al.*, 1975). Although there may be less emphasis on mollusciciding as a control strategy, there will remain a need to incorporate realistic assumptions about the snail intermediate host into whole life-cycle models (mentioned below) to determine the relative effects of different control strategies.

Those models for the prevalence of infection in humans tend to be refinements of catalytic models described by Muench (1959). This method was used to study *S. japonicum* in the Philippines (Hairston, 1965b). Recent work has involved the use of non-linear multiple regression to estimate some parameters as functions of other factors, such as population size and areas of possible contact (Rosenfield, 1975). While not attempting to 'explain' transmission biologically, such models may be of value in well-studied situations where guidelines to a specific question are sought.

It is convenient to consider models for the intensity of infection in humans and whole life-cycle models together. Although one does not imply the other, a particular branch of modelling has involved both and warrants attention. One approach to modelling the whole cycle (Hairston, 1962 and 1965a) involved life-table methods to calculate the reproductive rate of the helminth. Macdonald (1965) employed a differential equation to study the dynamics of infection. Considerable attention was paid to the allowance of pairing and to a property of the model called 'breakpoint' behaviour. Macdonald noted some differences between asexual and sexual populations and that, in particular, growth for sexual populations was slower at low intensities where few worms meant few worm pairs. As a result, if a population of worms could be sufficiently lowered, then an insufficient number of pairs would form to sustain transmission and the population of worms would spontaneously die out. The critical number of worms (or, equivalently, the mean worm load in a fixed number of human hosts) below which the infection could not sustain itself was termed the 'breakpoint'. Later a mathematically rigourous form of this model was developed in two dimensions (one for the infection in humans, the other in snails) and it was noted that 'breakpoint' behaviour need not exist (Nasell and Hirsch, 1973). For some ecological complexes, transmission can be sustained and will only be sustained if the mean worm load exceeds this criterion. In other complexes, no transmission can be sustained, regardless of the mean worm load which might be introduced. Thus, where transmission occurs, there are two control options: either to lower the mean worm load to below the critical level, or to alter the ecological complex so that transmission cannot be sustained. As the complex is altered (by, say, mollusciciding or provision of water supplies) a 'threshold' is passed, beyond which transmission (with 'breakpoint' behaviour) is impossible.

Nasell has elaborated on the above model by allowing for latency (Nasell, 1976) and the immigration of infection (Nasell, 1975). The former enables a more valid comparison with field data, as patently infected snails are readily counted. The latter notes that if there is sufficient immigration of infection, worm pairs are more readily formed, and the transmission dynamics may resemble those of an asexual disease: the breakpoint phenomenon need not necessarily exist. Macdonald (1965) and Nasell and Hirsch (1973) assumed that the distribution of worms in humans followed a Poisson distribution. A negative binomial distribution was investigated where some individuals could be very heavily infected and many more only lightly infected than assumed by the Poisson formulation. It was seen that dynamics were strongly affected by this 'clumping' effect (May, 1977; Bradley and May, 1978). From studying a modification of the Nasell–Hirsch model that makes no allowance for pairing effects but does allow for heterogeneity in exposure, it was shown that lighter levels of infection in snails can sustain transmission than those predicted with homogeneous exposure (Barber, 1978).

In the above whole-cycle models, some biological phenomena are described by mathematical relationships. Unfortunately, some other aspects of their qualitative behaviour do not agree with empirical evidence. Firstly, the level of infection in snails required by the models to sustain transmission usually exceeds snail infection rates from field data. The allowance for latency and heterogeneity goes some way in lessening this difference, but more realistic treatment of snail populations seems warranted. Secondly, such models predict a uniform increase in prevalence and intensity of infection with age, but survey results consistently display a peak in the teenage years. This may be accounted for by either an immune effect or a reduced exposure in older ages. These shortcomings are an important product of mathematical modelling: the factors considered to date are insufficient to explain some of the basic phenomena, and thus transmission depends on other factors.

Macdonald (1965) chose to compare 'control' methods by depositing a mathematical system with fixed values of parameters, changing different parameter values, and then following the model's numerical predictions. A more cautious attitude persists now, and while some conclusions can be drawn about the relative benefits of control strategies, there is a reluctance to expect accuracy in numerical predictions. Interest centres more on qualitative than quantitative behaviour, in particular the relative effects of control methods on changing thresholds or reaching breakpoints. We have not yet reached the point where there is general agreement as to which method is preferred.

Following a delay phase in the development of mathematical models for schistosomiasis in the 1960s, we are currently experiencing an exponential growth which is bound to continue. For those wishing to study this area in greater detail, a fuller summary of the various models is available with a useful bibliography (Cohen, 1977).

REFERENCES

Akpon, C. A. and Warren, K. S. (1975). *J. Infect. Dis.* **132,** 6.

Amorin, J. P. de, da Rosa, D. and de Lucena, D. T. (1954). *Revta Bras. Malar. Doenç. Trop.* **6,** 13.

Anderson, L. A. and Cheever, A. W. (1972). *Bull. Wld Hlth Org.* **46,** 233.

Ansari, N. (1973). *Epidemiology and Control of Schistosomiasis (Bilharziasis).* S. Karger, Basel, New York.

Awad El Karim, M. A., Collins, K. J., Brotherhood, J. R., Dore, C., Weiner, J. S., Sukkar, M. Y., Omer, A. H. S. and Amin, M. A. (1980). *Am. J. Trop. Med. Hyg.* **29,** 54.

Barber, A. D. (1978). *Trans. R. Soc. Trop. Med. Hyg.* **72,** 6.

Barbosa, F. S. (1975). *Ann. Trop. Med. Parasit.* **69,** 207.

Barbosa, F. S., Barbosa, I. and Arruda, F. (1962). *Science* **138,** 831.

Barbosa, F. S., Dobbin, J. E. and Coelho, M. V. (1953). *Publ. Avuls. Inst. Aggeu Magalhaes* **2,** 43.

Barbosa, F. S. and Voss, H. (1969). *Bull. Wld Hlth Org.* **40,** 966.

Barreto, A. C., Santos, I. and Oliveira, V. S. (1964). *Revta Inst. Med. Trop. S. Paulo* **6,** 233.

Berberian, D. A., Paquin, H. O. Jr. and Fantuzzi, A. (1953). *J. Parasit.* **39,** 517.

Bina, J. C., Tavares-Neto, J., Prata, A. and Azevedo, E. S. (1978). *Hum. Biol.* **50,** 41.

Blair, D. M. and Husting, E. L. (1965). *Cent. Afr. J. Med.* **11,** 243.

Blair, D. M., Weber, M. D. and Clarke, V. de V. (1969). *Cent. Afr. J. Med.* **15** (Suppl. 11), 2.

Bradley, D. J. (1965). *Ann. Trop. Med. Parasit.* **59,** 355.

Bradley, D. J. and McCullough, F. S. (1973). *Trans. R. Soc. Trop. Med. Hyg.* **67,** 491.

Bradley, D. J. and May R. M. (1978). *Trans. R. Soc. Trop. Med. Hyg.* **72,** 262.

Cameron, T. W. M. (1928). *J. Helminth.* **6,** 219.

Camus, D., Bina, J. C., Carlier, Y. and Santoro, F. (1977). *Trans. R. Soc. Trop. Med. Hyg.* **71,** 182.

Carney, W. P., Masri, S., Salludin and Putrali, J. (1974). *S.E. Asian J. Trop. Med. Publ. Hlth* **5,** 246.

Carney, W. P., Masri, S., Sudomo, M., Putrali, J. and Davis, G. M. (1975). *S.E. Asian J. Trop. Med. Publ. Hlth* **6,** 211.

Cheever, A. W. (1968). *Am. J. Trop. Med. Hyg.* **17,** 38.

Cheever, A. W. (1969). *Trans. R. Soc. Trop. Med. Hyg.* **63,** 781.

Cheever, A. W. and Duvall, R. H. (1974). *Am. J. Trop. Med. Hyg.* **23,** 884.

Cheever, A. W., Erickson, D. G., Sadun, E. H., von Lichtenberg, F. (1974). *Am. J. Trop. Med. Hyg.* **23,** 51.

Cheever, A. W., Kamel, I. A., Elwi, A. M., Mossimann, J. E. and Danner, R. (1977). *Am. J. Trop. Med. Hyg.* **26,** 702.

Cheever, A. W., Kamel, I. A., Elwi, A. M., Mossimann, J. E., Danner, R. and Sippel, J. E. (1978). *Am. J. Trop. Med. Hyg.* **27,** 55.

Cheever, A. W., Torky, A. H. and Shirbiney, M. (1975). *Am. J. Trop. Med. Hyg.* **24,** 284.

Cheever, A. W., Young, S. W. and Shehata, A. (1975). *Trans. R. Soc. Trop. Med. Hyg.* **69,** 410.

Chernin, E. and Antolics, V. M. (1973). *J. Parasit.* **59,** 589.

Chernin, E. and Perlstein, J. M. (1971). *J. Parasit.* **55,** 500.

Christie, J. and Upatham, E. S. (1977). *Am. J. Trop. Med. Hyg.* **26,** 894.

Chu, K. Y. (1978). *Bull. Wld Hlth Org.* **56,** 313.

Chu, K. Y. and Dawood, I. K. (1970). *Bull. Wld Hlth Org.* **42,** 575.

Chu, K. Y. and Klumpp, R. K. (1978). *Proc. Int. Conf. Schisto. Cairo* **1,** 85.

Chu, K. Y., Massoud, J. and Sabbaghian, H. (1966). *Bull. Wld Hlth Org.* **34,** 135.

Chu, K. Y. and Vanderberg, J. A. (1976). *Bull. Wld Hlth Org.* **54,** 411.

Clark, W. D., Cox, P. M., Ratner, L. H. and Correa-Coronas, R. (1970). *Ann. Int. Med.* **73,** 379.

Clarke, V. de V. (1966). *Cent. Afr. J. Med.* **12** (6) Suppl., 30.

Clarke, V. de V. and Blair, D. M. (1966). *Cent. Afr. J. Med.* **12,** 25.

Cline, B. L., Rymzo, W. T., Hiatt, R. A., Knight, W. B. and Berrios-Duran, L. A. (1977). *Am. J. Trop. Med. Hyg.* **26,** 109.

Cohen, J. E. (1977). *Rev. Ecol. System.* **8,** 209.

Collins, K. J., Brotherhood, R. J., Davies, C. R. M., Dore, C., Hackett, A. J., Imms, F. J., Musgrove, J., Weiner, J. S., Amin, M. A., El Karim, M., Ismail, H. M., Omer, A. H. S. and Sukkar, M. Y. (1976). *Am. J. Trop. Med. Hyg.* **25,** 410.

Cook, J. A., Baker, S. T., Warren, K. S. and Jordan, P. (1974). *Am. J. Trop. Med. Hyg.* **23,** 625.

Coutinho, A. B. and Coutinho, F. A. B. (1968). *Bull. Math. Biophys.* **30,** 553.

Coutinho, A. B., Dobbin, J. E. and Dacosta, D. P. P. (1973). *Revta Ass. Med. Bras.* **19,** 267.

Crofton, H. D. (1971). *Parasitology* **62,** 179.

Crossland, N. O. (1962). *Bull. Wld Hlth Org.* **27,** 125.

Dalton, P. R. (1976). *Bull. Wld Hlth Org.* **54,** 587.

Dalton, P. R. and Pole, D. (1978). *Bull. Wld Hlth Org.* **56,** 417.

Damian, R. T., Green, N. D., Meyer, K. F., Cheever, A. W., Hubbard, W. J., Hawes, M. E. and Clarke, J. D. (1976). *Am. J. Trop. Med. Hyg.* **25,** 299.

Dazo, B. C., Hairston, N. G. and Dawood, I. K. (1966). *Bull. Wld Hlth Org.* **35,** 339.

Diem, K. & Lentner, C. 1970. In *Scientific Tables* p. 537. 7th Ed. J. R. Geigy, S. A. Basle, Switzerland.

Domingo, E. O. and Warren, K. S. (1968). *Am. J. Path.* **52,** 369.

Edington, G. M., von Lichtenberg, F., Nwabuebo, I., Taylor, J. R. and Smith, J. M. (1970). *Am. J. Trop. Med. Hyg.* **19,** 982.

El Gindy, M. S. and Rushdi, M. Z. (1962). In *Bilharziasis: A Ciba Foundation Symposium*, p. 81. Eds G. E. W. Wolstenholme and M. O'Connor. Churchill, London.

Farooq, M. (1967). *W.H.O. Chron.* **21,** 175.

Farooq, M. and Mallah, M. G. (1966). *Bull. Wld Hlth Org.* **35,** 377.

Farooq, M. and Samaan, S. A. (1967). *Ann. Trop. Med. Parasit.* **61,** 315.

Fenwick, A. (1969). *Trans. R. Soc. Trop. Med. Hyg.* **63,** 557.

Forsyth, D. M. (1969). *Bull. Wld Hlth Org.* **40,** 771.

Forsyth, D. M. and Bradley, D. J. (1964). *Lancet* **ii,** 169.

Forsyth, D. M. and Bradley, D. J. (1966). *Bull. Wld Hlth Org.* **34,** 715.

Forsyth, D. M. and Hughes, M. (1973). *Trans. R. Soc. Trop. Med. Hyg.* **62,** 671.

Forsyth, D. M. and Macdonald, G. (1965). *Trans. R. Soc. Trop. Med. Hyg.* **59,** 171.

Forsyth, D. M. and Macdonald, G. (1966). *Trans. R. Soc. Trop. Med. Hyg.* **60,** 568.

Foster, R. (1967). *J. Trop. Med. Hyg.* **70,** 185.

Fuller, G. K., Lemma, A. and Haile, T. (1979). *Trans. R. Soc. Trop. Med. Hyg.* **73,** 121.

Gelfand, M. (1950). *Schistosomiasis in South Central Africa: a clinico-pathological study.* Juta & Co, Capetown.

Gerber, J. H. (1952). *J. Trop. Med. Hyg.* **55,** 52.

Ghandour, A. M. and Webbe, G. (1973). *Int. J. Parasit.* **3,** 789.

Gibson, M. and Warren, K. S. (1970). *Bull. Wld Hlth Org.* **42,** 833.

Goddard, M. and Jordan, P. (1980). *Trans. R. Soc. Trop. Med. Hyg.* **74,** 185.

Goldsmith, E. I. and Kean, B. H. (1969). *Am. J. Trop. Med. Hyg.* **18,** 382.

Goldsmith, E. I., Luz, F. F. C., Prata, A. and Kean, B. H. (1967). *J. Am. Med. Ass.* **199,** 275.

Goodgame, R. W. and Bartholomew, R. K. (1978). *Am. J. Trop. Med. Hyg.* **27,** 779.

Gremillion, D. M., Geckler, R. W., Kuntz, R. E. and Marroro, R. V. (1978). *Am. J. Trop. Med. Hyg.* **27,** 924.

Hadidjaja, P. and Sudumo, M. (1976). *S.E. Asian J. Trop. Med. Publ. Hlth* **7,** 227.

Hairston, N. G. (1961). *Bull. Wld Hlth Org.* **25,** 731.

Hairston, N. G. (1962). In *Bilharziasis: A Ciba Foundation Symposium*, p. 36. Eds G. E. W. Wolstenholme and M. O'Connor. Churchill, London.

Hairston, N G. (1965a). *Bull. Wld Hlth Org.* **33,** 45.

Hairston, N. G. (1965b). *Bull. Wld Hlth Org.* **33,** 163.

Hairston, N. G. (1971). In *Review of Human Schistosomiasis*, by P. Jordan and G. Webbe. *Am. J. Trop. Med. Hyg.* **20,** 164.

Hamilton, P. K., Hutchinson, H. S., Jamison, P. W. and Jones, H. L. (1959). *Am. J. Clin. Path.* **32,** 18.

Hiatt, R. A. (1976). *Am. J. Trop. Med. Hyg.* **25,** 808.

Hiatt, R. A., Cline, B. L. and Knight, W. B. (1978). *Am. J. Trop. Med. Hyg.* **27,** 535.

Hill, D. M. and Onabamiro, S. D. (1960). *Brit. Vet. J.* **116,** 145.

Hira, P. R. (1969). *Nature, London* **224,** 670.

Hira, P. R. (1972). *E. Afr. Med. J.* **49,** 526.

Hira, P. R. (1975). *Trop. Geogr. Med.* **27,** 83.

Hoffman, D. B. Jr., Lehman, J. S. Jr., Scott, V. C., Warren, K. S. and Webbe, G. (1979). *Am. J. Trop. Med. Hyg.* **28,** 249.

Husting, E. L. (1965). *Cent. Afr. J. Med.* **11,** 330.

Husting, E. L. (1970). *Cent. Afr. J. Med.* **16,** 5.

Iwanaga, Y., Santos, M. J. and Blas, B. L. (1977). *Hiroshima J. Med. Sci.* **26,** 5.

Jobin, W. R. and Michelson, E. H. (1967). *Bull. Wld Hlth Org.* **37,** 657.

Jobin, W. R. and Ruiz-Tiben, E. (1968). *Bol. Asoc. Méd. P. Rico* **60,** 279.

Jones, S. B. (1932). *J. Trop. Med. Hyg.* **35,** 129.

Jordan, P. (1963). *E. Afr. Med. J.* **40,** 250.

Jordan, P. (1972). *Br. Med. Bull.* **28,** 55.

Jordan, P., Cook, J. A. and Davis, A. (1974). *Trans. R. Soc. Trop. Med. Hyg.* **68,** 340.

Jordan, P. and Randall, K. (1962). *J. Trop. Med. Hyg.* **55,** 1.

Jordan, P. and Webbe, G. (1969). *Human Schistosomiasis*. Heinemann Medical Books, London.

Kagan, I. G., Negron, H., Arnold, C. J. and Ferguson, F. F. (1966). *A Skin Test Survey of the Prevalence of Schistosomiasis in Puerto Rico*. US Department of Health, Education and Welfare, Atlanta.

Kamel, I. A., Elwi, A. M., Cheever, A. W., Mossimann, J. E. and Danner, R. (1978). *Am. J. Trop. Med. Hyg.* **27,** 931.

Katz, N. and Brener, Z. (1966). *Revta Inst. Med. Trop. S. Paulo* **8,** 139.

Khattab, M., El-Gengehy, M. T. and Sharaf, M. (1968). *J. Egypt. Med. Ass.* **51,** 245.

Kieser, J. A. (1947). *S. Afr. Med. J.* **21,** 854.

Kitkoon, V. and Schneider, C. R. (1976). *S.E. Asian J. Trop. Med. Publ. Hlth* **7,** 238.

Kitkoon, V., Schneider, C. R., Sornmani, S., Harinasuta, C. and Lanzo, C. R. (1973). *S.E. Asian J. Trop. Med. Publ. Hlth* **4,** 350.

Klumpp, R. K. and Chu, K. Y. (1977). *Bull. Wld Hlth Org.* **55,** 715.

Kloetzel, K. (1962). *Am. J. Trop. Med. Hyg.* **11,** 472.

Kloetzel, K. (1963). *Am. J. Trop. Med. Hyg.* **12,** 334.

Kloetzel, K. (1964). *Am. J. Trop. Med. Hyg.* **13,** 541.

Kloetzel, K. (1967). *Trans. R. Soc. Trop. Med. Hyg.* **61,** 803.

Kloetzel, K. and Da Silva, J. R. (1967). *Am. J. Trop. Med. Hyg.* **16,** 167.

Kloos, H. and Lemma, H. (1977). *Am. J. Trop. Med. Hyg.* **26,** 899.

Kuntz, R. E. (1952a). *J. Parasit.* **38,** 24.

Kuntz, R. E. (1952b). *Proc. Helminth. Soc. Wash.* **19,** 123.

Lehman, J. S., Mott, K. E., Marrow, R. H., Muniz, T. M. and Boyer, M. H. (1976). *Am. J. Trop. Med. Hyg.* **25,** 285.

Long, E. G., McLaren, M. L., Goddard, M. J., Bartholomew, R. K., Peters, P. and Goodgame, R. (1981). *Trans. R. Soc. Trop. Med. Hyg.* **75,** 365.

Lucas, A. O., Adeniyi-Jones, C. C., Cockshott, W. P. and Gilles, H. M. (1966). *Lancet* **i,** 631.

Macdonald, G. (1965). *Trans. R. Soc. Trop. Med. Hyg.* **59,** 489.

Macdonald, G. and Forsyth, D. M. (1968). *Trans. R. Soc. Trop. Med. Hyg.* **62,** 766.

McCullough, F. and Bradley, D. J. (1973). *Trans. R. Soc. Trop. Med. Hyg.* **67,** 475.

McLaren, M. L., Long, E. G., Goodgame, R. W. and Lillywhite, J. E. (1979). *Trans. R. Soc. Trop. Med. Hyg.* **73,** 636.

Magendantz, M. (1972). *Bull. Wld Hlth Org.* **47,** 331.

Mahon, R. J. and Shiff, C. J. (1978). *J. Parasit.* **32,** 64.

Maldonado, J. F., Acosta-Matienzo, J. and Thillet, C. J. (1949). *Puerto Rico J. Publ. Hlth Trop. Med.* **25,** 153.

Manson-Bahr, P. E. C. (1958). *E. Afr. Med. J.* **35,** 401.

Martin, L. K. and Beaver, P. C. (1968). *Am. J. Trop. Med. Hyg.* **17,** 382.

May, R. M. (1977). *Mathl. Biosci.* **35,** 301.

Memoranda (1974). *Bull. Wld Hlth Org.* **51,** 553.

Michael, A. I., Awadalla, H. N. and Farag, H. F. (1979). *Tropenmed. Parasit.* **30,** 62.

Miller, J. H. (1959). *E. Afr. Med. J.* **36,** 56.

Miller, J. H. (1960). *Trans. R. Soc. Trop. Med. Hyg.* **54,** 44.

Most, H. and Levine, D. I. (1963). *J. Am. Med. Ass.* **186,** 453.

Muench, H. (1959). *Catalytic Models in Epidemiology.* Harvard Press, Cambridge, Mass.

Nasell, I. (1975). *Proc. 8th Int. Biomet. Conf. 1974, Constanta, Romania,* p. 123. Stockholm.

Nasell, I. (1976). *Theoret. Popul. Biol.* **10,** 47.

Nasell, I. and Hirsch, W. M. (1973). *Commu. Pure Appl. Math.* **26,** 395.

Nelson, G. S. (1960). *Trans. R. Soc. Trop. Med. Hyg.* **54,** 301.

Nelson, G. S. (1974). In *Parasitic Zoonoses,* p. 273. Ed. E. J. L. Soulsby. Academic Press, New York, San Francisco, London.

Nelson, G. S. and Saoud, M. F. A. (1968). *J. Helminth.* **42,** 339.

Neves, J., Marinho, R. P., de Araujo, P. K. and Raso, P. (1973). *Trans. R. Soc. Trop. Med. Hyg.* **67,** 782.

Okpala, I. (1961). *West Afr. Med. J.* **10,** 402.

Olivier, L. J. and Schneiderman, M. (1956). *Expl Parasit.* **5,** 109.

Ongom, V. L. (1970). *Symposium on Schistosomiasis,* p. 47. Organization of African Unity, OAU/STRC Publications Bureau, Addis Ababa.

Ongom, V. L. and Bradley, D. J. (1972). *Trans. R. Soc. Trop. Med. Hyg.* **66,** 835.

Pan, C. T., Williams, R. R. and Ritchie, L. S. (1954). *Am. J. Trop. Med. Hyg.* **3,** 136.

Paoli, A. C. de (1965). *Am. J. Trop. Med. Hyg.* **14,** 561.

Pereira, F. E. L., Bortolini, E. R., Carneiro, J. L. A., Da Silva, C. R. M. and Neves, R. C. (1979). *Trans. R. Soc. Trop. Med. Hyg.* **73,** 238.

Pesigan, T. P., Farooq, M., Hairston, N. G., Jauregui, J. J., Garcia, E. G., Santos, A. T., Santos, B. C. and Besa, A. A. (1958). *Bull. Wld Hlth Org.* **18,** 345.

Pimental, D., Gerhardt, C. E., Williams, E. R., White, P. C. and Ferguson, F. F. (1961). *Am. J. Trop. Med. Hyg.* **10,** 523.
Pitchford, R. J. (1959). *Trans. R. Soc. Trop. Med. Hyg.* **53,** 213.
Pitchford, R. J. and Visser, P. S. (1960). *Ann. Trop. Med. Parasit.* **54,** 237.
Pitchford, R. J. and Visser, P. S. (1962). *Trans. R. Soc. Trop. Med. Hyg.* **56,** 126.
Pitchford, R. J. and Visser, P. S. (1965). *Bull. Wld Hlth Org.* **32,** 83.
Polderman, A. M. (1974). *The Transmission of Intestinal Schistosomiasis in Begemder Province, Ethiopia.* Leiden University.
Powell, S. J., Englebrecht, H. E. and Welchman, J. M. (1968). *Trans. R. Soc. Trop. Med. Hyg.* **62,** 231.
Powers, K. G. and Cheever, A. W. (1972). *Bull. Wld Hlth Org.* **46,** 295.
Prata, A. and Schroeder, S. (1967). *Gaz. Med. Bahia* **67,** 93.
Pugh, R. N. H. and Gilles, H. M. (1978). *Ann. Trop. Med. Parasit.* **72,** 471.
Purvis, A. J., Ellison, I. R. and Husting, E. L. (1965). *Cent. Afr. J. Med.* **11,** 368.
Radke, M. G., Ritchie, L. S. and Rowan, W. B. (1961). *Expl Parasit.* **11,** 23.
Rijpstra, A. C. and Swellengrebel, N. H. (1962). *Trop. Geograph. Med.* **14,** 279.
Rosenfield, P. (1975). *Development and verification of a schistosomiasis transmission model.* PhD dissertation, Johns Hopkins University, Baltimore.
Rowan, W. B. (1958). *Am. J. Trop. Med. Hyg.* **7,** 374.
Rowan, W. B. (1964). *Am. J. Trop. Med. Hyg.* **13,** 572.
Sadun, E. H., von Lichtenburg, F. and Bruce, J. I. (1966). *Am. J. Trop. Med. Hyg.* **15,** 705.
Sadun, E. H., von Lichtenberg, F., Cheever, A. W., Erickson, D. G. and Hickman, R. L. (1970). *Am. J. Trop. Med. Hyg.* **19,** 427.
Salam, A., Mahmoud, A. A. F., Ishaac, S. and Civil, R. H. (1979). *J. Immunol.* **123,** 1829.
Sandt, D. G. (1973a). *Bull. Wld Hlth Org.* **48,** 27.
Sandt, D. G. (1973b). *Bull. Wld Hlth Org.* **48,** 35.
Saoud, M. F. A. (1965a). *J. Helminth.* **39,** 101.
Saoud, M. F. A. (1965b). *J. Helminth.* **39,** 363.
Schwetz, J. (1956). *Trans. R. Soc. Trop. Med. Hyg.* **50,** 275.
Shiff, C. J. (1964a). *Ann. Trop. Med. Parasit.* **58,** 94.
Shiff, C. J. (1964b). *Ann. Trop. Med. Parasit.* **58,** 106.
Shiff, C. J. (1964c). *Ann. Trop. Med. Parasit.* **58,** 240.
Shiff, C. J., Evans, A., Yiannakis, C. and Eardley, M. (1975). *Int. J. Parasit.* **5,** 119.
Siongok, T. K. Arap, Mahmoud, A. A. F., Ouma, J. H., Warren, K. S., Muller, A. S., Handa, A. K. and Houser, H. B. (1976). *Am. J. Trop. Med. Hyg.* **25,** 273.
Slobodkin, L. B. (1962). *The Growth and Regulation of Animal Populations,* 184 pp. Holt. Rinehart and Winston, New York.
Smith, J. H., Elwin, A., Kamel, I. A. and von Lichtenberg, F. (1975). *Am. J. Trop. Med. Hyg.* **24,** 806.
Smith, J. H., Kamel, I. A., Elwin, A. and von Lichtenberg, F. (1974). *Am. J. Trop. Med. Hyg.* **23,** 1054.
Smith, J. H., Warren, K. S. and Mahmoud, A. A. P. (1979). *Am. J. Trop. Med. Hyg.* **28,** 220.
Southwood, T. R. E. (1966). *Ecological Methods with Particular Reference to Insect Populations.* Methuen, London.
Stirewalt, M. A. (1953). *Amer. J. Trop. Med. Hyg.* **2,** 867.
Stirewalt, M. A. (1956). *J. Parasit.* **42,** 565.

Sturrock, R. F. (1973a). *Int. J. Parasit.* **3**, 175.

Sturrock, R. F. (1973b). *Int. J. Parasit.* **3**, 165.

Sturrock, R. F. (1975). *Bull. Wld Hlth Org.* **52**, 267.

Sturrock, R. F., Cohen, J. E. and Webbe, G. (1975). *Ann. Trop. Med. Parasit.* **69**, 133.

Sturrock, R. F. and Webbe, G. (1971). *J. Helminth.* **45**, 189.

Sudomo, M. and Carney, W. P. (1974). *Bull. Hlth Studies, Indonesia* **2**, 51.

Swellengrebel, N. H. and Rijpstra, A. C. (1965). *Trop. Geograph. Med.* **17**, 80.

Tanaka, H., Santos, M. J., Matusuda, H., Hambre, R. S., Iwango, Y., Shimomura, H., Blas, B. L. and Santos, A. T. Jr. (1978). *Japan J. Expl. Med.* **48**, 193.

Teesdale, C. and Nelson, G. S. (1958). *E. Afr. Med. J.* **35**, 427.

Theron, A. (1979). *Bull. Wld Hlth Org.* **57**, 971.

Theron, A., Pointier, J. P. and Combes, C. (1978). *Ann. Parasit. (Paris)* **53**, 223.

Upatham, E. S. (1972a). *J. Helminth.* **46**, 271.

Upatham, E. S. (1972b). *J. Helminth.* **46**, 277.

Upatham, E. S. (1973a). *Int. J. Parasit.* **3**, 289.

Upatham, E. S. (1973b). *S.E. Asian J. Trop. Med. Publ. Hlth* **4**, 367.

Upatham, E. S. (1973c). *Trans. R. Soc. Trop. Med. Hyg.* **6**, 884.

Upatham, E. S. (1974a). *Ann. Trop. Med. Parasit.* **68**, 343.

Upatham, E. S. (1974b). *Parasitology* **68**, 155.

Upatham, E. S. (1976). *Int. J. Parasit.* **6**, 239.

Upatham, E. S. and Sturrock, R. F. (1973). *Parasitology* **67**, 219.

Upatham, E. S., Sturrock, R. F. and Cook, J. A. (1976). *Parasitology* **73**, 239.

Usborne, V. (1954). *E. Afr. Med. J.* **31**, 451.

Walker, A. R. P. (1977). *S. Afr. Med. J.* **51**, 541.

Wallerstein, R. S. (1949). *Am. J. Trop. Med. Hyg.* **29**, 717.

Warren, K. S. (1967). *Trans. R. Soc. Trop. Med. Hyg.* **61**, 795.

Warren, K. S. (1969). *Gastroenterology* **57**, 697.

Warren, K. S. and Domingo, E. O. (1970). *Am. J. Trop. Med. Hyg.* **19**, 292.

Warren, K. S., Kellermeyer, R. W., Jordan, P., Littel, A. S., Cook, J. A. and Kagan, I. (1973). *Am. J. Trop. Med. Hyg.* **22**, 189.

Warren, K. S., Mahmoud, A. A. F., Cummings, P., Murphy, D. J. and Mouser, D. B. (1974). *Am. J. Trop. Med. Hyg.* **23**, 902.

Warren, K. S. and Peters, P. A. (1967). *Ann. Trop. Med. Parasit.* **61**, 294.

Webbe, G. (1962a). *Bull. Wld Hlth Org.* **27**, 59.

Webbe, G. (1962b). In *Ciba Foundation Symposium on Bilharziasis*, p. 7. Eds G. E. W. Wolstenholme and M. O'Connor. Churchill, London.

Webbe, G. (1965a). *Bull. Wld Hlth Org.* **33**, 147.

Webbe, G. (1965b). *Bull. Wld Hlth Org.* **33**, 55.

Webbe, G. (1966). *Ann. Trop. Med. Parasit.* **60**, 78.

Webbe, G., James, C., Nelson, G. S., Ismail, M. M. and Shaw, J. R. (1979). *Trans. R. Soc. Trop. Med. Hyg.* **73**, 42.

Webbe, G., James, C., Nelson, G. S., Smithers, S. R. and Terry, R. J. (1976). *Ann. Trop. Med. Parasit.* **70**, 411.

Webbe, G. and Jordan, P. (1966). *Trans. R. Soc. Trop. Med. Hyg.* **60**, 279.

Weisbrod, B. A. and Helminiak, T. W. (1978). *Proc. Int. Conf. Schisto., Cairo (1975)* **1**, 37.

Wilkins, H. A. (1977). *Ann. Trop. Med. Parasit.* **71**, 53.

Wilkins, H. A. and El-Sawy, M. (1977). *Trans. R. Soc. Trop. Med. Hyg.* **71**, 486.

Wilkins, H. A. and Scott, A. (1978). *Trans. R. Soc. Trop. Med. Hyg.* **72,** 397.

Winslow, D. J. (1967). In *Bilharziasis*, p. 230. Ed. F. K. Mostofi. Springer-Verlag, Berlin.

Wolfe, M. S. and Quartey, J. M. K. (1967). *Trans. R. Soc. Trop. Med. Hyg.* **61,** 90.

Woodstock, L., Cook, J. A., Peters, P. A. and Warren, K. S. (1972). *J. Inf. Dis.* **124,** 613.

World Health Organization (1967). *Tech. Rep. Series*, Number 349. WHO, Geneva.

Wright, C. A. (1967). In *Bilharziasis*, p. 3. Ed. F. K. Mostofi. Springer-Verlag, Berlin.

Yeo, D. (1962). *Bull. Wld Hlth Org.* **27,** 183.

Young, S. W., Farid, Z., Bassily, S. and El-Masry, N. A. (1973). *Trans. R. Soc. Trop. Med. Hyg.* **67,** 379.

Zilberg, B., Sanders, E. and Lewis, B. (1967). *S. Afr. Med. J.* **41,** 598.

11 Control

Gerald Webbe and Peter Jordan

Transmission of infection requires contact with water harbouring snail intermediate hosts in an area where sanitation is at a low level and there are infected persons.

Control of transmission thus involves measures aimed at (i) reducing the risk of exposure to infected water, and (ii) reducing the level of environmental contamination with schistosome ova and, more specifically, contamination of water.

Each of these objectives can be attained by 'disease-specific' and 'non-specific' methods (Table 11.1).

Table 11.1 Classification of control methods.

	'Disease specific'	'Non-specific'
Reduced exposure to infected water	Reduced infection in water: control of snails and free-living stages of parasite	Reduction in exposure: (i) water supplies; (ii) reduce water contact by fences, bridges etc.
Reduced contamination	Chemotherapy	Latrines

Specific measures of control—chemotherapy and snail control—generally have little or no impact on other health conditions, though effective chemotherapy will reduce morbidity, cure at least some cases of schistosomal disease and prevent the development of other cases. Specific measures are likely to be a direct charge to a health schistosomiasis control budget.

Non-specific measures are associated with improved standards of living and are the aim of all developing countries. They may be more acceptable environmentally than chemical control of snails and, although less dramatic than specific measures in their effects, having other social and medical benefits they may be more popular with public health administrators. Costs should be shared between health and community development budgets.

When non-specific measures and snail control are effective, there is a slow reduction in prevalence and intensity of infection and this leads secondarily to reduced morbidity and disease. Chemotherapy, however, in addition to having a direct disease preventive role can quickly reduce prevalence and intensity of infection and therefore transmission.

The United Nations has declared that attempts must be made in the 1980s to provide all people with safe water and acceptable means of disposing of human waste. It is hoped this will be achieved; if it is, some measure of schistosomiasis control can be expected, but every endeavour must be made in areas where the infection is endemic to encourage—in addition to safe drinking water—other facilities *to prevent contact* with infected water.

In the last decade, schistosomiasis control was synonymous with snail control, which was generally considered to offer the most effective and rapid means of reducing transmission (Farooq *et al.*, 1966), although the opinion was based as much on theoretical considerations and the failure of other methods as on demonstrated success of snail control. It was, however, not until 1972 that there was 'convincing evidence of the effect of mollusciciding on transmission' (Anon, 1973).

Drugs suitable for administration on a community basis have only recently been introduced and, although oxamniquine is being used in Brazil, St Lucia and Egypt, and metrifonate in Egypt and Ghana in research and public health schemes, their place in transmission control has yet to be clarified, particularly in relation to who should be treated and how often. It is, however, apparent that in transmission control they will only be effective where the population is co-operative and there is little immigration of infected persons.

Given alone (and repeated as necessary in order to keep the worm burden low in selected segments of the population), chemotherapy might also be used as a disease preventive measure, but this also requires further investigation (Kloetzel, 1974).

Integrated control strategies will probably be necessary in the intensive phase of transmission control campaigns but may be followed by a less costly follow-up or consolidation phase with a single method—chemotherapy or snail control. Alternatively, with medium- or long-term planning, habitat control through environmental changes and engineering—water supplies and sanitation—and health education may be successful in preventing a resurgence of transmission (Webbe, 1978).

Each method of control has particular advantages and disadvantages and the composition of any control programme will necessarily vary with the emphasis placed on different approaches depending on local conditions, the goal of the control effort, available resources and feasible strategy.

The ultimate object of control is to prevent schistosomal disease—epidemiologically related to high levels of prevalence and intensity of infection. Our knowledge of this relationship does not, however, indicate those levels of egg output (or prevalence) associated with defined rates of splenomegaly or hydronephrosis, nor lower levels with minimum disease which might serve as aims for control. As a result, all too often control schemes have only a generally ill-defined objective to reduce prevalence and intensity to lower levels—the lower the better. This should perhaps be revised, for while it may (in some endemic areas) be comparatively easy with intensive control to reduce a high prevalence to a low level, to reduce a low rate further is difficult and it may be uneconomical to attempt. The aim then should be to prevent a resurgence of transmission by a cost-effective follow-up strategy, accepting an inevitable low level of endemicity but with little disease. What this low level should be depends on other health problems in the area. In a few situations—in oases or on islands—it may be realistic to consider the long-term goal as eradication after a sustained intensive effort.

Those responsible must appreciate that long-term planning and recurrent expenditure are required—even for control. However, it is hoped that new strategies of intensive intervention with a follow-up or consolidation phase will eventually lead to lower costs.

DISEASE-SPECIFIC METHODS OF CONTROL

Control of the molluscan intermediate host

Control of snail intermediate hosts is an effective means of reducing transmission of schistosomiasis; its efficiency can be enhanced if combined with other methods of control. In planning snail control measures and evaluating their impact, knowledge of the ecology, bionomics, population trends and dynamics of the molluscan host are clearly essential (see Chapters 2 and 10). Climatic changes, many of which are seasonal, influence the life-cycles of snail intermediate hosts, their infection and the subsequent transmission of infection. Cognisance of these relationships must, therefore, form the basis of timing and application of any considered measures directed against snails for the purpose of controlling transmission. Transmission of schistosomiasis is characterised by its variability, and direct extrapolation of data on snail populations and their infections from one area to another, or data on human ecology, may not always be valid, even for closely adjacent areas. The failure to obtain a successful measure of control is usually attributable to a lack of such basic information and frequently to the dissipation of applied efforts through wrong emphasis or mistiming.

Seasonal fluctuations in the abundance of snails and of concomitant cercarial infections have already been discussed in relation to local climatic conditions (see Chapter 10). The number of infected snails that survive the winter or carry infections from one wet season to the next after aestivation, the rate of infection of a new generation of snails, and the length of time of development of the cercariae are all pertinent to the nature and timing of measures directed towards the control of snails.

In many tropical areas, fluctuations in snail population density and in the production of cercariae are as great as in temperate conditions, and transmission may be very limited and consequent upon the presence of water only during certain periods of the year. Appropriate snail control measures may be necessary, therefore, at particular times of the year and for limited periods. In some areas, however, where the hydrology and temperature remain stable, snail populations and production of cercariae are maximal throughout the year, and chemical measures directed against snails must be applied regularly or permanent measures involving habitat modification may be called for. In many endemic areas, the 'focal' nature of transmission is becoming increasingly recognised and the development of more cost-effective 'transmission control' methodology with concentration of effort at these sites is being achieved.

Snail control procedures

Methods which are applicable for species of *Biomphalaria* and

Bulinus in aquatic habitats differ in emphasis from those for the amphibian *Oncomelania* species.

Environmental control

This approach involves changes in the environments of both the definitive and intermediate hosts of the schistosomes. Prevention of contact with snail-infested waters is the principal objective in the case of the former, while for the molluscan intermediate hosts relatively drastic changes in ecology of the habitat are usually necessary in order to prevent further breeding. In order to effectively change the ecology of a snail habitat to render it unacceptable, data on the ecological requirements of the snail must be available. If the specific ecological requirements are known, then relatively small changes may be sufficient, but fundamental alterations are generally required in order to achieve the desired permanent result.

The ecology of snail intermediate hosts was discussed in Chapter 2 and their tolerance of relatively wide limits of different physical, chemical and biological factors emphasised. It is difficult to alter any one of these many factors sufficiently to effect adequate control, although alterations of one factor may subsequently influence others and achieve the desired effect.

In relation to any aquatic habitat, the removal of water is the most effective measure and, if it can be made permanent without adversely affecting local requirements, it is certainly the best available method. If, however, removal of water is only a temporary measure, as it must be in the case of irrigation systems, its efficiency will depend upon the ability of the snails in question to withstand desiccation. The marked capacity of aquatic planorbid and bulinid snails to survive periods of drying should be considered in this respect.

In natural breeding sites, alternatives to drainage which will contribute much to reduction of snail breeding (one of the most effective measures against aquatic snails) include filling, increasing velocity of flow, stream straightening, deepening of marginal areas, elimination of pools, removal of vegetation and prevention of pollution. Control of the rate of flow and the means to fluctuate the level of water in storage dams, reservoirs, and irrigation systems, are important assets and efficient water management is an essential adjunct to any attempt to control transmission. The cost and justification of the permanent alteration of an environment to effect control, however, must of course be established and the role of different habitats either as active transmission foci or as reservoirs of snails for other active foci should be known. This may apply in cases where fish culture or rice growing is an important local activity and where the co-operation of the indigenous population must be sought if effective measures are to be instituted (Ansari, 1973).

Water management and agricultural practices

The method of reducing habitats in control of snails was first put forward in Egypt by Leiper in 1916, but discouraging results have been obtained in most attempts made to use environmental techniques because of the primitive nature of irrigation and agricultural practices often used in endemic areas (McMullen, 1962).

There are, however, examples in the Philippines and in Japan where control of irrigation water, improved agricultural methods and adequate drainage have proved successful (Okabe, 1957; Pesigan, Farooq *et al.*, 1958; Hairston and Santos, 1961; Pesigan and Hairston, 1961). In many cases, habitats have been eliminated or are now amenable to control by molluscicides, and valuable areas of reclaimed land have been established.

In arid and semi-arid areas, the provision of water by irrigation, or the conversion of basin and partial irrigation to perennial irrigation, usually results in an increase in the prevalence and intensity of schistosomiasis, because the same factors which make an endemic area more satisfactory for man also make it more suitable for the molluscan intermediate hosts (McMullen *et al.*, 1962). In a few places in Iraq, Kenya, Ghana and Tanzania, however, there is some evidence that well-designed and constructed irrigation systems with efficient drainage, correctly prepared land, sound water management, adequate maintenance and good agricultural practices have prevented the usual increase of schistosomiasis.

The conditions encountered in many other schemes, however, including low-gradient canal systems with much silt and vegetation, unsatisfactory water management schedules employed for conveyance systems, poor drainage channels with night storage dams and temporary pools, are such as to provide suitable habitats for snail intermediate hosts. These factors, together with a lack of piped-water supplies for domestic purposes, proper sanitation and the siting of dwellings near irrigation canals, must result in a considerable increase in the incidence of infection (Webbe, 1963; Sturrock, 1965). The design of schemes should be such that these conditions do not develop.

In many areas, schistosomiasis, like malaria, is a man-made disease. Numerous breeding sites are created by careless engineering practices associated with road and rail construction, bridges, causeways, and general industrial activity, and the resulting ditches, borrow-pits, quarries and pools frequently provide ideal snail and mosquito breeding sites and ultimately active transmission foci. The elimination of such habitats is the responsibility of the construction authority and would usually involve little extra work or expense (Jobin and Ippen, 1964; Jobin and Michelson, 1969; Jobin, 1970; McJunkin, 1970; Santos *et al.*, 1970).

Man's interference either in relation to changes in the flow of a watercourse, resulting in the creation of suitable habitats for the amphibious *Oncomelania* spp., or to the building of dams for water storage and soil conservation, resulting in the formation of suitable habitats for aquatic snails, must also be considered.

During the last 10 years public health problems associated with man-made lakes in Africa have become significant and all such lakes now contain snail intermediate hosts of human schistosomiasis.

On the shores of Lake Kariba in game plains, and Lake Nasser in the desert, unsupervised immigrant populations exist in sufficient numbers to contaminate the lakes and, while *S. haematobium* transmission is occurring in the latter, the main impact of Lake Nasser is the result of perennial irrigation in upper and middle Egypt, and the water-logging of large areas due to increased irrigation and the high water table. In Lakes Volta and Kainji, fishing villages now exist and *S. haematobium* is transmitted, as well as *S. mansoni* in the latter (Brown and Deom, 1973).

The completion of the Cabora Bassa Dam in Mozambique, the Tafilalet Dam in Morocco, developments in the Mekong valley in south-east Asia and in the San Francisco valley in north-east Brazil will entail health hazards from snail-borne and insect-transmitted infections both in the impoundments and in associated irrigation systems.

The changing ecology of impoundments must be closely observed and human settlements and activities considered if improvements in human ecology and water management are to be made as a basis for feasible long-term control of the problem of schistosomiasis and other water-borne infections.

Control in natural habitats

In all endemic regions, many natural habitats provide important foci of transmission and their diversity calls for considerable ingenuity in devising different methods to effectively eliminate or, at any rate, reduce them. In planning any environmental control measures, in order to map all apparent and potential snail habitats, adequate topographical, hydrological and geological data must be obtained and wet and dry season surveys made. The watershed should be examined in planning such measures, beginning in the upper reaches of an area and working systematically through it. Consideration must be given to large rivers, small perennial streams, seasonal streams, seepages, lakes, marshes, swamps, ponds and temporary pools, and careful attention should be paid to basic ecological factors including velocity of flow, flooding, aquatic vegetation, pollution and the existence of microhabitats.

Drainage and filling may not always be practicable, or only partially successful, and periodic pumping from channels or wells may prove satisfactory in drying out marshes and swamps; in some localities marshes have been eliminated by constructing ponds and using the excavated earth as fill; the method has been effectively used in the case of sluggish streams with swampy edges in Leyte to control *O. quadrasi* (Hairston and Santos, 1961). This snail cannot live in such ponds, and fertile soil is thus made available for cultivation. Small ponds are frequently important transmission foci of *S. haematobium*, being used for domestic purposes and as watering points for animals. The most satisfactory method of control would be filling-in, but this is usually impracticable, as is fencing, particularly if no alternative safe water supply is available for local needs.

Habitat reduction and control of S. japonicum

In a lengthy campaign in the five areas of Japan where *S. japonicum* was endemic before 1950, considerable success has been achieved in reducing disease and the extent of *O. nosophora* habitats. Irrigation ditches have been lined with concrete and maintained clear of silt, vegetation and detritus. Land reclamation by drainage and filling has proceeded rapidly and the rice fields have been displaced by fruit. Molluscicides have been extensively used in conjunction with intensive habitat reduction. The use of faeces as manure has been displaced by chemical fertilisers which will also affect snail populations. Improved water supplies and excreta storage facilities are now widespread and many small settlements have swimming pools. Reservoir host cattle have been replaced by tractors. General education is widespread and includes the natural histories of diseases and their prevention. This is undoubtedly a highly effective programme at very high per capita cost and several components were not primarily antischistosome measures. The socio-economic factors, such as rising living standards, and the effects of urbanisation and industrial activity must also be considered (Yokogawa, 1972).

In mainland China, on the other hand, available information suggests that *S. japonicum* has been greatly reduced in prevalence by methods which have included destruction of snail habitats by labour-intensive measures at low capital cost. The main techniques have been to bury snails by relining canals or filling them in completely after placing the infected surface layer at the bottom of the channel. New channels are then dug parallel to the old. An improved system of faecal processing has been widely adopted whereby raw material does not come into contact with irrigation water, and faecal storage, until the ammonia from urine has killed the schistosome eggs, takes place in sealed earthenware containers not subject to flooding. It would appear that the strict community discipline has produced an effective control programme at low per capita cost.

The advantages of reduction or control of snail habitats by environmental changes and the reason why attention is now being focused upon them have been recently considered. These advantages include: the effect is persistent without continual re-application; health benefits may extend to other infective diseases; benefits outside the field of health may sometimes accrue, as in increased agricultural production; evidence of success in controlled epidemiological studies has accumulated; labour and funds are more interchangeable than in mollusciciding or chemotherapeutic programmes; the approach lends itself to local or small-scale use; and environmental concern has made people unenthusiastic about chemical control. In considering the introduction of ecological methods of control, the timescale of expenditure is an important issue and the relationship between capital and recurrent costs must be balanced according to local resources for expenditure on materials and labour. The time-scale of benefits is also of vital importance, because although environmental changes may result in reduced transmission, infections will persist for many years and it may be some time before the benefits are apparent to the inhabitants of the area in which they are applied. Their application may also be more demanding of the local population than in mollusciciding, and chemotherapy will, of course, give immediate results. Ecological methods are the long-term hope for schistosomiasis control and should be applied steadily and often in conjunction with other methods of more rapid effect, such as chemotherapy and mollusciciding. Concomitant inputs of education are important and maintenance of any environmental work is essential (Bradley and Webbe, 1978).

Biological control (*see also* Jordan, Christie and Unrau, 1980) Another ecological approach to schistosome control involves the use of organisms to attack the snail intermediate host, while schistosome larvae may also be attacked in the aquatic environment or by competition within the snail host.

During the past decade, increasing concern has arisen in relation to the use of pesticides because of their broad-spectrum activity, detrimental effects on desirable species, accumulation in the environment to destruction levels, and their increasing costs. It is, therefore, important that alternative methods of reducing snail populations are researched.

The successful control of any species must depend upon certain fundamental intrinsic properties of the species and of its quantitative interaction with other organisms in the environment as well, of course, as extrinsic factors such as the carrying capacity of a particular habitat (see Chapter 10). The most useful measure of the ability of a species to increase is the intrinsic rate of natural increase 'r', which should be calculated under density-independent conditions. It is the most accurate measure of the condition under which a population can or cannot maintain itself (Birch, 1953). It can be used to predict what will happen following the application of a short-term measure, or the ability of the target organisms to recover quickly from a failure of a biological control agent to continue its effectiveness. The qualities usually shown by a potentially good biological control agent have been reviewed (De Bach, 1974).

There are numerous records of the harmful effects of different parasites, predators and competitors on snail intermediate hosts, and species of bacteria, fungi, protozoa, fish, birds and other animals affect snails directly or indirectly (Michelson, 1957;

Ferguson, 1972, 1978; Hairston *et al.*, 1975). Very few of these agents, however, have been adequately tested under field conditions.

Competition
This is of considerable importance in determining the abundance of many species and, if a competing species is successfully introduced, the population of the target species will be reduced. According to the theory of 'competitive exclusion', if the requirements of the two species are very similar, and if the introduced species is really superior to the target species in obtaining requirements, complete elimination of the target species will result. The number of such introductions has apparently been impressive, particularly on oceanic islands, but many of these have had undesirable consequences. It is felt, however, that given adequate preliminary research, more such introductions should be undertaken (Hairston *et al.*, 1975). Competitive species of snails including *Marisa cornuarietis*, *Helisoma duryi*, *Pomacea haustru*, *Potamopyrgus jenkinsi*, *B. tropicus* and *Tarebia* (*Thiara*) sp. have been studied. The effectiveness of *Marisa* has been demonstrated in Puerto Rico in certain habitats, particularly ponds, as a competitive feeder and an incidental predator on the ova and juveniles of *B. glabrata*. The introduced *Marisa* had no adverse effects, but continuous effort was required to maintain the snail in transmission sites, with recurrent costs estimated at about one-third of the cost required to apply molluscicide (Ruiz-Tiben *et al.*, 1969; Jobin and Berrios-Duran, 1970). *H. duryi* may also prove to be a useful competitor under certain conditions, and available evidence suggests that competition for food, growth inhibiting factors, mechanical effects on egg masses and superior biotic potential may be involved in this process (Frandsen and Madsen, 1979).

Predation and parasitism
Several species of mollusc-eating fish have been studied as biological control agents, including *Tilapia melanopluera*, *Serranochromis* sp., *Astatoreochromis alluadi* and *Clarisa* sp., but adequate field evaluation of their effectiveness is wanting. Reports indicate that *Gambusia* sp. may also effect similar reductions in snail populations in certain habitats, as does the 'shell cracker' fish *Lepomis microlophus*. Other organisms of potential value include the aquatic *Lemipteran* (*Limnogeton fieberi*), an obligatory but

non-specific feeder on snails, and the larvae of sciomyzid flies (Berg, 1953; Veolker, 1968; McMahon *et al.*, 1977).

In the past decade, detailed studies have been made on the interaction of the larval stages (rediae) of certain trematodes (echinostomes) infecting the same snail (Lim and Heyneman, 1972; Lie, 1973). The antagonism may take the form of direct predation by one species on another, or may be indirect, acting by chemically induced degeneration of the other species. Some small-scale field trials have been undertaken in which variable degrees of success were achieved. The results emphasise that a very abnormal infection rate of the antagonistic species (70% or more) must be achieved in snails. It would seem that the efficiency of the system must be improved considerably in order for it to be of practical value.

Genetic manipulation and non-susceptible strains
Consideration has been given to genetic manipulation for control purposes and, in a few instances, undesirable insect species have been eliminated by the liberation of very large numbers of sterile males. However, this approach is unlikely to be practicable in the case of the aquatic planorbids—which are hermaphrodite. *Oncomelania* does have separate sexes but the populations which have been studied did not show changes in numbers of a sufficient magnitude to make the 'sterile male' technique feasible as a potential control measure.

The existence of non-susceptibility is of interest, and genetic analyses of susceptibility have been carried out on *Biomphalaria* (Richards, 1970, 1973; Richards and Merritt, 1972) and on *O. hupensis* (Davis and Ruff, 1973). It is considered that because non-susceptible strains interbreed with susceptible ones, the result of their introduction into natural populations would probably be that they would be swamped genetically by the local strain. The prospects for effective control of transmission of schistosomiasis by this means seem to be poor (Hairston *et al.*, 1975).

Some of the laboratory and limited field observations suggest that certain biological agents may be of value in combination with other methods in controlling transmission of schistosomes. In every biocoenosis, however, an eventual balance is reached. An obligatory snail-eating fish will ultimately be limited by a shortage of food in a natural habitat, so that the populations of fish and snails present will each fluctuate in density, but the density level of snails below which transmission will be stopped is unlikely to be maintained permanently, even if it is reached at all. This will also be the case if the fish predator is only a facultative mollusc feeder, which so many of those reported, in fact, are. It is imperative, therefore, that any biological control agent should be 'density-independent', leading to an unbalanced age-structure of the target organism and its ultimate elimination.

Successful biological control methods may prove to be highly cost-effective, but much more research is required into the feasibility and practicability of applying organisms of potential value in the field. Careful evaluation under field conditions is necessary together with thorough cost analysis. The capacity of any biological agent to transmit parasites of medical or veterinary importance should be thoroughly evaluated before an attempt is made to use it for the control of snail intermediate hosts of schistosomes, and such an agent should not be introduced into an exotic geographical area before exhaustive testing of its potential capacity to compete with, or destroy, animals or plants of economic importance (Anon, 1980).

Further researches should be encouraged in the Tropics for obligatory snail predators with a high search efficiency for the snail intermediate hosts of schistosomes and greater effectiveness in water more than a few centimetres deep. A search for agents or methods of biological control which can be used in flowing water is also necessary.

Chemical control

Available and candidate molluscicides
In the past decade, no outstanding development of a novel molluscicides has taken place and interest in the necessary research by industry has been, at best, sporadic and generally diminishing because of high development costs and the lack of an assured market.

Many available compounds have broad-spectrum activity and these biocidal properties are unfortunately possessed by the few molluscicides of accepted effectiveness.

For snail control, the conditions in which the chemical has to be applied are variable and a variety of formulations is desirable to meet these requirements. The efficacy of a particular compound may vary according to the method of application and the particle size of the active ingredients in the case of water-dispersible powder formulations. Diluted emulsions prepared from emulsifiable oils based on different solvents and emulsifiers also give different biological activities (Webbe, 1974). The development of a formulation for field use must, therefore, embrace a knowledge of many different factors. While much experimental work has been carried out on granules, capsules, slow-release matrices, oil-bound solids, pastes, solutions having high spreading properties, electrolytically released copper, baits, molluscicidal soaps and micronised powders, very few formulations are in fact available for field use—which is in part related to development costs, the present nature of most large-scale operations and, therefore, market potential.

Nearly all the compounds which have been developed and used in the field during the past 10 years have a low solubility in water compared with the high solubility of copper sulphate and sodium pentachlorophenate, and the newer products have the same toxic effects as sodium pentachlorophenate but at much lower Ct (concentration × time) products (Anon, 1973; Ansari, 1973).

Niclosamide (Bayluscide®, Mollutox®)
Niclosamide-2′5-dichloro-4′-nitro-salicylanilide is highly toxic to snails and their eggs, and to schistosome cercariae; it is not toxic to man and has limited biocidal effect. It is non-corrosive, reasonably persistent but not permanent and is degraded by sunlight into harmless organic chemicals. It is biodegradable and several micro-organisms, especially bacteria, metabolise it. Its disadvantages are its high cost and its lethal effects on fish and some other aquatic animals. It is stable in storage but may deteriorate in two to three years. For 24- and 1-hour exposures the mg/1 per h values are approximately the same, but with 6-hour exposures the efficiency is less. Loss by chemical or physical absorption is moderate, and it is not affected by the range of pH values recorded in most natural waters (optimum pH 6–8). The recommended field dosage for aquatic snails is 4–8 mg/1/h, and for amphibious snails on moist soils 0·2 g/m². It is available as a wettable powder containing 70% active ingredient (Bell *et al.*, 1966; Anon, 1973).

It is now also available as an emulsion concentrate (Clonitralide®) with 25% active ingredient. This formulation has given satisfactory results although it is more expensive. It appears to be more efficient and easier to apply and may prove to be cheaper in some circumstances on a cost/efficiency basis. The LC_{99} was 0·3 mg/l for *B. pfeifferi* and 0·55 mg/l for *B. (P.) globosus* (figures that are three times better than those for the wettable powder). For *Biomphalaria* sp. on St Lucia, the LC_{50} for a 24-hour exposure and a 48-hour recovery period ranged from 0·02 mg/l to 0·04 mg/l, i.e. the same range as with the wettable powder; the LC_{90} was about 0·06 mg/l. This formulation has strong piscicidal activity. Niclosamide is currently used in large-scale control operations and is available in two proprietary compounds, Bayluscide® and Mollutox®, the latter compound being made in Egypt.

*N-tritylmorpholine-Frescon®-Triphenmorph**
This is the most active molluscicide known, with active concentrations ranging from 0·1 mg/l to 0·5 mg/l for 1-hour exposures, and from 0·01 mg/l to 0·05 mg/l for 24-hour exposures. In these concentrations it is not toxic to snail eggs, but it has now been shown that, with prolonged exposures, it is ovicidal. It has no effect on schistosome cercariae. Large-scale trials in several countries have demonstrated its efficacy in controlling snails with very short exposures (4 mg/l for 15 min) and with prolonged applications (0·07 mg/l for 15 days). Most of the available data indicate that bulinid species are less susceptible to triphenmorph than *Biomphalaria*. Plants, insects and micro-fauna and flora are unaffected by such treatments, and in certain circumstances it has proved possible to control snails without harming fish populations. Laboratory and field studies show that mud, vegetation and light have little effect on the activity of triphenmorph, but hydrolysis to triphenyl carbinol, with loss of activity, may occur in acidic water, depending upon the initial concentration of the compound. The rate of hydrolysis is relatively high at low pH values (<7·0), but decreases logarithmically as the pH increases. Certain observations show that the compound may be absorbed by silt particles and a relatively short half-life (20–30 h only) has been observed in waters containing moderate silt loads. The breakdown of the compound and its residues in soil and rice has been studied and it is not considered likely to present a toxic hazard to man or animals (Anon, 1973).

* *See also* The Toxicology of Molluscicides Trifenmorph. Duncan, J. (1981) *Pharmac. Ther.* **14,** pp. 67–68.

Triphenmorph is available as a 16·5% w/v emulsion concentrate. The compound has not fulfilled its early promise and it is no longer readily available (Amin and Fenwick, 1977; Warley, 1978).

NaPCP (Sodium pentachlorophenate)
This compound is highly effective against both aquatic and amphibious snails and their eggs, but both show reduced susceptibility with age, particularly as exposure time is reduced. Good penetration has been noted in watercourses and it is used for other purposes (weed control); it is readily available and relatively cheap. Time–concentration studies show that 1- and 6-hour exposures do not give maximum efficiency and better results are obtained with 24-hour exposures, while the use of prolonged low dosages holds some promise. Its stability is adequate under storage conditions, but sunlight has an adverse effect—which is less in turbid waters. Absorption of the compound by mud takes place but does not appear to be very serious. It is very irritating to snails and may cause them to leave the water and thus escape a lethal concentration. The compound is highly irritating to man and extremely dangerous if carelessly handled. Its application requires strict supervision, particularly for the powder formulations. It is available also in the form of pellets and briquettes containing 70% active ingredient. The recommended dosage for aquatic snails in flowing water is 50–80 mg/1/h and 0·4–10 g/m^2 for amphibious snails on moist soil. Pentachlorophenol is widely used in China and copper-pentachlorophenate in Venezuela.

Copper sulphate
This compound, which has been used widely for many years, is effective at low pH and is less toxic to fish than other chemicals. It kills snails and their eggs, but its action is variable under field conditions. It is not phytotoxic at the concentrations usually applied but it is adsorbed by organic matter and soil and is ineffective at high pH. It is usually used as $CuSO_4.5H_2O$ and the recommended dosages are 15–30 mg/1 for application in impounded waters, and 20–30 mg/1/h in flowing water. It is generally safe to handle but is corrosive to equipment and the relatively high concentrations applied increase costs because of the bulk required. It is, however, readily available in many places and now substantially cheaper than other synthetic

compounds. Removal of vegetation is usually necessary, but continuous application is used as a vegetation control method.

Copper compounds of low or slow solubility
These have received some laboratory and field evaluation and may be of value where the properties of persistence and low toxicity to other forms of aquatic life are desirable. Copper carbonate has proved to have a good residual effect in slow-flowing streams. Like the soluble copper sulphate, insoluble copper compounds act through their copper (II) ions. Because of their low solubility and high specific gravity, however, they are likely to be toxic only to organisms ingesting them on the bottom of water bodies and, therefore, comparatively harmless to other aquatic life. They are freely available throughout the world as commercial fungicides, formulated as small-sized particles and easily applied with conventional equipment (Anon, 1973).

Other molluscicides
Yurmin 3,5 dibromo-4-hydroxy-'4'-nitroazobenzene has been in practical use in Japan, where it was shown to be 16–18 times as active as NaPCP against *O.h. nosophora*. The 5% granular formulation is used at the rate of 5 g/m^2. The lethal concentration is a little higher for fish than for snails. No apparent toxic hazards to man or vegetation were detected. Its manufacture has now ceased.

B-2-sodium, 2,5-dichloro-4-bromphenol (named B-2) has been evaluated for application in the field as a molluscicide against *O. nosophora*. B-2 was applied either as a 25% liquid or in a 10% granular form to each of 5 m^2 quadrats in an *O. nosophora* habitat in the Yamanshi Prefecture, Japan: 10 g/m^2 of the 25% liquid gave over 95% mortality of snails, which was not improved by increasing the dose; 25 g/m^2 of the 10% granular formulation was needed to achieve a similar mortality of snails. The residual concentration of B-2 in the soil decreased rapidly. The level in the rice grains harvested from the treated paddy field did not exceed 0·03 ppm (Kajihara *et al.*, 1979).

Tin and lead compounds (*see also* Duncan, 1980)
A large number of these compounds have shown appreciable molluscicidal activity in the laboratory and in small-scale field trials. The high activity against *B. glabrata* of a number of

organotins, including bis (tri-n-butyltin) oxide (TBTO) (Hopf *et al.*, 1967), has received extensive evaluation in slow-release formulations. Triphenyl lead acetate showed promise in field trials in Ethiopia.

The field use of these compounds has been impeded by concern about their toxicity. It is necessary to distinguish between inorganic tin and its salt and organotin compounds. The former have a low toxicological risk which is generally associated with poor adsorption after ingestion. The mono-alkyltins appear to be of low toxicity, while the tetralkyltins are inactive *in vitro*, but are converted *in vivo* to trialkyltin by the liver. Of the dialkyltins and trialkyltins, the latter are apparently the more toxic. In view of available toxicological data on organo-metals and, in particular, bis (tri-n-buyltin) oxide (TBTO) and because of inadequate information on their long-term cumulative effects in the aquatic environment, it was considered that the use of such compounds as molluscicides and for larvicides could not be recommended (Anon, 1980).

Nicotinanilides
Nicotinanilide and its 3′- and 4′-chloro-analogues have been reported to give effective molluscicidal activity in water at about 0·2 mg/l, but their ovicidal activity is apparently variable, although it has been reported that many ova surviving treatments were either under-developed or abnormal. When the three compounds were applied at dosages between 2 mg/l and 5 mg/l to fish ponds, no obvious effects were noted on fish, frogs, tadpoles or water weeds. The half-life in water of a solution of 4′-chloronicotinanilide was 10 days (Dunlop, 1976). It is considered that these compounds offer the possibility of selective control of snails and that their future development will involve laboratory and field trials of slow-release formulations, the investigation of field methods for analysis of low concentrations in water and, of course, market evaluation and commercial production (Duncan, personal communication).

Vegetable molluscicides
Endod (*Phytolacca dodecandra*) is a compound which has received extensive laboratory and field evaluation (Lemma, 1965, 1970). It has been shown to give promising results in the control of *B. pfeifferi* in Ethiopia but was considered to be less cost-effective than Bayluscide (Lemma *et al.*, 1978). It is a saponin and not a

selective molluscicide, but it might have value for local self-help schemes. Its widescale use would depend upon properly organised harvesting of the native bush for local use or adequate commercial production. This has not been undertaken.

There are numerous other vegetable molluscicides, including *Jatropha* spp. and *Ambrosia maritima* (Daffalla, 1973; Sherif and El Sawy, 1977). Their effective use requires organisation and attention must be given to their potential toxicity in the same way as the use of synthetic compounds.

Application of molluscicides

Little precise evidence exists that the snail intermediate hosts of schistosomes have acquired chemical resistance, but niclosamide resistance in *B. truncatus* from Iran has been suggested (Jelnes, 1977). In Sudan, *B. truncatus* from field populations exposed to triphenmorph for more than five years appear to exhibit resistance and take up the chemical more slowly than snails from an untreated area (Daffalla and Duncan, 1979). On the other hand, *B. glabrata*, from colonies exposed regularly for nine years to niclosamide in St Lucia, showed no evidence of resistance when compared with snails from colonies from other parts of the island never subjected to chemical treatment (Barnish and Prentice, 1981). A molluscicide resistance test kit is currently being assembled and evaluated (Duncan, personal communication). In the application of available molluscicides, the term mg/l/h (milligrams per litre × hours or concentration × time, Ct product) has been used. This expresses the concentration of chemical applied and the duration of application. Within limits, these components are of equal importance in relation to response to their application, but there are theoretical and practical limits to both parts of the concept, which is not a fixed entity and may vary under different circumstances. Such variables include the chemical and physical properties of the molluscicide, the nature of its action, chemical and physical consistuents of the water, the species of snail, ecological requirements, microhabitat etc. It is normally calculated on the basis of a 24-hour exposure period, and because appreciable differences in Ct values may exist over the range of times and concentrations used, the figures may not be realistic if applied to short exposure periods of 1–2 h (Ansari, 1973).

The diversity of snail habitats requires that a careful choice be made of the chemical and of the method of application to be used. The final choice of compound and method of application will be largely decided by the nature of the habitat, but the cost of the work in relation to the efficacy of the molluscicide must also be considered.

It is desirable that a molluscicide is thoroughly dispersed in water, and natural as well as mechanical means must be relied upon to ensure this. Particular attention should be paid to impounded waters where stratification due to vertical temperature differences may occur and the habitat may be too small for wave action and turbulence to help in mixing the chemical. In watercourses, a molluscicide may be carried along well in the main channel, but it may also fail to penetrate lateral pools and marginal vegetation harbouring many snails. Attention should also be given to the 'attenuation' of a chemical in flowing water, since the farther it penetrates the more diluted it becomes, and in long watercourses or channels it may be necessary to add further quantities of the molluscicide at lower points. Different colorimetric methods are available for determining chemical concentrations, but bioassay methods are also used (Haskins, 1951; Strufe, 1961; Webbe, 1964).

Reports have been made that certain molluscicides are degraded by bacterial action and this may be important in certain types of habitat (Etges *et al.*, 1965; Bell *et al.*, 1966), but many other factors already discussed also cause loss of activity. It is, however, important to know the duration of activity of a molluscicide, and in flowing water this is essential, since dilution will increase the loss of activity.

Two general strategies for snail control are in current use: focal control and area control. The former approach may be valuable where transmission is limited to particular foci, but area control is likely to be the only practical approach if transmission is widespread in a watershed or irrigation system.

Focal control depends upon a knowledge of the transmission foci, and periodic mollusciciding must be continued. In the control of an area or watershed unit, all snail habitats must be treated and, while initially it may prove more difficult than focal control, the result may be longer lasting and therefore more economic.

An analysis of the economics of applying molluscicides to flowing water has been made and attention given to their efficient application, but without taking labour costs into account (Jobin, 1968). The process of 'detoxication' of a molluscicide or the 'total pattern of chemical decay' is approximated 'by the generalised first order differential equation (1):

$$\frac{dC}{dt} = -kC$$

where C is the molluscicide concentration at any time (t).' The rate of decay for each molluscicide under specified field conditions is characterised by the 'half-life (a) which is calculated as 0·69/k, independent of Co, the concentration of molluscicide applied at time t = 0'. The toxic concentration Ct, which may be determined for snails under local conditions (being a value giving almost complete kill, e.g. LD 99·5), will produce this mortality at the point of application, but the mortality will soon decrease as the molluscicide moves downstream. The question is, what concentration should be applied as Co?

The most economical application value for Co can be calculated by finding 'the concentration which gives the maximum benefit-to-cost ratio (BCR)', in which the benefit is proportional to the length of stream penetrated by the toxic concentration; the cost being determined by the quantity of chemical required for the application.

'For the pattern of detoxication specified in equation-(1) the BCR can be written as the ratio of T, the time of effective downstream treatment to the initial concentration of chemical Co. Co is directly proportional to the cost of the chemical, and

$$T/Co = BCR \ldots$$

at maximum BCR,

$$\frac{Co}{Ct} = e = 2\cdot7'$$

Jobin (1968) concludes that in irrigation systems where the cost of chemical is likely to be the most important factor owing to the large amounts of water treated at each application, 'it is most economical to use Co/Ct of 2·7 unless smaller values are dictated by short travel times to the end of the canal' and that 'in general, the ratio of 2·7 can be used whenever the travel time to the end of the canal is greater than the half-life of the chemical'. Where labour costs are high, however, in natural drainage systems, 'it is best to use a Co/Ct of about 5, which is still only 12 per cent less efficient than the theoretical maximum'.

Available data show that mollusciciding is most cost-effective where the volume of water to be treated per caput at risk is small. It is, therefore, well suited to arid areas where transmission is seasonal and confined to relatively small habitats such as, for example, in Saudi Arabia and the Yemen Arab Republic. It may, however, be unsuitable in large rivers and lakes unless transmission is focal in distribution, as has now been established in Lake Volta, Ghana. Where the population density is high and the volume of water per person is, therefore, low, mollusciciding may be cost-effective, however, although the total volume may be large (Anon, 1973). Irrigation schemes where controlled water management is practised and where population density is high (e.g. Egypt, Sudan, China) are well-suited to cost-effective mollusciciding in the control of transmission.

Snail control by periodic area-wide mollusciciding is now being successfully carried out in several major control programmes based upon irrigation and controlled water management. 'Transmission control' based upon the essential focality of transmission is also being successfully prosecuted by mollusciciding and surveillance. This may be a highly cost-effective approach based upon accurate knowledge of human water contact patterns and it may result in a considerable saving of expensive chemical. It must be realised, however, that 'focal transmission control' may be totally impracticable in a flowing water system with a high population density and diffuse domestic and occupational human water contact. Further, it is labour intensive and will require considerable supervision with adequate logistic support. On a very large scale these requirements may prove costly and offset the savings made on chemical.

Delivery of molluscicides
The number of formulations of the available molluscicides and the methods used to apply them are relatively limited. In flowing water habitats, both wettable powder suspensions and emulsion concentrates are usually applied using a form of constant head dispenser to deliver a particular concentration for the required period of time. Impounded waters and delimited foci within them, the tail-ends of irrigation ditches and drains, swampy conditions, seepages and paddies usually require spraying and different types of knapsack and motor sprayers are currently used (Figs. 11.1 and 11.2; Ansari, 1973).

Aerial application of molluscicides has been carried out in different endemic areas with varying degrees of success but apparently with high cost-effectiveness in the Sudan (Barnish and Shiff, 1970; Sturrock and Barnish, 1973; Amin and Fenwick, 1977).

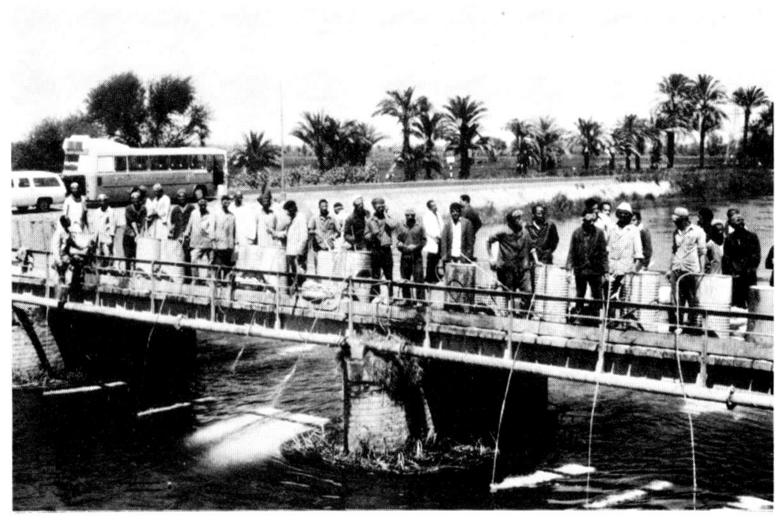

Fig. 11.1 The application of molluscicide to a large irrigation canal in Egypt by drip feed dispensers.

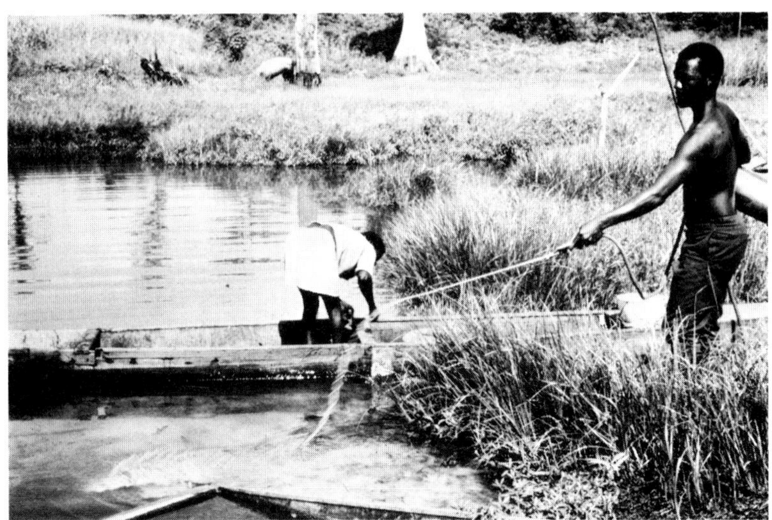

Fig. 11.2 The focal application of molluscicide by knapsack spraying in a water-contact site on Lake Volta.

Recognition of the 'focality' of transmission in many situations has prompted attempts to devise cost-effective methods of application and, in particular, slow-release formulation of a number of molluscicides (Cardarelli, 1974, 1977). Compounds which have been included in slow-release matrices (rubber sheets, baits, pellets) include copper salts, organotins, organoleads, niclosamide and triphenmorph (Anon, 1973). Field trials with bis-(tri-n-butyltin) oxide (Biomet SRM®), the commercially available formulation containing 6% TBTO, have been reported. The pellets were effective in controlling snails when applied at 20 g/m², and no adverse effects were noted in the case of other biota in the treated area. It is believed that the molluscicide is confined to the depths of a water body and exerts a selective action on snails (Shiff, 1974; Shiff and Evans, 1977). Other very successful field trials of TBTO have been carried out in St Lucia (Prentice, personal communication).

There has been little success in formulating niclosamide or triphenmorph in slow-release matrices, and slow-release copper formulations appear to be of little value (Christie *et al.*, 1978). The future of slow-release organometals, either as larvicides or molluscicides, appears to be questionable, however, unless more convincing toxicological information can be established.

The use of gelatin granule formulation of niclosamide has been reported in St Lucia, as have other locally made formulations (Upatham and Sturrock, 1977; Prentice, personal communication). Field trials of a slow-release glass formulation have recently been carried out in Ghana, and the material appears to have some advantages compared with elastomeric matrices, but its use appears to be confined to the use of inorganic molluscicides, e.g. copper (Duncan, personal communication).

More adequate strategies and delivery systems are required to optimise the cost-effectiveness of mollusciciding. There is a need to explore further the potential of new formulations of available compounds, and to examine the possibilities of developing molluscicides from natural products of local origin in endemic countries, if adequate agronomic back-up is feasible. Costs of molluscicides are high, and are likely to increase, usually requiring much-needed foreign exchange. The possibilities of local manufacture of the more sophisticated compounds should be examined such as, for example, 'Mollutox', although the costs of importing essential basic constituents may prove expensive.

The application of snail population parameters in control of intermediate hosts

When calculated from field data, the net reproductive rate (R_0) can be used to check the fecundity and survival of snails. It is possible to calculate that the snail population in an area studied doubled itself every two months (Webbe, 1962), and this can also be calculated independently from the estimates of mortality and reproduction indices in the data. Using a population parameter, it is also possible to predict the maximum possible rate of repopulation of snails following a control measure. The intrinsic rate of natural increase (r) can be calculated for the most favourable conditions encountered in the field, if age-specific reproduction and survival data are known for different seasons (Dazo *et al.*, 1966). Dazo and his colleagues calculated that under optimum field conditions *B. truncatus* and *B. alexandrina* can double their populations in 14–16 days, and considered that any control operations should take advantage of the information on population parameters.

The maximum expected average rate of repopulation can be calculated from an equation of exponential growth:

$$N_t = N_o e^{rt}$$

where N_o is the starting population, N_t is the expected population after time t, and e is the base of natural logarithms (Slobodkin, 1962). If an estimate of the percentage kill achieved by a particular control procedure is obtained, then it should be possible to establish the level at which the snail population might again require attention, and from this and the calculation on the rate of repopulation, an estimate of the required frequency of application of the selected method (Pesigan, Hairston *et al.*, 1958; Dazo *et al.*, 1966).

The model described above was found to be less effective in describing the behaviour of natural snail populations of *B. glabrata* in St Lucia than a second model (Smith, 1952).

$$N_t = \frac{K}{I + \dfrac{K - N_o\, e^{-rt}}{N_o}}$$

based on the Verhulst–Pearl equation (Pearl and Reed, 1920). For this model $K = 100$.

There is, in fact, little to choose between the two models if kills above 95% are achieved (this may not be the case in natural habitats) and if r does not exceed 0·4. 'The probability of poorer kills and of an opportunistic species (MacArthur, 1960) like *B. glabrata* with *r* values greater than 0·4 indicate that the second model would be preferable to the first one for St Lucian conditions' (Sturrock, 1973). Both models over-simplify the actual events occurring in the field and more sophisticated models (Jobin and Michelson, 1967) would give more accurate predictions if all the data were available.

A reduction in transmission may be achieved by lowering snail population density and altering its age structure, even though complete eradication is not accomplished (Webbe, 1962, 1965a). It is not known at present, however, to what level a snail population must be reduced in order to interrupt transmission, since the precise probability of a miracidium infecting a known density of snails is unknown. Available evidence suggests that in an area of high endemicity the 'threshold' below which snails will not become infected is probably close to complete eradication of the snail population (Chernin and Dunavan, 1962).

It is important in evaluating control measures to consider the period for which they are likely to remain effective. Few, if any, of the available methods of control involving the use of chemicals are likely to result in complete eradication of snails, and their high 'intrinsic rate of natural increase' is likely to result in the rapid restoration of damaged populations. Prevention of breeding may therefore be more important than success in killing snails, and a permanent result may require an alteration of the environment and, in turn, of the ecology of the population (Pesigan, Hairston *et al.*, 1958). The 'intrinsic rate of natural increase' will not be affected by such a change, of course, but the 'actual or realised rate of increase' will be influenced. If environmental resistance is so increased and the 'carrying capacity' of the population lowered, population density will ultimately be decreased. The change produced in the environment to bring this about may cause reproduction to slow down, or it may reduce the survival rates. In either case, an unbalanced age structure will result and whatever factor is chosen it is desirable that it should be 'density independent' and lead to complete elimination of the population (Webbe, 1965b).

CHEMOTHERAPY

Whereas there are innumerable different ecological situations affecting the interrelationship between the intermediate snail host and parasite and detailed pre-control studies are required for scientifically planned snail control projects, chemotherapy requires a minimum of pre-control studies.

Even before the introduction of the new drugs, attempts had been made to use chemotherapy in control. In Egypt, tartar emetic and Fouadin were used between 1953 and 1959 in a compulsory treatment project (Abdullah, 1973); Astiban was used in a mass suppressive management regime in 1964–5 (Sherif *et al.*, 1970); tartar emetic and niradazole were used, in conjunction with Bayluscide, in the Egyptian Fayoum project in 1968–71 (Abdullah, 1973); and niradazole was used in Tanzania (Eyakuze, 1972) and, with Frescon, in the Malagasy Republic (Degremont, 1973). In all these schemes prevalence of infection fell, but the use of toxic and multidose drugs meant, inevitably, that optimum population coverage was not obtained and the cost of drug administration was high.

With the advent of single-dose drugs—first, hycanthone in 1965—the prospects of adequate population coverage improved and control schemes in Egypt, Brazil and St Lucia were initiated. Although hycanthone quickly became unacceptable— for reasons discussed in Chapter 9—other drugs, oxamniquine and metrifonate, were available and were used on a large scale in Brazil, Egypt and Ghana even before pilot projects had clarified how best they could be delivered; praziquantel has now been developed and will no doubt be the drug of choice for *S. japonicum* and for mixed *S. haematobium* and *S. mansoni* infections.

Case detection

The new drugs are relatively free from toxic and side-effects, but for economic and ethical reasons it is generally considered that diagnosis of an active schistosome infection should be made prior to treatment. This necessitates parasitological examination rather than immunodiagnostic techniques which, at the present time, are unsatisfactory (see Chapter 7).

Methods used need to be low cost, quick and reliable but the sensitivity required might vary with the aim of the control programme, i.e. transmission control or disease prevention. Where transmission control is the aim, a high level of sensitivity may be important for case detection prior to treatment to reduce to a minimum the chance of snails becoming infected from undetected and untreated cases; if the aim is disease prevention through treatment of heavily infected persons at risk of developing schistosomal disease, then a lower level of sensitivity is acceptable.

The modified Kato–Katz smear is recommended for *S. mansoni* and *S. japonicum* infections and the filtration technique (with a nuclepore polycarbonate filter) for *S. haematobium*. The sensitivity of each of these techniques can be varied by changing the volume of the sample examined—if small volumes are examined, only high intensities of infection will be detected. These techniques require microscopy but intense *S. haematobium* infections can be detected very rapidly with urinalysis reagent strips using a combined criteria of haematuria and 30 mg/100 ml or more of protein (Wilkins *et al.*, 1979; Pugh *et al.*, 1980).

Delivery systems

Transmission control

'Mass' treatment of the whole population is rarely carried out although in the Special Schistosomiasis Control Programme in Brazil everyone was given treatment if prevalence was greater than 20% amongst 7- to 14-year-old children; if between 4% and 20%, persons between 5 and 25 years of age were treated, and when prevalence was less than 4%, only children found infected were treated. In other major schemes in Ghana, Egypt, Sudan and St Lucia, treatment is given only to infected persons—selective population chemotherapy (SPC).

Although proposals have been made for treatment of children only (Jordan, 1963) or heavily infected persons (Warren and Mahmoud, 1976)—both groups responsible for a high proportion of potential contamination—these approaches have not been evaluated for transmission control.

If population participation is good, a rapid fall in prevalence can be expected (Fig. 11.3; Cook *et al.*, 1977), but the degree of transmission control achieved depends on the extent of the reservoir of infection remaining in the community. This depends on (a) the co-operation of the population in respect of providing specimens for case detection and in respect of accepting treatment, (b) the sensitivity of the parasitological examination technique, (c) the 'cure' rate after treatment, and (d) the extent of immigration of infected persons.

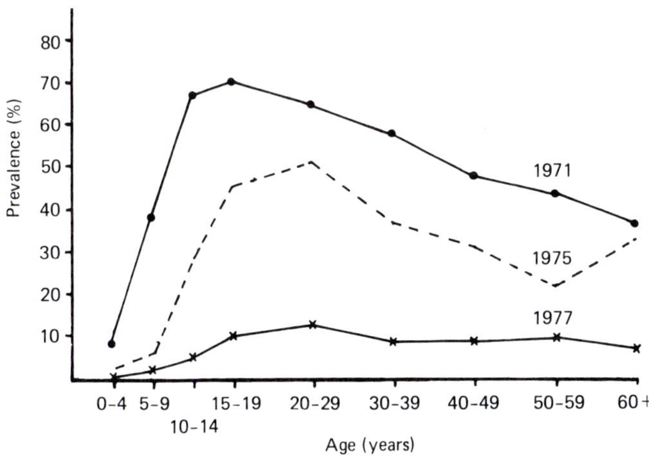

Fig. 11.3 Declining *S. mansoni* prevalence in all age groups following four years of snail control (1971–5) followed by a rapid fall after chemotherapy in 1975 and 1976. (St Lucian data: Jordan, Barnish *et al.*, 1978 and Jordan, Cook *et al.*, 1980.)

Unco-operative persons—refusing to be examined—were considered the most important factor in the remaining reservoir of infection in one project in St Lucia (Jordan, Cook *et al.*, 1980) where males are generally less co-operative than females, as are the 20–29 year age group amongst both sexes. Co-operation falls the longer control schemes operate, i.e. with each survey when four annual treatments were given. The compliance rate—the proportion accepting treatment—may vary with the delivery system and success of any health education programme, although it appears that the drugs now available are acceptable in most endemic areas.

The need for a sensitive parasitological technique to detect as many infected persons as possible has been stressed above. While it can be argued that light infections play little part in transmission, and need not therefore be treated, the risk of snail infections occurring from many, widely dispersed, lightly in-fected persons may be greater than from a few heavily infected individuals.

The drugs now available are very effective and in full doses high rates of 'cure' and of egg reduction can be expected; lower rates will occur when multiple doses of drugs are needed—e.g. with metrifonate in *S. haematobium* infections, and possibly with praziquantel in *S. japonicum* and oxamniquine with some north African strains of *S. mansoni*.

Population movement can be on a massive scale, as in the Sudan where thousands of immigrant workers enter the Gezira each year for seasonal cotton picking, and in Tanzania a population change of over 60% occurred within a three-year period after a chemotherapy-based control scheme (Ruyssenaars and McCullough, 1973). In other places population movement might be on a smaller and local scale.

The extent of the reservoir of infection remaining after chemotherapy and the local dynamics of transmission will determine when retreatment is required—this will also be governed by the goal of the programme.

In the Special Schistosomiasis Control Programme in Brazil the aim was to reduce prevalence throughout the country to below 4% and to achieve this, stools of children were examined every six months and treatment given as indicated above.

On the other hand, in less ambitious programmes, re-examination and treatment are usually given yearly. This, however, may not be necessary if prevalence and intensity of infection fall significantly after treatment. In one study in Brazil (Bina and Prata, 1970), three years after treatment stopped prevalence was still at a low level (Fig. 11.4) and the risk of disease developing was minimal. In St Lucia no infected sentinel or wild snails were found for two years (Christie and Upatham, 1977) after a selective population chemotherapy campaign. Wild snails subsequently became infected, transmission recurred and prevalence increased. However, after three years it was still much lower than its original level. In other studies four years after treatment, intensity of infection amongst those treated was only a third of the initial level (Kloetzel, 1967a). Unspecific as well as acquired and concomitant immunity (more effective in adults than children) were considered to influence the maintenance of low infection rates, and worm burdens after specific treatment of *S. mansoni* (Katz *et al.*, 1978)—but water-contact patterns must also have some influence on this.

As prevalence and intensity build up, chemotherapy must be repeated or some other control measure (i.e. snail control) can be used in a consolidation or follow-up phase. In spite, however, of the risk of re-infection amongst those treated, the worm burden and the number of eggs retained in the tissues will have been lowered, thus reducing potential morbidity and disease. In

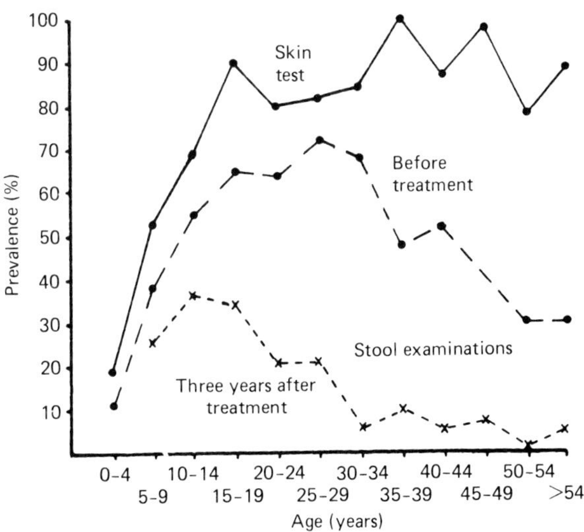

Fig. 11.4 Difference in prevalence in *S. mansoni*, as assessed by skin test and stool examination before intensive hycanthone treatment campaigns, and prevalence three years after. (Derived from Brazilian data: Bina and Prata, 1970.)

addition, progression of early schistosomal disease will have been stopped.

For disease prevention
In contrast to the widespread use of drugs to control transmission (and, secondarily, disease), targeted therapy for those at greater risk of developing disease has not been used extensively. Since in general, schistosomal disease is associated with high worm burdens and high levels of egg excretion, it was suggested that children between the ages of 7 and 10 years excreting more than 500 *S. mansoni* eggs/g of faeces should be treated to prevent hepatosplenomegaly: not one of 60 children so treated developed splenomegaly in the following four years and splenic enlargement disappeared or diminished in 21 of 23 cases after treatment (Kloetzel, 1967a). The level of 400 eggs/g was suggested after work in Kenya (Siongok *et al.*, 1976).

Although such targeted treatment will do much to prevent disease in those treated (Kloetzel, 1967b), children who at the time of examination are found with low levels of egg excretion (but who previously had heavy ones) will not be treated and may still be liable to develop late complications—which can also develop in some individuals with light infections.

A similar approach, but based on the detection by urinalysis reagent strips of individuals with heavy *S. haematobium* infections, has also been suggested (Pugh *et al.*, 1980).

High egg excretors are comparatively few in infected communities—but they may be responsible for a high proportion of potential contamination (see Table 10.8). Treatment of these persons alone will, however, leave a considerable reservoir of infection, and transmission will almost certainly continue so that re-examination and retreatment will probably be necessary annually.

Other regimes

Treatment of all children has been advocated as they are potentially responsible for a high proportion of contamination (Jordan, 1963; see Chapter 10) and are at risk of developing disease; infection in adults, on the other hand, is spontaneously declining in most endemic areas. The approach would prevent disease and, in theory, have a greater effect on transmission than treatment only of those with high levels of egg excretion: it has not, however, yet been evaluated although it is basically the routine in Brazil for areas where prevalence is between 4% and 20%. In many of the developing countries, a high proportion of children attend school and can readily be examined and treated—if necessary annually, but every two or three years may be enough to keep levels of egg excretion at a low level, thus reducing the risk of disease. More frequent treatments may be required in areas of intense transmission and very high prevalence and intensity.

Suppressive management (Freidheim and de Jongh, 1959) involves the periodic administration of subcurative doses of drug to produce a marked reduction in egg excretion and the risk of disease. The regime was developed when toxic antimonial drugs were the only ones available, but this form of management was extensively used only once and then for transmission control in Egypt (Sherif *et al.*, 1970). With the new drugs there is probably little need now for this approach but metrifonate at the standard dose of 7·5 mg/kg has been given successfully as a prophylactic at monthly intervals for five months (Jewsbury *et al.*, 1977); in the few infections that did occur, intensity of infection was low.

At present, insufficient studies have been carried out to compare the effects of different regimes. Such studies are urgently required to define the most cost-effective approach to transmission and disease control programmes or both.

Cost

The main costs in a chemotherapy campaign involve (a) case detection (containers, collection of specimens) and their examination, and (b) treatment (cost of drug and its distribution). Both aspects of the campaign require transport, administrative back-up and capital investment, vehicles, microscopes, etc.

Plastic bags are probably the cheapest containers for urine specimens but were not acceptable for faecal specimens when tried in St Lucia, where waxed cardboard of plastic containers are used. These, however, are costly (9·7 US cents each) and in an unco-operative population many are not returned, thus adding to the campaign cost. (All too frequently they are used in the home for storing sugar or butter!) This type of container may be unnecessary with the new techniques, where small volumes can be examined. When serodiagnosis is acceptable for case detection, the collection of blood spots on filter paper will be cheaper than the collection of stool or urine specimens.

The technique used for examining urine or stool can affect the cost of a programme—quantitative techniques are more time consuming than qualitative methods but the newer filtration techniques for urine examination and the 'modified Kato' for stool examination are significant advances in the field of case detection.

The cost of case detection can be reduced if—as in Brazil—the treatment regime is based on the results of examining children only. Further savings can be made if random samples of children are examined but, in both cases, drug costs will be unnecessarily high owing to uninfected persons being treated. Selective population chemotherapy requires identification of infected persons in all age groups. As this usually requires house-to-house visits for specimen collection, it is costly, but the expenditure of local currency benefits the employed nationals and, since only those infected are treated, foreign currency expenditure on drugs is kept to a minimum.

Further savings on drug charges accrue if only those with high egg loads are treated, but case detection in this regime involves examination of all individuals and quantitative evaluation of infected persons. This may be more costly (time consuming) than qualitative microscopy for selective population chemotherapy, though detection of heavy *S. haematobium* infections by urinalysis reagent strips may overcome this.

The treatment of children—particularly if this is done through schools—is probably the most cost-effective approach since they require less drug than adults, are responsible for a high proportion of the eggs excreted in the community (see Table 10.7), are most easily contacted and, in addition, are at greatest risk of developing disease. Treatment of school children should facilitate health education programmes and, in a public health scheme (as distinct from a research approach), is more realistic than a scheme based on house-to-house visits for collection of urine or stool samples—and non-attenders can probably be summoned for screening.

Drugs available and delivery system

The cost of drugs varies from country to country. The cost of hycanthone can be reduced by using a lower dose—1·5 mg/kg instead of 2·5–3·0 mg (Cook *et al.*, 1976; Warren and Mahmoud, 1976)—but even with this less toxic, but still effective dose, medical supervision is necessary. Because of this, the need to administer it by injection, and its suspected mutagenicity, hycanthone is unlikely to be used in any large-scale chemotherapy campaign now that other drugs are available.

Trained health personnel are used to administer metrifonate oxamniquine and praziquantel. Metrifonate is the cheapest schistosomicidal drug available. Unfortunately, delivery costs are high owing to the necessary three treatments at fortnightly intervals and, although in Kenya good results were obtained at four months with a single 10 mg/kg dose (Siongok *et al.*, 1978), results with this regime were unsatisfactory in Ghana (Davis, personal communication) and the Gambia (Wilkins and Moore, 1980), but two 10 mg/kg doses at 14-day intervals were effective in mild to moderate infections (Davis, personal communication).

The use of combined niridazole (25 mg/kg) and metrifonate (12·5 mg/kg) in a single dose gave good results (Pugh, 1978), but the demonstrated mutagenicity and carcinogenicity of niridazole (see Chapter 9) make it unlikely that such a combination will be widely used.

The optimum method of drug delivery will vary with local conditions but, wherever possible, the existing health personnel infrastructure should be used, although initially it might be necessary to have drug administration by mobile teams. Treatment can be given during house-to-house visits but this raises the problem of finding the patient 'at home', particularly when adults are involved. In St Lucia, a central point in a village is chosen and those to attend for treatment are notified. This approach is probably more economical than house-to-house visiting but treatment of children at school is certainly the least costly.

The frequency of treatments in any regime requires clarification. However, if treatments are repeated annually, the proportionate costs of different aspects of the campaigns are likely to change. With fewer cases to detect (as control becomes established), it is probably uneconomical to treat without examination but the cost of detecting a decreasing number of cases forms an increasingly greater proportion of the total costs (Table 11.2); therapy absorbs a correspondingly smaller proportion—an important factor when foreign exchange is involved.

Table 11.2 Costs (in US dollars) of four selective chemotherapy campaigns using hycanthone. (The fewer the cases detected, the higher the proportionate cost of their detection compared with the costs of therapy.)

	1973	1974	1975	1976
Stools examined	2911	2523	2170	2510
Stools positive	734	164	96	78
Number of treatments	709	159	96	78
Case detection costs (US$)*	1946 (46)	1849 (73)	1809 (82)	2279 (87)
Therapy costs: drugs and materials*	1226 (29)	440 (17)	234 (11)	200 (8)
salaries, transport etc.*	1056 (25)	254 (10)	154 (7)	131 (5)
Total cost	4228	2543	2197	2610
Cost (US$) per: stool examined†	0·67	0·73	0·83	0·91
case detected‡	2·65	11·27	18·85	29·21
treatment‡	5·96	15·99	22·90	33·46
person protected	1·36	0·82	0·70	0·84

* Figures in parentheses are percentages of total estimated cost.
† Increasing cost of stool examination reflects increasing inflation.
‡ With few cases to detect but the same screening required, cost per case found and per treatment increases.

Apart from identifying those for treatment, the detection of cases serves an additional purpose, as periodic surveys monitor the state of transmission.

NON-SPECIFIC METHODS OF CONTROL

Reduce exposure

Measures that prevent or reduce human contact with cercarial-infested water will reduce infection. While this is accepted, safe water supplies have not been seriously considered as a method of control owing to cost, maintenance difficulties and the belief that rural people would not accept the change from the age-old river or pond washing to washing from a piped water supply.

For social and medical reasons, water is now being supplied to an increasing number of rural communities in developing countries. Health benefits are usually thought of in relation to bacterial and viral intestinal infections and for this reason there is emphasis on the provision of safe drinking water with usually no facilities for washing, bathing or recreation—major causes of water contact associated with schistosome infection—and transmission continues. However, in Egypt it was noted that 'even the partial use of protected water markedly lowers the rates of (schistosome) infection'. The effect was greater with *S. mansoni* than *S. haematobium* (Farooq *et al.*, 1966). The first serious attempts at controlling transmission by reducing exposure to infected water were made in Zimbabwe (Pitchford, 1970b); contact was prevented by fencing, as well as the provision of piped water, and simple swimming pools. In Brazil, washing units, communal supplies obtained from a dug well and fitted with hand pumps, latrines and health education were shown to reduce transmission (Barbosa *et al.*, 1971).

A community standpipe system had little effect on transmission in St Lucia, as the infected river was still the main site for washing clothes and bathing; but with laundry shower units (Fig. 11.5) and health education, water contact and transmission fell.

In areas with an experimental individual household water supply, transmission was markedly reduced (Jordan *et al.*, 1975; Unrau, 1975; Jordan, Bartholomew *et al.*, 1978). Laundry and shower units and simple swimming pools supplemented the household supply. A health education programme was needed to obtain maximum benefit from the facilities provided. The scheme indicated age-old customs (such as washing clothes in the river) *can* be changed so that children accompanying their mothers when washing played alongside the washing unit instead of getting infected in the river. The response to water

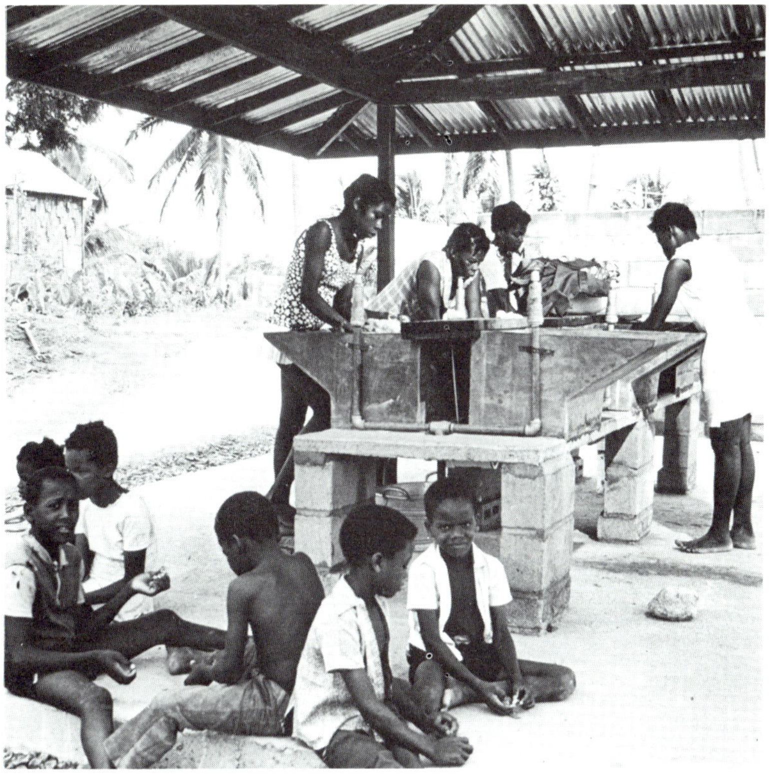

Fig. 11.5 Laundry unit in St Lucia with showers in background. Laundry tubs fitted with Fordilla taps (faucets) to prevent the wasting of water. (Photograph by courtesy of M. A. Prentice.)

supplies and health education will depend on the attractiveness of pre-existing supplies—a clear, sparkling river may be more attractive than a wash tub, but the latter may be a delight if the alternative is a small dirty pond.

When alternative water supplies and facilities are provided and accepted by the community, reduced contact with previously favourite sources of water may lead to less contamination. However, in St Lucia there was evidence of the reverse— when a local stream was no longer needed for domestic purposes it was used as a latrine and snail infection rates increased.

Owing to high capital costs, water supplies are unlikely to be installed as a measure to control transmission of schistosomiasis. However, it is emphasised that where safe water is being provided—as it is in so many rural areas—then those special facilities to reduce *water contact* should be added to the scheme to ensure greater health and social benefits of the water.

Water supplies are more likely to be provided in areas of dense or moderately dense populations, but in areas of low population simple water supplies can be provided from protected springs, bore holes etc., and simple hand pumps can operate the delivery system (Fig. 11.6). However, whether this be simple or more sophisticated, adequate maintenance service must be ensured.

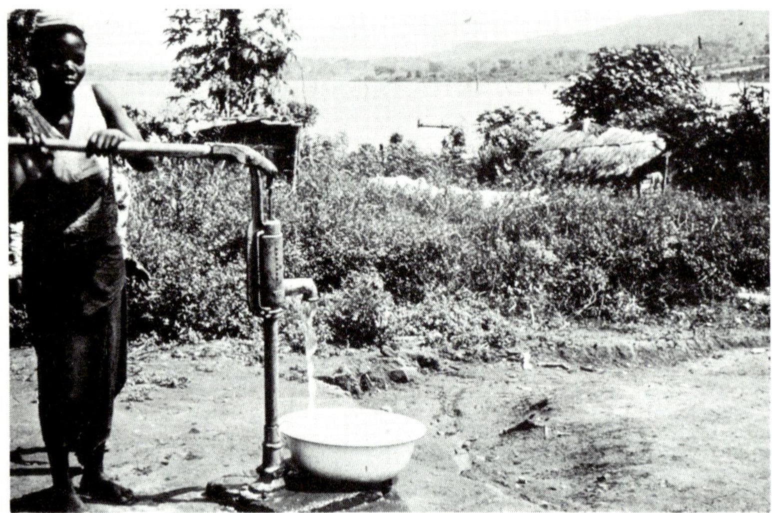

Fig. 11.6 Domestic water supply in a village on Lake Volta installed to reduce domestic water contact and exposure to infection.

Water outlets should be conveniently sited with an abundant supply of reasonably clean water. This is more important than a limited supply of high quality water. With limited-flow taps, or faucets, and other water-saving devices, 60 litres per head of population is adequate; with ordinary taps, up to three times this amount may be required owing to wastage associated with them.

Schools should have a good water supply so that health education in relation to cleanliness will have real meaning; similarly, adequate latrine facilities are essential to emphasise the importance of health relative to sanitation.

Water supplies can reduce contact and exposure to schistosome infection; other methods of achieving this include physical barriers, such as fences and bridges, and the siting of new villages as far as possible from any lake, river or canal and providing a piped water supply.

Water—quality and quantity

Engineering aspects of water supplies are outside the scope of this monograph, but obtaining 'safe' from 'unsafe' water is not—it is paradoxical that the very source of infection (i.e. infected water) can be made safe and distributed as a means of schistosomiasis control.

Water containing schistosome cercariae can be made safe by storage, filtration or chemical treatment.

In the laboratory, infectivity of cercariae was reduced by more than 90% 14–15 h after emergence from the snail. As conditions in the field are always more rigorous, it was concluded the half-life is probably only a few hours even in the absence of predators.

Water stored for a minimum of 24 h can therefore be considered non-infective. The storage of water in a rural system has the added benefit of being available in case of a breakdown in the system and other organisms apart from cercariae may be killed.

Sand and diatomaceous earth filters remove cercariae but they must be properly designed, constructed, operated and maintained. Horizontal filters using sand of 0·35 mm diameter or smaller were highly effective, but with larger particles and rapid water flow cercariae passed through (Bernade and Johnson, 1971).

Alum in the strongest concentrations used does not destroy cercariae and, although it has been shown to affect them, this is due mainly to the high pH never reached in normal water treatment (McJunkin, 1970).

Chlorination is effective but pH is important. Cercariae are killed within 30 min by 1 ppm chlorine residual in the pH range 7·5–8·9, 0·3 ppm at pH 5, and 5 ppm at pH 10 (McJunkin, 1970). Lower residuals are effective over longer periods of time. Boiling water for drinking purposes is, of course, a standard recommendation in rural areas but is an impossible way of killing cercariae in large volumes of water. However, much lower temperatures are lethal to cercariae which succumb to 30-min exposure at 45°C (Krakower, 1940).

A safe water supply is essential, particularly where surface water is being used. Where water is being collected from a surface reservoir and supplied by gravity without treatment or storage, care must be taken that the supply is uninfected.

Prevention of contamination

As with water development, there is an increasing awareness of the need for people in developing countries to have acceptable means of disposing of their waste matter. This has stimulated recent meetings (Pacey, 1978) and useful publications (Rybenzynski *et al.*, 1978).

Latrines for use in rural areas have generally been regarded as unsatisfactory owing to fly and odour problems. Recent developments in design overcome many of these problems, which should result in their better acceptance. Improvements in ventilation and on offset squatting plate are essential features of the Reed Odourless Earth Closet (ROEC) used in Botswana (Rybenzynski *et al.*, 1978). The use of composting latrines, pit latrine derivatives, the aquaprivy (Blackmore *et al.*, 1978) and water seal latrines have all been reviewed recently (Morgan and Clarke, 1978; Unrau, 1978).

While in theory, efficient and safe disposal of human waste should do much to reduce transmission of schistosomiasis, many believe improved sanitation is of little value. It has been said 'Any number of them (latrines) will not prevent human beings urinating when they get into water nor will they stop indiscriminate defaecation when under normal circumstances the Bantu empty their bowels about three times a day' (Pitchford, 1970a).

While there may be some truth in this, it is no justification for not encouraging the development and use of latrines and a positive approach such as 'urinate before swimming' might be better than 'don't urinate while swimming'. While it is unlikely that field workers will go back 'home' especially to defaecate, it should be recognised that in most situations transmission occurs mainly in the village environment, not in the fields. Improved sanitation should be encouraged in spite of the frequently, unfortunately incorrectly, quoted work purporting to show sanitation failed to control transmission (Scott and Barlow, 1938; Weir *et al.*, 1952). The prediction made by Macdonald (1965) that sanitation will not reduce transmission was based on the false assumption that water bodies were 'saturated' with miracidia.

Any effect sanitation has is likely to be only slowly apparent, and may well be less with *S. japonicum* where animal reservoir hosts are important. However, in a limited trial in the Philippines (Pesigan, Hairston *et al.*, 1958), when latrines were provided the *S. japonicum* infection rate in nearby snail colonies fell. At the same time there was a rise in infection rate amongst snails near to houses not provided with latrines.

In the Brazilian National Schistosomiasis Campaign, improved sanitation is an important supplement to chemotherapy and snail control; sanitation and water supplies reduced transmission in an earlier pilot project (Barbosa *et al.*, 1971).

Even with a latrine, care must be taken that adequate treatment is carried out to kill schistosome eggs. Eggs containing mature miracidia live for two days at 24°–32°C in formed stool and for more than a week at 7°–10°C. In semi-formed or liquid stools they live for only 24 hours (Faust and Hoffman, 1934).

In pit latrines, schistosome eggs die, but with aquaprivies and septic tanks safety depends on the retention time, with septic tanks presenting a greater hazard than the aquaprivy as hatching is most unlikely in the waste matter of the latter. Transmission has resulted from passage of eggs in effluent into snail-infested streams.

Three types of sewage treatment were investigated—sedimentation, trickle filtration and activated sludge (Rowan, 1964a). No method was entirely safe, and chlorination of effluent to give a 15-min residual level of at least 2·5 mg/l was advocated (Rowan, 1964b).

In China, night-soil is collected into communal earthenware containers. When full, they are sealed and left for three to seven days for the generated ammonia from urine to kill schistosome eggs. When excreta are urgently needed as fertiliser, they are boiled or treated with chemical. Composting kills eggs due to the raised temperature (Cheng, 1971). Composting or ammonia treatment should be carried out if excreta are to be used on irrigated land.

Miracidia were found in the effluent liquid of Chinese biogas plants (Pacey, 1978).

COMMUNITY INVOLVEMENT AND HEALTH EDUCATION

The importance of involving the community in control is being increasingly appreciated now that chemotherapy, requiring the co-operation of the people, is being used; this contrasts with minimal community involvement with snail control.

In any scheme, whether research orientated or public health, the people should be told the nature of the work and what is involved. This is usually done by talks in schools and by meetings for adults when films or other visual aids on the parasite, its life-cycle, and the disease, are shown.

Apart from these semi-formal contacts, survey teams (whether for parasitological or biological studies) can help by explaining the programme to the people as they go about their work in and around the villages; probably the most effective way of educating people in health is by individual home contact. Although posters are often used, they are not considered to have much of an impact in developing countries, but radio and television programmes should, where appropriate, be encouraged.

Some schemes have advised the public of the work on special boxes or books of matches, or in information pamphlets, and in St Lucia two stories featuring a folklore hero, Brer Rabbit, were written for children.

Where chemotherapy is to be used, the health educator's job is to get the co-operation of the community so that stool or urine specimens are provided for case detection, and, further, so that people accept treatment.

In mollusciciding schemes, it is essential to warn the population that a chemical will be used in the water and that fish as well as snails will be killed—but the fish can sometimes be eaten.

People must have water and until alternative safe supplies are available it is pointless to try to educate people not to use the nearby river or pond. When water supplies are being provided, the community can be involved by digging pipelines while health education should concentrate on teaching how to get the best possible benefits from it—not only by staying out of river and ponds infected or potentially infected with schistosomiasis but also by improved cleanliness generally (hand washing after defaecation, washing fruits and vegetables before eating, etc.). The value of the water supply should also be emphasised so that waste may be minimised and the system not damaged.

Although latrines have not been effective in control schemes, they should, nevertheless, be encouraged in a general development programme and there may be a need for education as to their proper use and maintenance. For different reasons children are often not allowed to use them but, since they are potentially responsible for a high proportion of environmental contamination, they should be encouraged to do so.

It is important that where hygiene is taught in school there should be properly maintained and adequate water and toilet facilities at the school to emphasise classroom teaching.

ASSESSMENT OF CONTROL

Indirect evidence and an early indication of the efficacy of control measures may be obtained from various parameters in relation to the snail intermediate hosts.

An indication of the success of mollusciciding will be given by the reduced numbers or absence of snails, but the use of techniques to detect cercariae by animal exposures or filtration techniques will add support to such findings.

If pre-control data are available on the infection occurring in the intermediate snail host, then a reduction in the numbers of infected snails, after attempts to reduce contamination of water, may be indicative of reduced transmission. The 'sentinel snail technique' is currently being used in St Lucia and Ghana—reduced numbers of infected snails were found after chemotherapy. Where an animal reservoir of infection exists, evidence of successful control of transmission may be apparent from a lower prevalence and intensity of infection in the reservoir hosts (Massoud and Nelson, 1971).

Where the aim of control is to reduce contact with infected water, success or failure can be demonstrated by appropriate observation studies of human water contact.

However, lowering or changes in indices of infection in the human population must ultimately be demonstrated to provide evidence of reduced transmission. Changes in the incidence, prevalence and intensity of infection amongst children are of prime importance, but adults should also be investigated to ensure control is effective amongst all age groups.

Parasitological techniques of diagnosis may lack sensitivity and thus light infections can be missed; techniques are, however, specific and indicate active infections. They can be used to determine all indices of infection.

When satisfactory serodiagnostic techniques have been developed they may be of use in monitoring transmission in children. They will probably be of use for determining incidence of new infection (in seronegative children) and prevalence amongst this segment of the population, but unless the test is negative in persons with old inactive infections they will be of little use for prevalence data amongst adults.

In research-orientated control programmes, where detailed epidemiological studies are being made, children should be examined annually or bi-annually (if seasonal patterns of transmission are to be determined), whereas adults can be examined less frequently, e.g. after four or five years of control.

In public health control schemes, prevalence data from school children can be used for a less detailed evaluation.

Incidence of new infections

Incidence is the only true measure of the level of transmission and when chemotherapy is used in control its use is essential in the early years of evaluation. Its measurement has been described in detail in Chapter 10.

With successful control, fewer older children are infected; there will therefore be more of them, proportionately, than in pre-control groups. Appropriate statistical methods of analysis must therefore be used for comparing pre- and post-control data (Table 11.3).

Table 11.3 Changes in the rate of new infections (percentage incidence) associated with two annual chemotherapy campaigns. (From Cook *et al.*, 1977.)

Age (years)	1972/3		1973/4		1974/5	
	Number examined	Percentage positive	Number examined	Percentage positive	Number examined	Percentage positive
0–2	88	16	62	0	58	2
3–5	122	15	103	4	77	1
6–7	64	19	76	8	88	2
8–10	62	34	75	9	116	9
11–13	43	37	48	21	89	2
0–13	379	21	364	7	428	4

Conversion:reversion ratio

A reduced incidence of new infection after intervention will indicate some success in control, but a better indication of the level of control attained by measures other than chemotherapy comes from the conversion:reversion ratio.

With reduced transmission (and fewer re-infections), the number of lost infections increases and, when there are more lost infections (reversions) than new ones (conversions), the conversion:reversion ratio is less than 1. If this stage is continued, the infection gradually dies out.

Table 11.4 Change in status of schistosome infection in a cohort of children examined in 1974 and again in 1975 (after control had been operating for four to five years).

Age (years) in 1974	Number examined both years	Number (%) positive in 1974	Conver-sions*	Rever-sions	Number (%) positive in 1975
0–2	53	4 (8)	0	4	0
3–5	95	10 (11)	6 (7)	7	9 (9)
6–7	87	24 (28)	12 (19)	14	22 (25)
8–10	133	53 (40)	14 (18)	23	44 (33)
0–10	368	91 (25)	32 (12)	48	75 (20)

* Figures in parentheses indicate percentage incidence.

The ratio of conversions to reversions is 32:48 or 1:0·66 (cf. Table 10·6 where before control it was 1:2·1). The 1974 25% prevalence of the cohort fell to 20% in 1975 in spite of the children being a year older.

Cohort studies over one, two or more years indicate changes in a static population, whereas age-specific prevalence data may be affected by population movements.

Prevalence and intensity of infection

So long as population movement is not excessive, prevalence data can be used to indicate changes in transmission. Children are usually used for this purpose, as those born after the start of successful control will be free of infection. In addition, older children will have ceased to acquire new infections and any they had prior to control will gradually die out, leading to a reduced intensity of infection. Thus the 5–9 or 10–14 year age groups are useful for monitoring control (Fig. 11.7). In Puerto Rico, the stools of first grade (6 year old) school children were examined annually and a gradual decline in prevalence from 16% in 1953 to zero in 1966 was noted (Jobin, 1970).

Adults are less frequently examined in control schemes but in the absence of re-infection their worm burden is gradually reduced with a lowering of intensity of infection and prevalence. This is usually accompanied by a shift of the peak prevalence to an older age group (see Fig. 11.3).

Changes in the potential contamination of the environment with schistosome eggs can be shown as a result of reducing these two indices of infection and this may be reflected by changes in

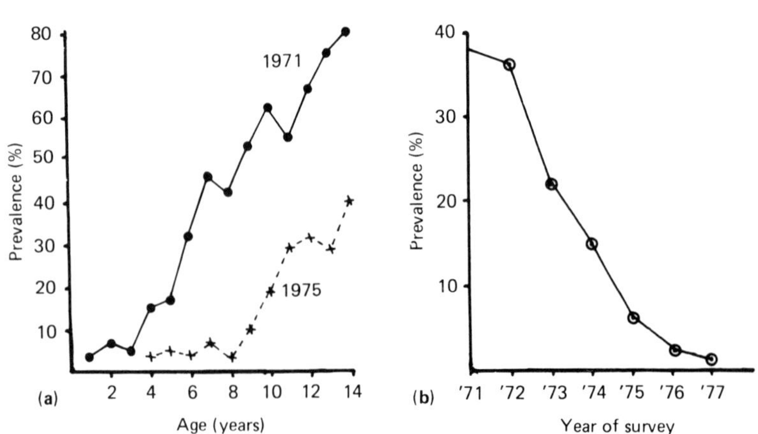

Fig. 11.7 The effect of snail control on prevalence of *S. mansoni* in children: (a) absence of infection in children born after control and loss of infection amongst those originally infected; (b) declining infection in 5–9 year olds after snail control supplemented by chemotherapy in 1975 and 1976. (St Lucian data, original.)

sentinel snail infection rates (Jordan, Bartholomew *et al.*, 1978). The percentage reduction in potential contamination gives an indication of the reduced worm burden of the population.

Health centre and hospital data may provide additional evidence of falling transmission, with a steady decline in the number of cases attending for treatment or being found on routine stool examination. Thus, amongst routine stool examinations in St Lucia, 15% were found to be *S. mansoni* positive in 1970—less than 1% (all adults) were positive in 1980.

ACHIEVEMENTS OF CONTROL PROGRAMMES

Schistosomiasis control programmes were reviewed by the Expert Committee of the World Health Organization (Anon, 1973) and it was noted that, in projects using molluscicides alone, a clear impact on 'incidence' of infection had been achieved, including the schemes in Ghana, Tanzania, Egypt and Japan. In others, where changes in 'prevalence' of infection were estimated, pronounced reductions were observed in Brazil (Paulini *et al.*, 1972) and in Zimbabwe (Shiff *et al.*, 1973). Other successful research, pilot and major control schemes in which combinations of methods (molluscicides and chemotherapy) have been employed include those in Malagasy (Degremont, 1973); Tanzania (Fenwick, 1972a, 1972b); West Cameroon (Duke and Moore, 1976a, 1976b, 1976c); Iran (Arfaa, 1976); Fayoum Governorate of Egypt and in Zimbabwe. Combined chemotherapy, mollusciciding, environmental control, sanitation, health education and legislative action have been applied in the long-standing control programme in Japan (Yokogawa, 1972) and in Venezuela (Anon, 1973), and in each country the programmes have resulted in a marked reduction in schistosomiasis as a problem of public health significance. The substantial and scientifically acceptable data which are available from many of these programmes show the efficacy of single and combined control measures and, in particular, of the valuable role of molluscicides in the control of schistosomiasis.

Recent and current research and pilot control programmes
St Lucia

Evaluation of the experimental mollusciciding programme to control *S. mansoni* transmission in St Lucia shows that, after four years of a surveillance/treatment snail control programme using an emulsifiable concentrate of niclosamide—25% active ingredient—(Bayluscide®)—the size and numbers of colonies of *B. glabrata* were substantially reduced; the incidence of *S. mansoni* infections in 0- to 10-year-old children fell from 22% to 4·3%, while in a comparison area the incidence remained at 20%. With reduced transmission over four years, the prevalence of infection in a cohort of children examined in 1971 and 1975 fell from 34% to 23%. The fall in prevalence and intensity of infection led to a reduction of 66% in the index of potential contamination, being reflected in the reduced rate of infection among sentinel snails and representative samples of *B. glabrata* collected during surveillance searches. The overall annual cost of the programme was US $3·24 per caput (Jordan, Barnish *et al.*, 1978).

Ghana

Investigations in northwestern Ghana followed by a pilot control project (Lyons, 1974) showed that selective, dry season molluscicidal control of *S. haematobium* foci can be effective in reducing transmission. Ponds and smaller riverine habitats were treated with Bayluscide (70% wettable powder) to give a concentration of 0·5 mg/l, with large habitats receiving a concentration of 1 mg/l active ingredient. The annual cost per caput of population in the villages protected was US $2·34.

In the Ghana Government UNDP/WHO project of Research on the Epidemiology and Methodology of Schistosomiasis Control in Man-made Lakes, on Lake Volta, Ghana, intervention measures which commenced in 1976 involving snail control by mollusciciding and/or removal of weeds in focal lake-shore transmission sites, together with selective population chemotherapy, health education and the provision of water supplies in selected villages, have resulted in a pronounced reduction in transmission with corresponding falls in prevalence and intensity of infection in the population of the study villages (Scott, personal communication). The essential focality of transmission which is seasonally predominant and correlated with the lake-level drawdown and related vegetation changes has been established (Klumpp and Chu, 1977). Transmission foci are treated monthly with Bayluscide (70% wettable powder) by spraying to achieve a concentration of 0·5 mg/l (Chu, 1978). Annual costs *per capita* for population chemotherapy were estimated in 1978 to be US $1·94; for snail control US $1·10; and for the combined measures protecting a lakeside population of 7000 and an additional hinterland community of 8000, a total per capita cost of US $3·04.

Sudan

In a pilot project area of 1000 km² in the Gezira Irrigated Area of the Sudan, the results from a series of applications of the molluscicide N-tritylmorpholine (Frescon—16.5% emulsifiable concentrate) have been used, since 1971, to formulate a regimen for snail control aimed at reducing the snail population by at least 95% of the population levels in untreated canals, in order to control the transmission of *S. mansoni*.

It was found that drip-feed application of the molluscicide failed except during the months September to December. At that time, water requirements were maximal but the molluscicide coverage of the system was incomplete and it was necessary to supplement each application with knapsack spraying of canal tail-ends.

It was subsequently established that aerial spraying is the most effective, quickest and cheapest application technique. The regimen employed consisted of five aerial sprays of all main, major and minor canals at 0·25 mg/l Frescon, per annum, i.e. early September, mid-November, late January, Mid-March and early June (Amin and Fenwick, 1977).

Epidemiological evaluation of the initial control measures using Frescon indicated equivocal results in terms of reduced 'incidence' of transmission. The new regimen is currently being evaluated and consideration given to alternative methods of control, including the use of an alternative molluscicide (Bayluscide), focal rather than blanket snail control, provision of water supplies, and chemotherapeutic measures. The total cost of the annual regimen of aerial spraying Frescon in the 1000 km² pilot area is estimated to be US $0·73 per caput of population protected.

National control programmes

Egypt

There have been several notable pilot control programmes, including those in the Dakhla Oasis in the Western Desert and at Warraq El-Arab north-west of Cairo, in which copper sulphate and sodium pentachlorophenate, respectively, were used and, of course, the Joint WHO/UNICEF/Egyptian Government Project in Baheira Governorate (Egypt 49), in which Bayluscide was employed (Gilles *et al.*, 1973; Ayad, 1976).

In 1968, large-scale control operations commenced in Fayoum Governorate (an irrigated area of 400 000 feddans with a population of 1 163 000 people and an overall prevalence of *S. haematobium* of 45·7%). The applied control strategy involved area-wide applications of Bayluscide (70% wettable powder) by dispensing, in the spring, summer and autumn, followed by surveillance and spraying as required, together with specific population chemotherapy in which tartar emetic and niridazole have been used. Epidemiological evaluation showed that prevalence dropped from 45·7% to 9·1% after five years of the applied control measures. In the present maintenance phase of this programme, two annual area-wide applications of molluscicide are made in the spring and autumn, from a single dispensing point, followed by surveillance and spraying if required. The present prevalence of *S. haematobium* is 12%, and metrifonate (Bilarcil®) has now been introduced for treatment of the remaining infected people. This programme costs annually approximately US \$0·5 per caput of population protected.

A major control programme has been operational in Middle Egypt since 1976, in an area of some 1 050 000 irrigated feddans, with a population of 4 500 000 people. The area is one in which a major tile-drainage programme is taking place in collaboration with the World Bank (IBRD). The control strategy involves area-wide applications of molluscicide (Bayluscide®) by dispensing in irrigation canals three times a year—spring, summer and autumn—with complementary spraying of all drains and static waters, and population chemotherapy for which metrifonate (Bilarcil®) is being used. The area to be controlled was selected because of the large-scale reclamation operations taking place which involved deepening and widening existing drains (777 km) as well as excavating some 865 km of new open drains, in order to reinforce the control operations in Fayoum Governorate, and to prevent the spread of the transmission of *S. mansoni* south of Cairo. Overall prevalence of *S. haematobium* in the area was estimated to be 34·3%, and more than 900 000 infected patients have now received treatment. Snail control operations are based upon synoptic data of the irrigation rotations being applied in the area and, as was found in the Fayoum control operations, the Bayluscide 70% wettable powder formulation is proving highly efficient, with carriage from single dispensing points over long distances through secondary and tertiary canals and in main drains. Concentrations of 1–2 mg/l active ingredient are being applied according to the prevailing water conditions. Preliminary epidemiological evaluation in a sample of 58 villages shows that overall prevalence has been reduced from 29·7% to 10·1% during the past three years and the annual cost of the programme is estimated to be about US \$1·0 per caput of population protected (Mobarak, personal communication).

In 1979, control operations, involving the same strategy as is applied in Middle Egypt, commenced in the irrigated area of 1 120 970 feddans between Aswan and Assiut which has a population of 5 099 000 people. These measures will consolidate the control operations in Middle Egypt and complete the control of *S. haematobium* transmission from Aswan to Giza. Perennial irrigation in Upper Egypt, which replaced basin irrigation when the High Dam became operational, resulted in a marked increase in prevalence of infection. It is considered important that transmission of *S. haematobium* be controlled and the prevalence and intensity of infection in the population reduced, since potential settlement populations for new townships on the shores of Lake Nasser may eventually be drawn from these areas in Upper Egypt (Mobarak, personal communication). Elsewhere in Egypt, limited snail control operations are being carried out involving the use of copper sulphate and niclosamide (Mollutox®), the latter compound being made in Egypt.

Saudi Arabia

The focal nature of schistosomiasis transmission (wells, small canals, cisterns, small swamps, temporary streams, residual pools and ponds) in most parts of the country offers the opportunity to reduce it by snail control operations, with an excellent prospect of good results (Arfaa, 1976; Davis, 1977). Control of *B. truncatus*, *B. beccarii*, *B. reticulatus wrighti* and *B. 'arabica'* populations is currently made using niclosamide Bayluscide® and Mollutox®.

Iran

Control measures covering the entire endemic area of Khuzestan Province commenced in 1966. Bayluscide has mainly been used, but snail control has also involved drainage of swamps and filling operations. Coupled with chemotherapy improvements in water supply, sewage disposal and some health education, the control measures have resulted in a marked reduction in prevalence of infection, at an annual estimated cost of about US $0·40 per caput of population protected.

Recent information indicates that applied control measures are not maintaining effective control of the problem in all situations, but the reasons for apparent failures are unknown to the authors. There are, however, preliminary data which suggest that *B. truncatus* from Dezful, where mollusciciding has been carried out for the past 10 years, may have developed resistance to Bayluscide (Jelnes, 1977).

Brazil

Very successful pilot control projects, using only mollusciciding with Bayluscide as the sole means of control, have been carried out in areas of natural drainage and some with primitive irrigation, in Belo Horizonte, Sao Laurenco and Taquarendi. A national control programme has now been launched with a budget of some US $157 million, for a four-year period, in which population chemotherapy (using oxamniquine), snail control measures by mollusciciding, improved sanitation and water supplies with health education, will be applied.

Philippines

A five-year schistosomiasis control plan has been formulated with a budget of some US $188 million, which will include: multiple control measures; population chemotherapy; environmental sanitation; snail control by land reclamation, 'agro' engineering, drainage, filling, etc. and application of molluscicides (Bayluscide and/or Biomet® in a rubber formulation—the latter formulation, which contains tributyltin oxide, being intended to serve as a cercariacide in streams in which workers are exposed during reclamation work); together with health education. It is estimated that some 3·9 million people are exposed to transmission of *S. japonicum* in 22 provinces, and that the programme will annually cost some US $9·64 per caput of population protected.

China

In the multiple control approaches applied in endemic areas, extensive use is made of a variety of molluscicides. The preferred compound is pentachlorophenol (PCP), which although water insoluble, is favoured because it is cheaper than sodium pentachlorphenate (NaPCP). The PCP is also much less costly than niclosamide and other synthetics. In different areas and at various times, other molluscicides have been used including niclosamide, tribenzylmethylmorpholine, N-tritylmorpholine (Frescon), 3, 5-dibromo-4-hydroxy-4-nitroazobenzene (Yurimin) and calcium cyanamide. Other compounds which are sometimes used are an extract of *Camelia oleosa* (tea-cake seeds) and ethylene diamine. Ethylene diamine is sprayed on the soil banks of fish ponds ($10-15$ g/m^2) and the saturated soil is then immersed in the water. A concentration of less than 100 mg/l is lethal to snails, while the lethal concentration for fish is 3200 mg/l, thus making it a most suitable compound for use in fish ponds.

A variety of snail control techniques is apparently employed, including: physical measures in which snails are buried; molluscicides are additionally sprayed both on water surfaces and on the snail habitats of the banks of canals, channels, ditches and rivers; PCP is used at 10 g/m^2. The mixture of bank weeds, soil and snails is moved below water level near the shoreline and the compacted mass is reported to retain a high concentration of PCP, with subsequent high mortality of snails both above and below the water level. Before the transplantation of young rice shoots, the fields are levelled by hand. Water is added and either calcium cyanamide 12·5 kg/m or PCP 1 kg/m (Davis, personal communication).

Puerto Rico

Control of schistosomiasis was initiated in Puerto Rico in five pilot schemes in 1953 and, as at present, is primarily aimed at control of the snail intermediate host *B. glabrata*. Initially, sodium pentachlorophenate (NaPCP) was used together with drainage of swamps and seepages by hand ditching. In 1958, acrolein was introduced in the larger irrigation canals, in the south, for weed and snail control, and Bayluscide replaced NaPCP in 1963.

In 1958, use of *M. cornuarietis* began in irrigation systems, farm ponds and big lakes for the biological control of *B. glabrata* (Ruiz-Tiben *et al.*, 1969; Jobin *et al.*, 1970 and 1977). The biological control programme is estimated to be some two orders of magnitude cheaper than chemical control, with a high level of effectiveness. In ponds and lakes it is 1% of the cost of chemical control.

The multiple control measures (including snail control by environmental, biological and chemical means, provision of improved public water supply, a latrine distribution programme and limited chemotherapy) applied during the past 25 years have cost some US $7 million, or approximately $1·0 per caput of population protected.

REFERENCES

Abdullah, A. (1973). *J. Egypt. Publ. Hlth Ass.* **48,** 290.
Amin, M. A. and Fenwick, A. (1977). *Ann. Trop. Med. Parasit.* **71,** 205.
Anon. (1973). Wld Hlth Org., *Techn. Rep. Ser.* No. **515,** 13.
Anon. (1980). Wld Hlth Org., *Techn. Rep. Ser.* No. **643,** 44.
Ansari, N. (1973). *Epidemiology and Control of Schistosomiasis (Bilharziasis).* S. Karger, Basel, New York.
Arfaa, F. (1976). WHP/Schisto/76. 41.
Ayad, N. (1976). *Egypt. J. Bilh.* **3,** 129.
Barbosa, F. S., Pinto, R. and Souza, G. A. (1971). *Trans. R. Soc. Trop. Med. Hyg.* **65,** 206.
Bernade, M. A. and Johnson, B. (1971). *J. Am. Wat. Wks. Ass.* **63,** 449.
Barnish, G. and Prentice, M. A. (1981). *Trans. R. Soc. Trop. Med. Hyg.* **75,** 106.

Barnish, G. and Shiff, C. J. (1970). *Rhodesia Agric. J.* **67,** 1.
Bell, E. J., Etges, F. J. and Jenelle, L. J. (1966). *Am. J. Trop. Med. Hyg.* **15,** 539.
Berg, C. O. (1953). *J. Parasit.* **39,** 630.
Birch, L. C. (1953). *Ecology* **34,** 698.
Bina, J. C. and Prata, A. (1970). *Revta Soc. Bras. Med. Trop.* **8,** 217.
Blackmore, M. D., Boydel, R. A. and Mbere, N. (1978). In *Sanitation in Developing Countries*, p. 56. Ed. A. Pacy. John Wiley & Sons, Chichester, New York, Brisbane, Toronto.
Bradley, D. J. and Webbe, G. (1978). In *Proc. Int. Conf. Schisto. Cairo 1975* **2,** 691.
Brown, A. W. A. and Deom, J. O. (1973). *Health aspects of man-made lakes, Knoxville, Tennessee, U.S.A. 1971*, Geophysical Monograph Series **17,** 755.
Cardarelli, N. F. (1974). In *Molluscicides in Schistosomiasis Control*, p. 177. Ed. T. C. Cheng. Academic Press, London.
Cardarelli, N. F. (1977). *Controlled Release Molluscicides*. University of Akron, Ohio.
Cheng, T. M. (1971). *Am. J. Trop. Med. Hyg.* **20,** 26.
Chernin, E. and Dunavan, C. A. (1962). *Am. J. Trop. Med. Hyg.* **11,** 455.
Christie, J. D., Prentice, M. A., Upatham, E. S. and Barnish, G. (1978). *Am. J. Trop. Med. Hyg.* **27,** 6161.
Christie, J. D. and Upatham, E. S. (1977). *Am. J. Trop. Med. Hyg.* **26,** 894.
Chu, K. Y. (1978). *Bull. Wld Hlth Org.* **56,** 313.
Cook, J. A., Jordan, P. and Armitage, P. (1976). *Am. J. Trop. Med. Hyg.* **25,** 602.
Cook, J. A., Jordan, P. and Bartholomew, R. K. (1977). *Am. J. Trop. Med. Hyg.* **26,** 887.
Daffalla, A. A. (1973). MSc Thesis, University of London.
Daffalla, A. A. and Duncan, J. (1979). *Pestic. Sci.* **10,** 423.
Davis, A. (1977). EM/SCHIS/66, EM/SAA/MPD/002. WHO, Geneva.
Davis, G. M. and Ruff, M. D. (1973). *Malacol. Rev.* **6,** 181.
Dazo, B. C., Hairston, N. G. and Dawood, I. K. (1966). *Bull. Wld Hlth Org.* **35,** 339.
DeBach, P. (1974). *Biological Control by Natural Enemies*. Cambridge University Press, Cambridge.
Degremont, A. A. (1973). *Mangoky Project: Campaign against schistosomiasis in the lower Mangoky (Madagascar)*. Swiss Tropical Institute, Basle.
Duke, B. O. L. and Moore, P. J. (1976a). *Tropenmed. Parasit.* **27,** 297.
Duke, B. O. L. and Moore, P. J. (1976b). *Tropenmed. Parasit.* **27,** 489.
Duke, B. O. L. and Moore, P. J. (1976c). *Tropenmed. Parasit.* **27,** 505.
Duncan, J. (1980). *Pharmac. Ther.* **10,** 407.
Dunlop, R. W. (1976). PhD Thesis, University of London.
Etges, F. J., Bell, E. J. and Gilbertson, D. E. (1965). *Am. J. Trop. Med. Hyg.* **14,** 846.
Eyakuze, V. M. (1972). *Proceedings of the East African Medical Research Council Scientific Conference, 1972*.
Eyakuze, V. M. and Rugemalila, J. B. (1978). *Proc. Int. Conf. Schisto. Cairo 1975* **1,** 291.
Farooq, M., Nielson, J., Samaan, S. A., Mallah, M. B. and Allam, A. A. (1966). *Bull. Wld Hlth Org.* **35,** 319.
Faust, E. C. and Hoffman, W. A. (1934). *Puerto Rico J. Publ. Hlth Trop. Med.* **10,** 1.
Fenwick, A. (1972a). *Bull. Wld Hlth Org.* **47,** 325.
Fenwick, A. (1972b). *Bull. Wld Hlth Org.* **47,** 573.

Ferguson, F. F. (1972). In *Schistosomiasis: Proceedings of a Symposium on the Future of Schistosomiasis Control*, p. 85. Ed. M. J. M. Miller. Tulane University, New Orleans.

Ferguson, F. F. (1978). In *The role of biological agents in the control of schistosome bearing animals*, p. 109. Department of Health and Education and Welfare Center for Disease Control, Atlanta, USA.

Frandsen, F. and Madsen, H. (1979). *Acta Trop.* **36,** 67.

Freidheim, E. A. H. and de Jongh, R. T. (1959). *Ann. Trop. Med. Parasit.* **53,** 316.

Gilles, H. M., Abdel Aziz Zaki, A., Soussa, S. A., Samaan, S. A., Soliman, S. S., Hassan, A. and Barbosa, F. S. (1973). *Ann. Trop. Med. Parasit.* **67,** 45.

Hairston, N. G. and Santos, B. C. (1961). *Bull. Wld Hlth Org.* **25,** 603.

Hairston, N. G., Wurzinger, R. H. and Burch, J. B. (1975). *WHO/Schisto* **75,** 40.

Haskins, W. T. (1951). *Anal. Chem.* **23,** 1672.

Hopf, H. S., Duncan, J., Beesley, J. S. S., Webley, D. J. and Sturrock, R. F. (1967). *Bull. Wld Hlth Org.* **36,** 955.

Jelnes, J. E. (1977). *Trans. R. Soc. Trop. Med. Hyg.* **71,** 451.

Jewsbury, J. M., Cooke, M. J. and Weber, M. C. (1977). *Ann. Trop. Med. Parasit.* **71,** 67.

Jobin, W. R. (1968). *Bull. Wld Hlth Org.* **38,** 322.

Jobin, W. R. (1970). *Am. J. Trop. Med. Hyg.* **19,** 1049.

Jobin, W. R. and Berrios-Duran, L. (1970). *Bull. Wld Hlth Org.* **42,** 177.

Jobin, W. R., Brown, R. A., Ferguson, F. F. and Velez, S. (1977). *Am. J. Trop. Med. Hyg.* **26,** 1018.

Jobin, W. R., Ferguson, F. F. and Palmer, J. R. (1970). *Bull. Wld Hlth Org.* **42,** 151.

Jobin, W. R. and Ippen, A. T. (1964). *Science* **145,** 1324.

Jobin, W. R. and Michelson, E. H. (1967). *Bull. Wld Hlth Org.* **37,** 657.

Jobin, W. R. and Michelson, E. H. (1969). *Am. J. Trop. Med. Hyg.* **18,** 207.

Jordan, P. (1963). *E. Afr. Med. J.* **40,** 250.

Jordan, P., Barnish, G., Bartholomew, R. K., Grist, E. and Christie, J. D. (1978). *Bull. Wld Hlth Org.* **56,** 139.

Jordan, P., Bartholomew, R. K., Unrau, G. O., Upatham, E. S., Grist, E. and Christie, J. D. (1978). *Bull. Wld Hlth Org.* **56,** 965.

Jordan, P., Christie, J. D. and Unrau, G. O. (1980). *Acta Trop.* **37,** 95.

Jordan, P., Cook, J. A., Bartholomew, R. K. and Auguste, E. (1980). *Trans. R. Soc. Trop. Med. Hyg.* **74,** 493.

Jordan, P., Woodstock, L., Unrau, G. O. and Cook, J. A. (1975). *Bull. Wld Hlth Org.* **52,** 9.

Kajihara, N., Horimi, T., Minai, M. and Hosaka, Y. (1979). *Jap. J. Med. Biol.* **32,** 225.

Katz, N., Zicher, F., Rosa, R. S. and Oliviera, V. B. (1978). *Revta Inst. Med. Trop. S. Paulo* **20,** 273.

Kawata, K. and Kruse, C. W. (1966). *Am. J. Trop. Med. Hyg.* **15,** 896.

Kloetzel, K. (1967a). *Trans. R. Soc. Trop. Med. Hyg.* **61,** 609.

Kloetzel, K. (1967b). *Bull. Wld Hlth Org.* **37,** 686.

Kloetzel, K. (1974). *Trans. R. Soc. Trop. Med. Hyg.* **68,** 344.

Klumpp, R. K. and Chu, K. Y. (1977). *Bull. Wld Hlth Org.* **55,** 715.

Krakower, C. A. (1940). *Puerto Rico J. Publ. Hlth Trop. Med.* **19,** 669.

Leiper, R. T. (1916). *Proc. R. Soc. Med.* **9,** 145.

Lemma, A. (1965). *Ethiop. Med. J.* **3,** 187.

Lemma, A. (1970). *Bull. Wld Hlth Org.* **4,** 597.

Lemma, A., Goll, P. H., Duncan, J. and Bahta Mazengia (1978). *Proc. Int. Conf. Schisto. Cairo 1975* **1**, 415.

Lie, K. J. (1973). *Expl Parasit.* **33**, 343.

Lim, H. K. and Heyneman, D. (1972). *Adv. Parasit.* **10**, 191.

Lyons, G. R. L. (1974). *Bull. Wld Hlth Org.* **51**, 621.

MacArthur, R. (1960). *Am. Naturalist* **XCIV**, 25.

Macdonald, G. (1965). *Trans. R. Soc. Trop. Med. Hyg.* **59**, 489.

McJunkin, E. (1970). *Engineering Measures for Control of Schistosomiasis*, p. 69. Washington DC, Agency for International Development.

McManon, J. P., Highton, R. B. and Marshall, I. F. de C. (1977). *Envir. Conserv.* **4**, 285.

McMullen, D. B. (1962). *Ciba Foundation Symposium on Bilharziasis*, p. 382. Eds G. E. W. Wolstenholme and M. O'Connor. J and A Churchill, London.

McMullen, D. B., Buzo, Z. I., Rainey, M. B. and Francotte, J. (1962). *Bull. Wld Hlth Org.* **27**, 25.

Massoud, J. and Nelson, G. S. (1971). *Trans. R. Soc. Trop. Med. Hyg.* **66**, 191.

Michelson, E. H. (1957). *Parasitology* **47**, 413.

Morgan, P. R. and Clarke, V. de V. (1978). In *Sanitation in Developing Countries*, p. 100. Ed. A. Pacey. John Wiley & Sons, Chichester, New York, Brisbane, Toronto.

Okabe, K. (1957). *J. Parasit.* **43** (suppl), 30.

Omer, A. H. S. (1978). *Brit. Med. J.* **2**, 163.

Pacey, A. (1978). *Sanitation in developing countries.* John Wiley & Sons, Chichester, New York, Brisbane, Toronto.

Paulini, E., de Freitas, C. A. and Aguirre, G. H. (1972). In *Schistosomiasis: Proceedings of a Symposium on the Future of Schistosomiasis Control*, p. 104. Ed. M. J. Miller. Tulane University Press, New Orleans.

Pearl, R. and Reed, L. J. (1920). *Proc. Nat. Acad. Sci. U.S.A.* **6**, 275.

Pesigan, T. P., Farooq, M., Hairston, N. G., Jauregui, J. J., Garcia, E. G., Santos, A. T., Santos, B. C. and Besa, A. A. (1958). *Bull. Wld Hlth Org.* **19**, 223.

Pesigan, T. P. and Hairston, N. G. (1961). *Bull. Wld Hlth Org.* **25**, 479.

Pesigan, T. P., Hairston, N. G., Jauregui, J. J., Garcia, E. G., Santos, A. T., Santos, B. C. and Besa, A. A. (1958). *Bull. Wld Hlth Org.* **18**, 481.

Pitchford, R. J. (1970a). *Cent. Afr. J. Med.* **16** (Suppl.), 31.

Pitchford, R. J. (1970b). *S. Afr. Med. J.* **44**, 475.

Pugh, R. N. H. (1978). *Ann. Trop. Med. Parasit.* **72**, 495.

Pugh, R. N. H., Bell, D. R. and Gilles, H. M. (1980). *Ann. Trop. Med. Parasit.* **74**, 597.

Richards, C. S. (1970). *Nature, London* **227**, 806.

Richards, C. S. (1973). *Am. J. Trop. Med. Hyg.* **22**, 748.

Richards, C. S. and Merritt, J. W. Jr. (1972). *Am. J. Trop. Med. Hyg.* **21**, 425.

Rowan, W. B. (1964a). *Am. J. Trop. Med. Hyg.* **11**, 630.

Rowan, W. B. (1964b). *Am. J. Trop. Med. Hyg.* **11**, 577.

Ruiz-Tiben, E., Palmer, J. R. and Ferguson, F. F. (1969). *Bull. Wld Hlth Org.* **41**, 329.

Ruyssenaars, G. van Etten, G. and McCullough, F. S. (1973). *Trop. Geog. Med.* **25**, 179.

Rybenzynski, W., Polprasert, C. and McGarry, M. (1978). *Low Cost Technology Options.* IDRC, Ottawa, Canada.

Santos, A. T. Jr., Blas, B. L., Redona, F. and Santos, M. J. (1970). *J. Philipp. Med. Ass.* **46,** 732.

Scott, J. A. and Barlow, C. H. (1938). *Am. J. Trop. Med. Hyg.* **27,** 619.

Sherif, A. F., El Sawy, M. F., Madary, S. A. and Barakat, R. M. (1970). *Alexander Med. J.* **16,** 169.

Sherif, A. F. and El Sawy, M. F. (1977). *Bull. High Inst. Publ. Hlth* **7,** 1.

Shiff, C. J. (1974). In *Molluscicides in Schistosomiasis Control*, p. 241. Ed. T. C. Cheng. Academic Press, London.

Shiff, C. J., Clarke, V. de V., Evans, A. C. and Barnish, G. (1973). *Bull. Wld Hlth Org.* **48,** 299.

Shiff, C. J. and Evans, A. C. (1977). *Cent. Afr. J. Med.* **23,** 6.

Siongok, T. K. A., Ouma, J. H., Houser, H. B. and Warren, K. S. (1978). *J. Infect. Dis.* **138,** 856.

Siongok, T. K. A., Mahmoud, A. A. F., Ouma, J. H., Warren, K. S., Muller, A. S., Handa, A. K. and Houser, H. B. (1976). *Am. J. Trop. Med. Hyg.* **25,** 273.

Slobodkin, L. B. (1962). *Growth and Regulations of Animal Populations*, p. 48. Holt, Rinehart and Winston, New York.

Smith, F. E. (1952). *Ecology* **33,** 441.

Strufe, R. (1961). *Bull. Wld Hlth Org.* **25,** 503.

Sturrock, R. F. (1965). *Bull. Wld Hlth Org.* **32,** 225.

Sturrock, R. F. (1973). *Int. J. Parasit.* **3,** 165.

Sturrock, R. F. and Barnish, G. (1973). *Bull. Wld Hlth Org.* **49,** 283.

Upatham, E. S. and Sturrock, R. F. (1977). *Ann. Trop. Med. Parasit.* **71,** 85.

Unrau, G. O. (1975). *Bull. Wld Hlth Org.* **52,** 1.

Unrau, G. O. (1978). In *Sanitation in Developing Countries*, p. 104. Ed. A. Pacey. John Wiley & Sons, Chichester, New York, Brisbane, Toronto.

Veolker, J. (1968). *Entomol. Mitcheil. Aus. Dem. Zool. Stattsint. und Zool. Mus. Hamburg* **3,** 1.

Warley, A. P. (1978). *Proc. Int. Conf. Schisto., Cairo 1975* **1,** 441.

Warren, K. S. and Mahmoud, A. A. F. (1976). *Trans. Ass. Phys.* **89,** 195.

Webbe, G. (1962). *Bull. Wld Hlth Org.* **27,** 59.

Webbe, G. (1963). *E. Afr. Med. J.* **40,** 235.

Webbe, G. (1964). *E. Afr. Med. J.* **41,** 508.

Webbe, G. (1965a). *E. Afr. Med. J.* **42,** 605.

Webbe, G. (1965b). *Bull. Wld Hlth Org.* **33,** 147.

Webbe, G. (1974). *Molluscicides in the Control of Schistosomiasis*, p. 41. Ed. T. C. Cheng. Academic Press, London.

Webbe, G. (1978). *Proc. Int. Conf. Schisto., Cairo 1975* **1,** 13.

Weir, J. M., Wasif, I. M., Farooq, Rick H., Attia, S. M. and Abdel Kader, M. (1952). *J. Egypt. Publ. Hlth Ass.* **27,** 55.

Wilkins, H. A. and Moore, P. J. (1980). *Trans. R. Soc. Trop. Med. Hyg.* **74,** 692.

Wilkins, H. A., Foll, P., Marshall, T. F. de C. and Moore, P. (1979). *Trans. R. Soc. Trop. Med. Hyg.* **73,** 74.

Yokogawa, M. (1972). In *Proceedings of a symposium on the future of schistosomiasis control*, p. 129. Ed. M. J. Miller. Tulane University, New Orleans.

Index